P9-APE-431

Excessive Appetites: A Psychological View of Addictions

Excessive Appetites: A Psychological View of Addictions

Jim Orford

*Department of Psychology,
University of Exeter*

and

*Department of Clinical Psychology,
Exeter Health Authority*

JOHN WILEY & SONS

Chichester · New York · Brisbane · Toronto · Singapore

Reprinted June 1986.
Reprinted December 1986.
Reprinted October 1987.

Library of Congress Cataloging in Publication Data:

Orford, Jim.
Excessive appetites: a psychological view of addictions

Includes index.
1. Substance abuse. 2. Gambling. 3. Psychosexual disorders. I. Title.
RC564.076 1985 616.86 84-22066
ISBN 0 471 10301 2

British Library Cataloguing in Publication Data:

Orford, Jim
Excessive appetites: a psychological view of addictions
1. Drug Abuse—Psychological aspects
I. Title
616.86 RC564

ISBN 0 471 10301 2

Phototypeset by Dobbie Typesetting Service, Plymouth, Devon.
Printed and bound in Great Britain

To Judith, Tim, Paul and Will.
Family of a workaholic.

Preface

The ideas contained in this book have been germinating for a long time and have been nourished by people and influences too numerous to mention. Those who stand out include the late David Davies who pioneered the Alcohol Education Centre Summer Schools in the late 1960s and who encouraged me to develop the ideas contained in my Summer School lecture on the Psychology of Alcoholism. My Ph.D. supervisor, Bram Oppenheim, of the London School of Economics, and my colleague at the Addiction Research Unit, David Robinson, were amongst those who helped me move towards a greater interest in social psychology and sociology. Another significant influence was meeting Gordon Moody, of the Churches' Council on Gambling, who introduced me to a number of former excessive gamblers and to people working in that field.

Principal amongst the many colleagues then and since to whom I owe a debt of gratitude for the stimulation and support which they have given me, is Griffith Edwards, Director of the Addiction Research Unit at the Institute of Psychiatry, London, where I worked from 1966 to 1976. Griff Edwards enlarged my horizons in two ways. First, he created a multidisciplinary research community which taught me how stimulating that kind of collaborative work could be and what folly it was to assume that one discipline had all the answers. Secondly, with his own capacity for realizing the relevance of disciplines not normally brought together, he showed me the importance of both the biological sciences, such as physiology and pharmacology, and the social sciences such as history and economics.

I am glad to be able to acknowledge his permission to use, in a modified form, my paper on hypersexuality which appeared in the *British Journal of Addiction*, which he edits, in 1978. I am also pleased to acknowledge the following permissions to use extracts from published works: Academic Press (extracts from Janis and Mann, 1968); the *British Journal of Psychiatry* (Edwards *et al.*, 1973); Free Press (Janis and Mann, 1977); Marcu Dekker Inc. (Smart, 1971); Dr. Michael Russell (Russell *et al.*, 1974); the *Journal of*

Studies on Alcohol (Jessor and Jessor, 1977); The Kinsey Institute (Kinsey *et al.*, 1948); Paperjacks, Ontario (Miller and Agnew, 1974); Rand McNally & Company (Janis and Mann, 1968); and The Williams and Wilkins Co., Baltimore (Barker and Miller, 1968).

Finally, my sincere thanks to Margaret Topham and Hazel Hunt for typing draft and final versions of the manuscript.

Jim Orford
Exeter
June 1984

Contents

CHAPTER ONE

Introduction

> Intemperance—N. *intemperance*, immoderation, unrestraint; *excess*, excessiveness, luxury; *redundance*; indiscipline, incontinence; indulgence; addiction, bad habit; *habit*; full life, dissipation; *sensualism*; intoxication; *drunkenness*.
> Adj. *intemperate*, immoderate, exceeding, excessive; *redundant*; untempered, unmeasured, unlimited; spendthrift; *prodigal*; unascetic, unspartan, indulgent, unrestrained, uncontrolled, incontinent; *unsober*, wet; *drunk*. *(Roget's Thesaurus*, Penguin Edition, 1966, p.379.)
> Unfortunately, overeating, smoking and alcohol abuse are studied and treated separately. Few attempts are made by researchers in these separate areas to compile and share knowledge or to formulate general theories of addiction (Miller, P., 1979).

At one time people who indulged in consumption of a drug or engaged in some other form of activity to the point of social or physical damage, and continued with such behaviour despite contrary statement of intent, and despite recommendations from others, were said to be suffering from a form of mania such as dipsomania, narcotomania, kleptomania, or pyromania (Stekel, 1924). The people so afflicted were in the grip of 'morbid appetites' or were suffering from 'diseases of the will'. Although such language is now largely out-dated, the phenomena to which it referred have continued unabated, and an adequate understanding of them is of the utmost importance both to public health and to theoretical psychology.

Although such apparently paradoxical behaviour raises uniquely puzzling questions about volition and motivation, central topics within psychology, the only way to understand such behaviour which commands widespread acceptance at present is one which proposes that repetitive but damaging behaviour of an appetitive kind constitutes a form of disease. 'Alcoholism' and 'drug addiction' are the clearest examples. Not only has acceptance of such behaviours as diseases had little or no impact on the general level of drinking, drug, and other appetitive behaviour problems, but also little advance in theoretical understanding of these forms of behaviour has followed from the view of them as diseases.

Seeley (1962) recommended a disease view of 'alcoholism' because 'crime' and 'sin' were the only alternatives. Indeed, the 'alcoholism as disease' movement was humanistic in its attempt to remove serious excessive and problematic drinking from the realms of morality and the law. But Seeley recommended acceptance of the disease view only on a trial basis, and there is a widespread feeling now that the disease view has stood trial for long enough. Its replacement, however, still waits upon the acceptance of a satisfactory alternative.

It will in fact be the major argument of this book that such an alternative already exists if we care to piece together fragments of knowledge and theory concerning a range of excessive appetitive behaviours. Indeed, part of the problem has been the failure to relate the study of excessive drinking and drug-taking to the study of other forms of behaviour, both moderate and excessive. The way in which 'alcoholism' became a specialty, divorced from the general study of behaviour, was perhaps inevitable but regrettable. When it has been linked with other kinds of behaviour at all, it has most usually been placed alongside 'drug addiction', a marriage which has emphasized the pharmacological basis of behaviour, and which has encouraged a disease view and discouraged genuine alternatives. Equally, if not more useful, parallels are to be drawn between drinking, gambling, and sexual behaviour, although comparisons between excessive forms of these behaviours have scarcely been explored at all. The triad of drink, sex, and gambling share many features. According to public morality they are acceptable in moderation or within limits, but meet with disapproval if taken to excess. Each can prove troublesome, damaging, or even fatal if uncontrolled, and each is universally the subject of forms of formal and informal social control which have varied widely from place to place and from time to time. As we shall see, each has given rise to fascinating and similar logical and semantic problems when attempts have been made to view their excessive forms as diseases.

The rest of this book is divided into two parts. In Part 1, as a necessary background against which to develop a more adequate psychological view of excessive appetitive behaviour, five forms of excessive behaviour are briefly introduced in turn. My purpose is to show that each of these forms of behaviour can lead to excess, and that the phenomenology described by people affected is remarkably similar. The comparison of these five also illustrates the many points of similarity in terms of definition—addiction, dependence, habituation, abuse, excess, compulsion—and in terms of social control policy. Although my sources are admittedly second or third hand, I have also attempted in places to introduce historical and anthropological perspectives because they can aid comparisons. For example, whilst modern Western tobacco-smoking is difficult to equate with urban heroin addiction, it is easier to see the comparison with English nineteenth-century opium-taking, or with Peruvian twentieth-century coca use.

The five excesses which together make up Part I are drinking, gambling, drug-taking, eating, and sex. The inclusion of alcohol and gambling needs little justification: both are acceptable in our society in moderation and their potential for excess is not in dispute (although the way that excess is construed is controversial). When it came to drug-taking, however, I seriously considered including tobacco but excluding the opiates and other illicit drugs on the grounds that the psychology of their use would be very different from the psychology of activities such as drinking and gambling. Even a very cursory reading of what has been written about drug use historically and in different cultures shows how very narrow this view would have been. Prevailing attitudes and laws in one part of the world turn out to be very arbitrary: drinking, gambling, and tobacco-smoking have all been illegal somewhere at some time, and the use of opium and opiates has been permitted in the United Kingdom in very recent history, and in 1984 is permitted under certain circumstances and in certain forms. Indeed, it turns out that forms of drug-taking with potential for excess are so varied—some 'hard' some 'soft', some illicit and some not, some recreational and some medicinal—that a study of drug-taking in all its variety raises in itself all the same questions of definition, prevention and treatment of excess, and psychological theory, which are posed by comparing drinking, drug-taking, gambling, eating, and sex.

Some may question the inclusion of eating because, unlike drinking, drugs, and gambling, it is not only acceptable in moderation but is a necessity, and because excessive forms of eating do not meet with the same degree of social reaction and forms of social control that arise in the case of the other excessive appetites. Again, a study of the subject shows how short-sighted this view would have been. For one thing, the phenomenology of some forms of excessive eating is very similar to that of excessive drinking and gambling. Indeed, many over-eaters remark themselves on the similarity with 'alcoholism' or 'drug addiction'. It also turns out that over-eating, or at least obesity (which, as we shall see, are not the same thing), meets with considerable social disapproval, even though governments have not felt impelled to try and prevent it. Much point has been added to the inclusion of a chapter on eating by a recent change of direction in theorizing about excessive eating. Attention has shifted from obesity, which is physical, to 'restrained eating', which is psychological. Since restraint is one of the core concepts around which the psychological model of excessive appetites presented in Part II is constructed, the inclusion of excessive eating has been a particular asset. Another advantage is that excessive eating, or at least concern about it, has been more common amongst women than men. This helps redress an imbalance that might be created by an over-emphasis on forms of excessive behaviour which have been more common amongst men. There are also immediate parallels to be drawn with the idea of 'nymphomania', which reflected the greater concern that was felt about excessive sexuality in women than in men, with some forms of drug-taking, such as tranquilizer use, that appear to be more common amongst women, and with recent changes in the balance of women and men amongst excessive drinkers.

Some may question the inclusion of a chapter on excessive sexuality. Its inclusion was however never in doubt. Problems, for individuals and for societies, of restraining an appetite which always threatens to get out of control, is perhaps clearest of all in the case of sex. It probably appears a strange companion to excesses such as excessive drinking and drug-taking because, whereas our understanding of the latter has been over-influenced by the presentation of these problems in clinical settings, excessive sexuality, although undoubtedly a psychological fact, rarely comes to the attention of doctors or other therapists. Its inclusion is thus one of the best aids to the development of a psychological view of excessive appetites which does not rest upon the idea of disease.

Why stop with these five? Other candidates for inclusion were kleptomania and pyromania, long-term survivors of the predilection for adding the suffix 'mania' to indicate an apparently irrational compulsion focused upon one object or activity. In German-speaking countries particularly, the concept of addiction has been extended, as witnessed by the terms *Geltungssucht* (literally status mania, or power mania), *Wandersucht* (wandering mania), and even *Arbeitssucht* (work mania) (Kielholz, 1973). Haberman (1969) also considered over-work as one of the self-indulgences which might be a complement or a counter-attraction to excessive drinking. Perhaps because there is not the same moral ambivalence about work that there is about the forms of behaviour included in the list of five, there is no evidence to this writer's knowledge that individuals have experienced the kind of conflict over excessive working which is the hallmark of excessive appetitive experience.

A particularly creative attempt to extend the concept of 'addiction' still further was made by Peele and Brodsky (1975) in their book, *Love and Addiction*. The core of their argument was that many relationships between couples have the quality of an addiction, particularly in a society that fails to foster a sense of security and self-sufficiency and which expects people to marry as the norm. In all the instances which they give of 'love addiction' they argued that the relationship had become one of increasing dependence on that experience as the only source of gratification, '. . . an increasingly closed, isolated, and mutually protected relationship' (p.84). Such relationships were valued for the protection they provided; they were growth-preventing rather than growth-enhancing. However, despite some insightful comments on the nature of 'addiction' generally, the relationships they described seem to be just rather unsatisfactory ones, entered into for the wrong reasons and difficult to get out of. There is some analogy with excessive appetitive behaviour, but in this writer's view it is not sufficiently close to compel the inclusion of 'interpersonal addiction' as one of our examples, other than that involving many partners (Chapter 6).

Finally, on the subject of the different excessive appetites that could have been included in the list, special mention should be made of two relative newcomers that have attracted much national and local press attention in very recent years. One is 'solvent abuse' (discussed again in Chapter 4). The other is excessive playing of electronic games which offer no possibilities of financial return. Because the latter are not gambling machines they will not be discussed with excessive gambling in Chapter 3. Nevertheless, reports have it that some young people are spending all their money, borrowing, stealing, and selling personal possessions in order to finance their electronic game 'habit', and that worried and angry parents are 'fetching home' their offspring from amusement arcades, remonstrating with arcade managers, and even, in one report, taking an axe to the machines. As with solvents, this appears to be an instance of new technology producing an activity that has the necessary features to give it potential for excess, and catching society unawares before it can anticipate the dangers and instigate the sorts of controls that have grown up around more traditional pursuits such as drinking alcohol or gambling. This well illustrates the fact that appetitive excess is a human potential, and is not merely a property of those substances and activities that have been with us for centuries or which have always been with us.

The larger part of this book, Part II, is devoted to the development of a psychological model of the excessive appetitive behaviours introduced in Part I. It is a model rather than a theory because it is a way of looking at excessive appetites which could lead to specific theories, rather than being a theory with definite predictions itself. The attempt has been to formulate a psychological understanding without recourse to the notion of disease. At the same time, an important consideration has been not to throw out the baby with the bath water, but to make it clear why excessive appetites have attracted the suffic 'mania' or 'ism' and formulations in terms of disease. No model that does not take account of the disease-like characteristics of excessive appetitive behaviour will suffice in this writer's view. Neither an extreme deviancy perspective, suggesting that the problem is created solely by the reactions of other people, nor an extreme psychotherapeutic orientation, claiming that excessive appetitive behaviour is merely a symptom of an underlying fault in individual personality or family dynamics, is adequate. The key concepts around which Part II is written are *inclination*, *restraint*, *attachment*, *conflict*, *decision*, and *self-control*.

PART I

The Excessive Appetites

CHAPTER TWO

Excessive Drinking

> Can you state any other evil effects which proceed from this habit of drunkenness?—Yes; it is not only a great vice in itself, but, from its very nature, directly or indirectly, it leads to almost every other. . . . It wastes the body, perverts the mind, and necessarily leads to misery and death. In fact, intemperance, like a destroying pestilence, is sapping the very foundation of society, and producing among the lower orders throughout the land disease, poverty and crime. (The Reverend David Ruall, giving evidence to the 1834 Select Committee *Inquiry Into Drunkenness*.)

Excessive drinking of alcohol provides the best known example of the type of behaviour which constitutes the theme of this book—namely apparent loss of control over a form of activity which, for most people, serves as a pleasurable and moderate indulgence. It forces upon our attention the major psychological issues with which this book attempts to deal, and at the same time illustrates how the same phenomenon can be viewed from totally different perspectives depending upon the fashion of thought at the time and the orientation of the observer. Such an excessive appetite may be viewed as non-problematic over-indulgence, as sinful behaviour, as crime, as disease, as maladaptive behaviour, or as deviance: there is no better illustration of this diversity of view than the recent history of thought concerning excessive drinking.

There have been many autobiographical accounts written by excessive drinkers and it is worth quoting briefly from just two of these in order to illustrate the point that individual people can and do describe experiencing intense personal suffering which they attribute to their own excessive drinking behaviour. In her book, *I'll Cry Tomorrow*, the American actress Lilian Roth (1978) describes sixteen years of existence in 'a nightmare world' of virtually continuous over-drinking and intoxication which culminated in her conviction that she was being driven insane. The final scenes depicted in her book are ones of degradation, of self-imposed solitary confinement, and of a serious risk of death from alcohol poisoning, suicide, or accident. Earlier in her book, however, there are significant descriptions of her behaviour which raise key issues about the very nature of the phenomenon of losing control over consumption. These are the very issues with which we are centrally concerned here and to which this book will return repeatedly. For example:

> Although beer by day and liquor by night satisfied me while I [had been] busy . . ., now my nerves demanded more. I switched from a morning beer to a jigger of liquor first thing after I awoke.
>
> It seemed a good formula. I improved upon it by pouring two ounces of bourbon into my breakfast orange juice so [my husband] was none the wiser (p.113).

Later on she described escalation to a new level of excess, and dated this from an occasion when a shopping expedition turned into a drinking session and a bartender advised her to carry drink with her in future:

> I realised that I could never go out of the house again without liquor. Orange juice and bourbon in the morning was not enough. The physical demand was growing. I would need liquor more often—not because I wanted it, but because my nerves required it.
>
> Soon I was slipping down doorways, vanishing into ladies' rooms, anywhere I could gain privacy, to take a swift drink. . . . The two-ounce bottles graduated to six-ounce, and then to a pint, and in the last years of my marriage . . . wherever I went, I carried a fifth of liquor in my bag (pp.113–4).

Quite apart from the overall theme of her account, which is the attribution of her problems to a growing addiction to alcohol, two features are particularly noteworthy and are typical of many such accounts. First, there is the use of the word 'demand'. She does not 'want' to behave in this way but something alien to her own wishes demands it. In her case the demand is ascribed to her 'nerves' and then later to a 'physical' need. The second feature is the growing secrecy of her behaviour, and her involvement in deceit. Both features indicate conflict, first within herself and secondly between herself and other people. An adequate psychological understanding of excessive appetitive behaviour must account for both these types of conflict—intrapsychic and interpersonal.

The second personal account is given by John Gardner (1964) in his book, *Spin the Bottle: the Autobiography of an Alcoholic*. In his case the conflict over excessive drinking was made the more acute by his training and practice as a clergyman. After years of drinking excessively off and on, he reached a point where he recognized that control over his drinking was lacking and that something should be done:

> At the beginning of Lent I made the supreme effort . . . Whatever else happened I really must give up the drink—as a sign of good faith—for the forty long days. On Ash Wednesday, crouching at the altar rail . . . I made the vow. Not a drop would pass my lips until Easter Day. On Sunday—legalising that Sundays did not fall within the official forty days of the penitential six weeks—I decided that just one, as a sort of refresher, would not hurt. The one became two. Three. Four and five: until I lurched happily and felt strength returning. Having vaguely admitted that I had a problem involving alcohol, I lost the first battle.
>
> This must have been the primary hint that control was passing out of my hands (p.97).

Later still, Gardner described the same kind of demand, of loss of capacity to choose whether to drink or not, which Lilian Roth also depicted:

> The stuff which had given so much pleasure and power was now starting to turn in on me; becoming not something to brighten the day, but a force as necessary as the air and the wind and the rain. However strong the will-power, the liquor in the bottle was stronger, because by now my body needed it; shrieking for the daily ration as a drug addict's nerve-ends scream for the needle. In junkie's parlance I was on main line (pp.97–8).

Among famous individual excessive drinkers of this century are the playwright Eugene O'Neill and the novelist F. Scott Fitzgerald. Both of these cases have been described by Goodwin (1970, 1971). According to the first of these accounts there was already by O'Neill's late teens 'no doubt' about his 'drinking problem'. From then until his cure at the age of thirty-seven he is said to have been a periodic binge drinker; his wife described mad and violent drunken outbursts; and he suffered 'monumental hangovers' for which he prescribed a diet of soup, milk shakes, and more drink. He wrote when on the wagon between drinking bouts. Two years after his brother 'died of alcoholism' O'Neill took a brief six weeks' psychoanalysis and thereafter, with a few temporary lapses, went on the wagon for the remaining twenty-eight years of his life. His play, *Long Day's Journey Into Night* (O'Neill, 1941), which shows a single family wracked by accusations and guilt about, amongst other things, the drinking of the father and the two brothers, has been described as largely autobiographical (Ghinger and Grant, 1982).

Goodwin describes Scott Fitzgerald as, 'an alcoholic *par excellence*'. By age twenty-three he was, 'getting drunk regularly and in earnest', and beginning to experience, '. . . the social, domestic, professional and finally medical problems that, coming singly or in flurries, characterize the natural history of alcoholism'. By his mid-twenties he was decidedly 'alcoholic': '. . . he recognised it and so did his friends'. By his late twenties his drinking was more a solitary than a social affair and he began regular attempts to control it although, unlike O'Neill, he never succeeded for longer than a few months at a time. He even hired nurses to watch him for his own good but he '. . . sneaked drinks when they were not looking'. He refused the psychiatric treatment which he was advised to accept and died of a heart attack aged 44.

These accounts, by a modern medical expert, are quite clear on two points: drinking behaviour in both cases was problematic, and in both cases the problem could be attributed to an understandable entity, 'alcoholism'. The latter is something which has a 'natural history'. It is something that can be recognized or not as the case may be; it is something for which treatment can be offered and which is best accepted, and it can cause death. This conception of excessive drinking as a disease-like entity is now the over-riding view, at least in countries with well-developed specialist health and welfare systems, and is embodied in the 1952 World Health Organization (WHO) definition of 'alcoholism':

> Alcoholics are those excessive drinkers whose dependence on alcohol has attained such a degree that it shows a noticeable mental disturbance or interference with their bodily or mental health, their interpersonal relations and their smooth social and economic functions, or who show the prodromal signs of such development. They, therefore, require treatment (World Health Organization, 1952).

Not surprisingly, given such a wide and imprecise definition, the literature on the subject is found to be full of arguments and counter-arguments about the appropriate usage of the term 'alcoholism' and related terms such as 'alcohol addiction' and 'alcohol dependence'. It is important to stay with this perplexed question of definitions for a while, and in particular to consider the thoughts on the subject of the psychiatrist E. M. Jellinek. Present-day medical acceptance of 'alcoholism' as a disease is often attributed to Jellinek and to his book, *The Disease Concept of Alcoholism*, published in 1960. The medical concept of 'alcoholism' is in fact a hundred or more years older than that, as Jellinek himself was at pains to point out. His book is instructive, however, for a number of reasons. He travelled widely for the WHO, and thus less hampered than most by a stereotype of the form excessive drinking might appear to take in his own culture, he was able to describe the different forms that it took in different parts of the world. His book is therefore still the best source of description of the variety of drinking phenomena with which a psychological account of excessive drinking must deal. Furthermore, he thought hard about the different forms of behaviour which were described to him and about the appropriateness of applying terms such as 'alcoholism' and 'disease' to them. Thus, although he was only concerned with excessive drinking, his thoughts on the subject are highly relevant to the attempt which is being made here to juxtapose different forms of excess which involve the consumption of alcoholic drinks, the use of other drugs, forms of gambling behaviour, eating, and sexual behaviour. Finally, despite his evident wisdom, it is possible to see parts of his book as sources of later confusion on the subject.

Jellinek's attempt to make sense of the diversity he found is shown diagrammatically in Figure 1. It is a brilliant attempt at classification, and his species of 'alcoholism' denoted by the first five letters of the Greek alphabet are still employed by some practitioners today. A few quotations from his book illustrate the subtlety of his approach. He started by stating that, 'In order to do justice to these international, as well as our own national differences, we have termed as *alcoholism any use of alcoholic beverages that causes any damage to the individual or society or both*' (1960, p.35, his emphasis). He went on: 'Obviously there are species of alcoholism—so defined—which cannot be regarded as illnesses . . .. We must be particularly definite about those forms

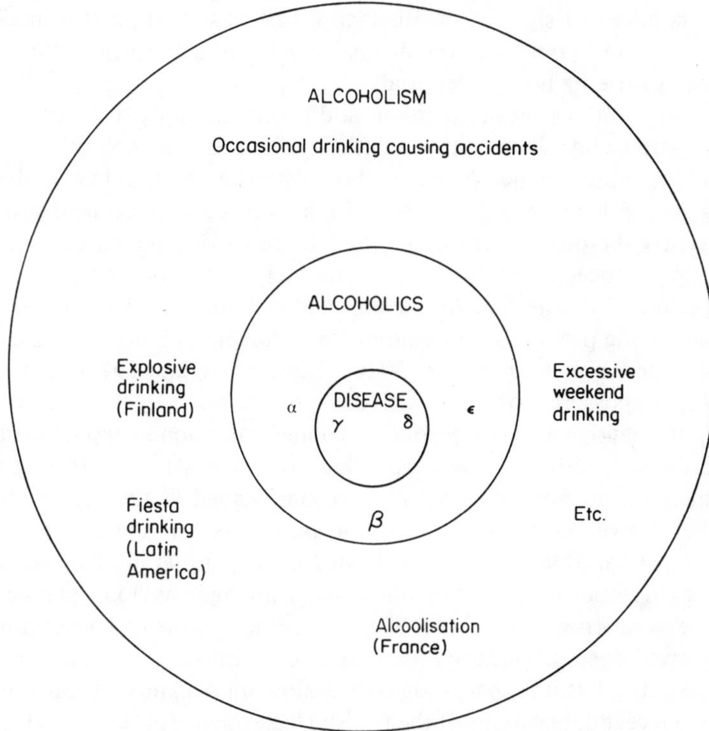

Figure 1 Jellinek's model of alcoholism (based on Jellinek, 1960, pp.35–41)

which we wish to examine as possibly constituting illnesses' (pp.35–6). Then he made an extraordinary statement which no doubt he understood, but which is too subtle and which puts the whole discussion on a parallel with similar arguments about such apparent entities as 'nymphomania' and 'compulsive gambling': 'Furthermore . . . we cannot say that alcoholics are those who suffer from alcoholism as defined above. We shall have to make a distinction between alcoholism and alcoholics' (p.36). He later admitted that the line he drew between the five types of 'alcoholic' (alpha to epsilon) and other forms of 'alcoholism' was an arbitrary one. Finally, he reserved the word 'disease' for the gamma and delta types, for only here did he believe there was a 'physio-pathological process' involving adaptation of cell metabolism, the acquisition of tissue tolerance, and the experience of withdrawal symptoms. Robinson (1972), a sociologist, has pointed out that Jellinek is much quoted but little read, that the experts have lost sight of the distinctions he was attempting to make, and that we have, 'lost control of the disease concept of alcoholism'. Such a state of affairs is little to be wondered at.

The distinction between 'alcohol addiction', roughly corresponding to Jellinek's gamma and delta types, and other varieties of 'alcoholism' or 'problem drinking', is quite frequently made. For instance, Wilkins (1974) drew this dividing line in a survey of excessive drinkers in general medical practice—until recently the only survey of its kind to be carried out in Britain. In his own group practice, with a list of approximately 12,000 patients, he recorded, over a period of 12 months, 46 'alcohol addicts' and 41 further patients with 'serious drinking problems' not amounting to 'alcohol addiction'. In contrast, a recent expert report from the WHO (Edwards *et al.*, 1977) finds such a distinction impossible to make. On the other hand a line is drawn in this latter report that seems to correspond to Jellinek's division between 'alcoholism' and 'alcoholics', although the terminology is quite different. In fact neither term, 'alcoholism' nor 'alcoholics', is recommended in the report. In place of Jellinek's five central varieties of 'alcoholic' is 'the alcohol dependence syndrome', a variable entity compounded of varying amounts of abnormal physiological response to alcohol, abnormal drinking behaviour, and abnormal subjective experience of drinking. This term, 'alcohol dependence syndrome', with its two-edged implication that excessive drinking can amount to an abnormal entity but one that is highly variable in its manifestations, has been adopted in recent publications of the British Department of Health (DHSS, 1981) and Royal College of Psychiatrists (1979) in preference to the term 'alcoholism' which is considered too imprecise for modern usage. The new term was accepted for the ninth revision of the *International Classification of Diseases* in preference to 'alcoholism'.

In place of Jellinek's wider concept of 'alcoholism' are 'alcohol-related disabilities', recognition of the apparent fact that a wide range of problematic social and medical incidents, such as traffic accidents, crimes of various sorts, and a range of illnesses, may be at least partially attributable to drinking without being part of an enduring and abnormal use and experience of alcohol on the part of particular individuals. Alcohol use can cause problems for people without those individuals necessarily having an enduring problem of excessive drinking.

It is clear then that present-day students of the subject have run into terminological and conceptual confusion over the nature of excessive drinking. How old, in fact, is the notion of excessive drinking as an individual trait involving an interference with freedom of choice to take or leave drink as the individual desires? Levine (1978), writing with particular reference to the United States, has argued for the emergence of this idea towards the end of the eighteenth and the beginning of the nineteenth centuries. Prior to that time drunken excess was well recognized as something that many American colonials indulged in sometimes and which some indulged in often, but was viewed as the result of free individual choice and not as something that constituted a problem in itself. Unlike Lilian Roth's and John Gardner's understanding of their excessive drinking, habitual drunkards were so because they liked it and chose to be that way. As Levine put it:

> In colonial thought, alcohol did not permanently disable the will; it was not addicting, and habitual drunkenness was not regarded as a disease. With very few exceptions, colonial Americans did not use a vocabulary of compulsion with regard to alcoholic beverages (1978, p.144).

This pre-addiction view was based, Levine pointed out, on the philosophical premise that it is impossible to differentiate between Desire and Will. As he so rightly said, this distinction is the kernel of the concept of 'addiction', and is much in evidence in Roth's, Gardner's, and other modern-day accounts of excessive drinking.

This is not to say that drunkenness was not viewed by some as either extremely troublesome or very sinful. Indeed, the early to middle eighteenth century in England offers a notorious example of alcoholic excess on a large scale. Economic and legislative factors seem, according to Coffey's (1966) account, to have been the major influences. French imports of wines and spirits were prohibited towards the end of the previous century and English brewers learnt to distil gin, which had been introduced from the Low Countries, from English grain. Total consumption of gin in England rose from half a million gallons in 1685 to 11 million in 1750. Controlling legislation was attempted in 1729 and 1736, but the first attempt was too weak to be effective and the second law, too repressive, was flouted. Effective legislation came in 1751 through limitations on the issue of retail licences and the introduction of stiff penalties for unlicensed retailing. Consumption dropped to under two million gallons within a decade and to around one million by 1790.

Much of the poverty and lawlessness of the period was, and has been since, attributed to gin-drinking, particularly by the London poor. Amongst other ill-effects, a staggeringly high infant mortality rate (75 per cent before age five according to one historian) was blamed upon a combination of maternal excessive drinking and the practice of dosing babies with gin either to quieten them or as a deliberate act of murder. Hogarth's print *Gin Lane*, depicting drunkenness, pawning, child neglect, starvation, emaciation, suicide, and a thriving trade of pawnbrokers and undertakers, may have been one of the influences for reform. By contrast, his print *Beer Street* is a portrait of restraint and prosperity. As in colonial North America, however, there appears to have been no generally accepted concept of 'addiction' or 'dependence' at this time in England. Those who gave evidence to the 1834 Select Committee's Inquiry into Drunkenness (1968), were still taking a largely moral view, particularly of drunkenness and the, '. . . . misery and immorality of the lower orders amongst the working classes . . .' (from the evidence given by J. R. Farre, Esq.), which was assumed to be the *result* of excessive drinking rather than its cause. Medical views were represented, but they were extreme. Dr. R. G. Dodds, for example, asked about maladies arising from intemperance, said:

> Apoplexy is a very common result from intemperance, insanity is not infrequent, mental delusions are often see, delirium tremens, and a most fearful disease, which though not very common, has been repeatedly witnessed, spontaneous combustion.

The change in thinking that occurred shortly thereafter Levine (1978) attributed to a total change in the philosophical climate of the times, associated with the emancipation of the new middle-class for whom self-control and self-restraint became cherished values that signalled and helped retain their position in society. Deviant excess was now an abnormality, which in an otherwise respectable person could only be ascribed to a sort of sickness, a disease of the will. Whether this view of history is right or wrong, it is generally held to be the case that writings on drunkenness with a modern 'addiction' ring to them began to appear at the end of the nineteenth century. Certainly the evidence given to the 1872 Select Committee on Habitual Drunkards (1968) strikes a very different note to that given to the Committee of 1834. The inclusion of the word 'habitual' in the title is itself an immediate indication of the recognition that individuals can acquire a special propensity to excess: we are now dealing not just with instances of drunkenness, but with people, unlike others, who are in the habit of getting drunk regularly. There was even recognition by some who gave evidence, of the variety of forms of excessive drinking which Jellinek was to note many years later. For example, a Mr Mould anticipated Jellinek's distinction between gamma and delta types:

> I should divide habitual drunkards into two classes; those who drink impulsively, and not continuously, and who are of the most violent and dangerous characters, and require immediate control and restraint; and those who continuously drink and get into a kind of soddened and muddled state.

And Dr Anstie recognized the epsilon type of bout drinking or 'dipsomania' as it was once called:

> I knew a man who was in an exceedingly good position . . . he always lived a sober and chaste life, except when the fit was upon him; he did not go far off to avoid scandal, but went to the nearest public-house, and consorted with loose women, and shut himself up in a back parlour and and drank brandy with them for six weeks, close to the village where he was an important man; he was a manufacturer, it was a very well-known case at the time.

A view from the prison service of that time could, with the exception of reference to the treadwheel, belong quite comfortably in the 1970s or 1980s:

> In your opinion what is the effect of the existing method of punishing the drunken, and the drunken and disorderly, by short terms of imprisonment?—I think that it is quite useless; I think that it does more harm than good . . . in the numerous cases of three, and five, and seven days, it is worse than useless; they are entirely useless in the prison, they are unfit to work, and in fact I make a point of not allowing them to go in amongst the regular prisoners until they get the drink worked out of them; they are unfit for it. If I were to put them on the treadwheel in the ordinary way, of course there are exceptions, but if the general run of those prisoners were put upon the treadwheel the day after they came in, they would faint, and would fall off (evidence of Mr H. Webster).

Thomas Trotter in Britain and Benjamin Rush in the United States are names particularly associated with the new way of thinking (Jellinek, 1960; Levine, 1978). The latter especially, better known now for his works on mental illness, is remembered as a forerunner of present-day medical specialists on the subject. According to the then editor of the *Quarterly Journal of Studies on Alcohol*—a research journal published at the Centre for Alcohol Studies at Rutgers University in New Jersey—Rush was responsible for the earliest American publication of any scientific note on the subject of 'inebriety'. Despite being first published, in all probability, in 1785, in many ways it bears remarkable similarities to many modern publications on the subject. It bore the title: *An Enquiry into the Effect of Spirituous Liquors Upon the Human Body and Their Influence upon the Happiness of Society*, and was reprinted by the editor of the *QJSA* in 1943. Dr Rush listed the chronic effects of ardent spirits as, '. . . a decay of appetite, sickness . . . and puking . . .', '. . . obstructions of the liver', 'jaundice and dropsy . . .', 'hoarseness', 'diabetes', 'redness, and eruptions on different parts of the body . . .', '. . . fetid breath', 'frequent and disgusting belchings', 'epilepsy', 'gout', and lastly 'madness' (Rush, 1943, pp.327–8). Furthermore, ardent spirits, '. . . impair the memory, debilitate the understanding, and pervert the moral faculties' (p.328). Later editions of his book included the 'moral and physical thermometer', which was to become quite famous and which looks remarkably like the forerunner of several modern lists or charts showing the progressively incurred 'symptoms' of 'alcoholism' (see Glatt, 1975, for one of the best known modern lists).

In at least two major details, however, modern views part company with those of the much respected Dr Rush. First, he was clear that the acute effects of ardent spirits, or the 'prompt' effects as he called them, merited the term 'disease'. Amongst the 'symptoms' of drunkenness in his list were 'profane swearing and cursing', '. . . a rude disposition to tell [others] . . . their faults', '. . . certain immodest actions' (which even occurred he was 'sorry to say', in women otherwise known for 'chaste and decent manners'), and 'certain extravagant acts which indicate a temporary fit of madness' (pp.325–6). This is a more important point than it may at first appear. It indicates that he was principally concerned with bodily and mental *effects*, whether prompt or chronic. He was an eighteenth-century medical practitioner and not a twentieth-century psychiatrist or psychologist, and was hence more concerned with medical symptoms than with behaviour *per se*. Modern conceptions of 'dependence' are more concerned with the functional role of alcohol for the individual and, on account of the development of tolerance to the drug, often view drunkenness and 'alcoholism' as unrelated, or even as inversely related.

Secondly, Rush confined his attack to 'ardent' or distilled spirits (principally rum in the United States of those days) and he viewed the consumption of wine and beer relatively favourably. Indeed, he considered that:

> The peasants of France who drink them [wines] in large quantities are a sober and healthy body of people. Unlike ardent spirits, which render the temper irritable wines generally inspire cheerfulness and good humour (p.331).

Recent views have been more informed by recognition of alcohol as a chemical substance common to many beverages, whether brewed, fermented, or distilled, and French wine-drinking habits have been considered particularly disposing towards excess.

Nevertheless the main hallmarks of the modern view of 'alcoholism' are there in Rush's Enquiry: compulsive loss of control over drinking as the essence of the condition; the appropriateness of the ascription 'disease'; and the prescribing of total abstinence as the only way to cure habitual drunkenness (Levine, 1978, p.152). Not that the introduction of an enlightened medical view of excessive drinking has gone unchallenged by the moralists, however. Jellinek (1960) reported that the *Journal of Inebriety*, when it first came out in the 1870s, met with much criticism from both clergymen and some doctors who, '. . . denounced the work as materialistic and an effort to excuse crime and dignify vice' (Crothers, 1911, cited by Jellinek, p.3). Nor had such views disappeared by the time Jellinek was compiling his book, although by then the language had changed in some cases. For example:

> Alcoholism is due to defective superego development and is therefore a moral question. In its destructive aspects, alcoholism must be viewed as a crime (Björk, 1950, cited by Jellinek, p.58).

Or:

> Alcoholism is no more a disease than thievery, or lynching; like these, it is the product of a distortion of outlook, a way of life bred of ignorance and frustration (McGoldrick, 1954, cited by Jellinek, p.59).

The nineteenth century was a century of temperance societies and workers in the United States (the movement in the United States has been described by numerous writers, including Jellinek, 1960, and Levine, 1978), in Britain (again numerous sources, but see especially Harrison, 1971, and Longmate, 1968), and in Ireland (for a recent brief account of temperance in Ireland see O'Connor, 1978, Ch.4). Part of Levine's argument was that the emerging medical view of habitual excessive drinking as 'addiction' and the temperance aim of reducing habitual drunkenness went hand in hand; but that the temperance movement, in the United States at least, became preoccupied with the political goal of total prohibition at the end of the century (the same was true in England also); and that the alliance of medicine and temperance only resurfaced in a new form with Alcoholics Anonymous (AA) and a renewed medical interest in the 1930s and 1940s. This is clearly to cut a very long story short. What is persuasive, however, is Levine's point that temperance (religious, non-scientific) and medical (supposedly scientific) approaches were by no means as antithetical as might be supposed. We shall see below that these two currents have been inextricably interwoven in recent times also.

One of the hallmarks of nineteenth-century temperance which finds its modern equivalent in certain aspects of AA procedure and in professionally directed group therapy for 'alcoholics' was the public announcement or confession and the taking of an abstinence pledge. One of the first such confessions recorded was made by James Chalmers of New Jersey who in 1795 made the following sworn and witnessed statement:

> Whereas, the subscriber, through the pernicious habit of drinking, has greatly hurt himself in purse and person, and rendered himself odious to all his acquaintances and finds that there is no possibility of breaking off from the said practice but through the impossibility to find liquor, he therefore begs and prays that no person will sell him for money, or on trust, any sort of spirituous liquors (Cherrington, 1920, cited by Levine, pp.153–4).

The loss of freedom or will-power where drink is concerned is clearly expressed in this statement and the confessor appeals to externally imposed restraint to help him overcome his lack of internal self-control.

The role of pledge-taking is nowhere better illustrated than in accounts of Father Mathew's campaign in Ireland. A whole chapter in Longmate's book, *The Water Drinkers* (1968), about the temperance movement in Britain, is devoted to this one man's influence on Irish drunkenness in the 1830s and 1840s. During his public tours of the country it is estimated that he administered two million pledges to nearly a quarter of the population (O'Connor, 1978). Longmate, who is well aware of the possibilities of exaggeration in the accounts of this campaign, declares:

> The transformation of Ireland during the Father Mathew years was by any test remarkable . . . By the end of 1841 it was claimed that there were at least five million on the teetotal roll in a population of eight million. Brewers and distilleries went out of business and publicans deserted their trade (1968, p.114).

For a variety of reasons, however, the effects of this campaign appear to have been short-lived in Ireland. Father Mathew was a charismatic leader who left little organization behind him, his movement was not linked directly to the Catholic Church, and furthermore Ireland was shortly to be preoccupied with the stress of the potato famine. By comparison, Father Cullen, the founder of the Pioneer Total Abstinence Association, was far better organized and established and the association he founded lives on in Ireland as a significant influence to this day (O'Connor, 1978). Nevertheless, there can be little doubt of the short-term effectiveness of Father Mathew's campaign, and the role of the pledge as an instrument of behaviour change is a theme to which this book will return in a later chapter.

Because of its apparent ability to reconcile the seemingly incompatible moral and medical views of excessive indulgence, and because many of its precepts have been borrowed by those who have wished to combine with others to help themselves overcome excesses of other kinds, Alcoholics Anonymous will be the object of quite close scrutiny later in this book. Its very existence, and its success in recruiting many tens of thousands of members (there were over 600 groups in England and Wales in 1976 according to Robinson, 1979) in well over a hundred countries, is probably the strongest testimony of all to the fact of personal concern over drinking excess. Its individual disease-of-the-will perspective has, arguably at least, laid the immediate foundations on which modern concern has been built.

Of this present-day concern there can be little doubt. The concept of a disease-like entity, and the term 'alcoholism' to describe it, have by now achieved widespread acceptance by members of the professions and the lay public, certainly in Britain and the United States. Like many other putative individual conditions or entities it has become a strong candidate for explaining a whole range of social and personal problems. This way it is argued that 'alcoholism' is much more prevalent than may appear, that it is often missed or misdiagnosed, and that it is often the 'real' problem underlying presenting medical or social problems. There now exists a whole range of categories of people and problems for whom excessive drinking is thought to provide at least a partial 'explanation'. These include the vagrant, single homeless (Edwards *et al.*, 1968; Archard, 1979), people convicted of public drunkenness offences (e.g. Gath, 1969), prison inmates serving both short- and long-term prison sentences (e.g. Hensman, 1969; Gibbens and Silberman, 1970), those experiencing marital or family disharmony (Paolino and McCrady, 1977), or family violence (e.g. Gayford, 1975), children with behaviour problems (Wilson, C., 1982), and some newborn infants with certain mental and physical abnormalities constituting the so-called foetal alcohol syndrome (e.g. Abel, 1980).

'Alcoholism' has been held to underlie a great range of medical and social problems which present themselves in a general medical practice setting (Wilkins, 1974) or in a general hospital (Murray, 1977). The better known medical conditions that have been linked to excessive drinking are cirrhosis of the liver, pancreatitis, gastritis and peptic ulcer, tuberculosis, cardiomyopathy, and peripheral neuritis. There is evidence that people diagnosed as suffering from 'alcoholism' are much more likely than the average person to commit suicide (e.g. Kessel, 1965), and high rates have been discovered amongst victims of accidents in the home, at work, and in traffic. Hence, accident and emergency services of general hospitals are said to deal with a very large number of people who are really 'alcoholics'. Overweight in men, and anxiety or depression in women, are amongst the many signs and symptoms of personal excessive drinking, or of excessive drinking in the family, which a general medical practitioner may overlook unless he or she is especially on the lookout for it (Wilkins, 1974). Any textbook of psychiatry will list neurological and psychological consequences of 'alcoholism', such as seizures and delirium tremens, depression, and dementia. The number of mental hospital admissions for 'alcoholism' is often said to be a considerable underestimate of the true rate amongst psychiatric patients.

In recent times particular concern has been expressed about excessive drinking in drivers (Department of the Environment, 1976) and amongst members of the work-force (Hore and Plant, 1981). It may be costly to the nation in quantifiable financial terms, both in lost productivity and the provision of accident services. Concern is particularly expressed about the possibility of disproportionately growing rates of 'alcoholism' amongst two major groups: women and the young. For various reasons, not least the existence of a double standard that makes excessive drinking more stigmatizing amongst women, it is said to be even harder to unearth the 'real alcoholism' that exists amongst women (e.g. Curlee, 1969; Otto, 1975). Finally, the possibility of excessive drinking in the young, as is true for excessive appetitive behaviour of any kind, is a highly emotive topic (O'Connor, 1978), and one which has excited a great deal of public and Press comment and concern in recent years.

Recent concern has by no means been confined to English-speaking countries. Table 1, adapted from Moser's (1980) international review for the World Health Organization, shows the widespread increase in alcohol consumption that occurred in most parts of Europe in the previous twenty to thirty years. The adverse effects of 'alcoholism', particularly upon family life, are noted in such countries as Germany, Switzerland, France, Yugoslavia, and the Scandinavian countries; indeed, wherever there are medical or social scientists with a special interest in the subject.

Table 1 Changes in consumption of alcoholic beverages in Europe 1950–1976

	1950	1976	% Change 1950–1976
France	17.2	16.5	− 4
Portugal	—	14.1	
Spain	—	14.0	
Luxembourg	6.8	13.4	+ 97
Italy	9.2	12.7	+ 38
Germany, Fed. Rep.	2.9	12.5	+331
Austria	5.0	11.2	+124
Hungary	4.8	10.7	+123
Switzerland	7.9	10.3	+ 30
Belgium	6.3	10.2	+ 62
Czechoslovakia	4.0	9.2	+130
Denmark	3.6	9.2	+156
Ireland	3.3	8.7	+164
United Kingdom	4.9	8.4	+ 71
Netherlands	2.1	8.3	+295
Germany, Dem. Rep.	1.2	8.3	+592
Poland	3.0	8.2	+173
Finland	1.7	6.4	+276
Sweden	3.6	5.9	+ 64
Norway	2.2	4.3	+ 95

Source: Moser (1980). Consumption expressed as average annual consumption of 100 per cent ethanol equivalent per annum.

The particular forms of concern and sometimes the language in which this concern is expressed vary from country to country. In Zambia, for example, where concern has been acute, the effect of parental 'alcoholism' upon malnutrition in children has been noted (Khan and Gupta, 1979). In Eastern Europe, on the other hand, there is greater anxiety about 'moral disorder in youth' (e.g. Jurek, 1974). Governments around the world have involved themselves in alcohol control in the twentieth century just as the British Government was forced to do in the eighteenth. Wilkinson (1970) provided a useful review of some European examples of control policies, particularly highlighting the example of Sweden which has experienced both a tightening and a later release of restrictions. As in several other countries, including Belgium, Denmark, and Britain, new restrictions were introduced in Sweden during or just after the First World War. They were unusually comprehensive, including a ration book (the motbok) system, taxation controls, licensing restrictions, and the empowering of temperance boards to forbid alcohol sales or driving licences to individuals whose drinking was excessive. Wilkinson concluded that these measures had no discernible effect, although the abolition of the motbok in 1955 did result in large increases in consumption and drunkenness offences.

One of the most drastic uses of taxation for alcohol control, a method that has been quite widely canvassed in Britain in recent years (e.g. Grant, 1979), occurred in Denmark in 1917 when the tax on spirits was increased 34-fold, and the price of aquavit increased 15-fold; the consumption of spirits dropped markedly. France provides a more modern instance of the employment of a concerted public health campaign to combat excessive drinking (Fleck, 1970) which may have been responsible for the fact that France is the only European country where alcohol consumption has not increased since the 1950s, albeit remaining at the highest level in Europe (Moser, 1980).

Heath (1976), reviewing a large body of anthropological work on alcohol, pointed out that its use had almost universally been subject to special rules and regulations which have had a strong emotional charge relating not only to drinking itself but also to drunkenness and 'drunken comportment'. Predominant feelings might be positive, negative, or ambivalent, depending upon the culture, but indifference was rare. One of the most dramatic examples of cultural response to, and control of, the use of alcohol is the story of the development of the abstinence norm in Arab countries after the rise of Islam. Baasher (1981) has related how successive Revelations of the Prophet Muhammed first urged good judgement and discrimination between useful and harmful practices, later warned about the dangers of strong drink, then prohibited drinking before prayer, and finally commanded that all should desist, not only from drinking, but also from brewing, carrying, serving, selling, or buying. These directives were backed up by a range of punishments including reprimanding, group scolding, and up to 40 lashes with palm branches. Baasher's account thus suggests that drinking attitudes and practices in Medina were transformed within a very few years and that from there prohibition spread to the rest of the growing Islamic world. The *Qur'ān*, he points out, '. . . besides being a religious doctrine . . . constitutes a code of civil and criminal law as well as social and behavioural codes' (p.234). The role of religion in the control of appetitive behaviour has been a pervasive one, as we shall see.

A major consequence of viewing drinking excess as a disease-like property of individuals, whether in Zambia, Sweden, or Britain, is that the matter becomes suitable for investigation by the methods of medical epidemiology. It becomes a question of 'recognizing cases' and of counting heads. It becomes reasonable to ask how many people suffer from *it*, and it becomes important to know the answer in order to plan preventive and treatment services. It goes without saying that the problems involved in such exercises are huge, particularly as it is supposed that many people are reluctant to seek help for problems associated with excessive drinking and that much of the problem remains hidden. Nevertheless, the ways in which epidemiologists have gone about this task of estimating the numbers of excessive drinkers in a community are most instructive if we wish to understand what they have meant by 'alcoholism' or a 'drinking problem'.

A popular but very indirect method to assess the number of 'cases' of 'alcoholism' in a population uses a formula, devised by Jellinek, for estimating the number of 'alcoholics' from the number of people in the same population dying each year from cirrhosis of the liver. Unfortunately, the formula requires for its accuracy the assumption of two constants. First, an assumption must be made concerning the proportion of cirrhotic deaths which are attributable to excessive drinking. Secondly, it has to be assumed that a certain constant proportion of 'alcoholics' die from this cause. Jellinek's formula has been severely criticized on these grounds (Popham, 1970). Nevertheless, estimates based upon his formula have proved to be less inaccurate than might have been expected when compared with more direct survey estimates. Incidentally, the estimate for Britain for the late 1950s was 11 people with serious drinking problems per thousand of the adult population. This estimate was still being used by the Department of Health in major planning and policy documents in the late 1970s, but has recently been revised upwards.

Examples of the use of more direct methods of estimation have been surveys carried out in the Camberwell area of South London by the Institute of Psychiatry's Addiction Research Unit team (Edwards *et al.*, 1972a, 1972b, 1973). The surveys were of two quite distinct types. One (Edwards *et al.*, 1973) was a reporting agency survey which relied for its estimates of prevalence upon the likelihood of 'alcoholics' being known to one or more of a number of agencies. The agencies involved are shown in Table 2. This list gives a good indication of the sites at which people who drink excessively would be expected to come to public notice in a modern, industrialized society with a well-developed health and social service system. The length and content of this list is itself a fact of considerable interest. The survey produced an overall figure of 4.7 'alcoholics' per thousand adults (8.6 for men and 1.3 for women) during a one-year period. Medical agencies alone reported 2.4 per thousand (4.1 for men and 0.8 for women).

These figures represent what might be termed the known or 'labelled' prevalence (Edwards *et al.*, 1973; Cartwright *et al.*, 1975) and are clearly unsatisfactory to the epidemiologist if a 'true' picture of actual prevalence is required. They do, however, give some indication of the extent to which the problem is visible. The second type of survey is the more familiar household survey, in the course of which a sample of the population is asked a series of pertinent questions. Such surveys are more germane in the present context, not just because they may produce a more 'accurate' prevalence estimate, but because in the course of such research the investigators must operationalize what they mean by 'alcoholism' or a 'drinking problem'. This provides us with invaluable insights into the nature of the concepts being employed, and hence

Table 2 Sources included in the Camberwell agency survey (reprinted, with permission from Edwards *et al.*, 1973, p.170)

1	Courts: magistrates' courts, Inner London Sessions, and the Central Criminal Court
2	Probation Service: at these courts
3	Local weekly newspapers
4	General hospital casualty departments
5	Clergy of seven different denominations
6	Local employers with more than 10 people on the payroll
7	Local government welfare agencies: education authorities, children's departments, welfare department, housing authorities, reception centre
8	Local government non-medical health agencies: mental welfare officers, health visitors, public health inspectors, district nurses
9	Voluntary welfare, non-specialized: university settlements, Samaritan organizations, old people's welfare agency, family casework agencies, counselling centres, children's agencies, ex-service agency
10	Voluntary alcoholism agencies: counselling centres and rehabilitation hostels
11	Alcoholics Anonymous
12	General practitioners
13	Psychiatric hospitals and psychiatric departments
14	General hospitals
15	Prison medical service
16	Coroners' records

is a necessary starting-point for seriously considering the underlying psychological processes at work.

In the Camberwell household sample survey interviewers asked the twenty-five standard questions shown in Table 3. Any respondent with five or more such 'symptoms' was 'arbitrarily defined a "problem" ' (Edwards *et al.*, 1973, p.175). This procedure resulted in a much greater prevalence rate of 31.3 problem drinkers per thousand adults (61.3 men and 7.7 women). The problems of aggregating items and of arbitrarily deciding cut-off points are immediately apparent and have been much discussed in the literature on drinking surveys (e.g. Room, 1977). Cartwright *et al.* (1975) carried out a survey in the same area almost ten years after that of Edwards *et al.*, and found a very similar but somewhat increased prevalence rate using essentially the same criterion.

Almost all of the questions listed in Table 3 concern harmful *consequences* of excessive drinking, rather than drinking behaviour *per se*. The same was true of the criteria for problem drinking used in the largest American survey of drinking practices and problems, a study involving several thousand respondents throughout the United States (Cahalan, 1970; Cahalan and Room, 1974). In the later of these two reports the authors concentrated on men between the ages of 21 and 59, this being the group with the highest prevalence of problems. They reported no less than 20 per cent of adult men having 'high current overall problems'. Certainly all estimates, including those based on the Jellinek formula, suggest that 'alcoholism' and 'problem drinking' rates are higher in the United States than in the United Kingdom, but Cahalan and Room's figure of 20 per

Table 3 Problem drinking questions in the Camberwell household survey (reprinted, with permission, from Edwards *et al.*, 1973, pp.175–6)

1	Have you ever felt that you ought to cut down on your drinking?
2	Have you ever spent more money than you ought to on drink?
3	Have you ever gone without drink for a period to prove you can do so?
4	Have you ever been 'under the influence'?
5	Have people annoyed you by criticizing your drinking?
6	Have you ever had trouble or quarrels with family or friends because of your drinking?
7	Have you ever had fights with members of family or friends after drinking?
8	Have you ever had financial problems due to drinking?
9	Have you ever been in trouble with the police due to a 'drunk' offence (other than 'drunk driving')?
10	Have you ever been in trouble with the police for 'drunk driving'?
11	Have you ever been in trouble with the police for anything else connected with drinking?
12	Have you ever been in a road accident (as a driver or pedestrian) because of drinking?
13	Have you ever been in other accidents (e.g. at home or at work) because of drinking?
14	Have you ever had difficulties at work because of drinking?
15	Have you ever arrived late at work due to a hangover?
16	Have you ever ever missed a day's work because of a hangover?
17	Have you ever lost a job through drinking?
18	Has your doctor ever advised you not to drink as much as you do?
19	Have you ever had health problems due to drinking?
20	After drinking have you ever found you can't remember the night before?
21	Do you ever find that when you start drinking you can't stop?
22	After drinking have you found your hands shaky in the morning?
23	Have you ever had a drink first thing in the morning to steady your nerves or get rid of a hangover?
24	Have you ever 'heard' or 'seen' things due to drinking?
25	Have you ever had special medical treatment for drinking?

cent was arrived at by a process even more arbitrary and difficult to interpret than that employed by Edwards *et al.* in Camberwell. In order to come within their 'high problem' category it was necessary to admit to having had a severe problem within the last three years in at least one of seven areas of life (with wife, relatives, friends or neighbours, job, police, health, or finances). Alternatively, minor problems in three of these areas could place a respondent in the 'high problem' category, or a moderate problem in one area and a minor problem in another, etc. However, it should certainly not be thought that the authors cited have been uncritical about these problems of definition and classification.

Although such investigations have principally been concerned with social problems caused by drinking, it is clear that they have taken an *individual* rather than a group or community perspective because they attempted to aggregate problems experienced by individuals and to come to some conclusion about the status of individuals. As Cahalan and Room themselves pointed out, the assumption is that different problems associated with drinking (or at least assumed to be) have enough in common so that 'alcoholism' or 'problem drinking' can be regarded as an entity, and furthermore that this entity is a *condition* and not just an occurrence. In other words, we assume there is a state of being liable to problems related to drinking and that this state has some continuity in time.

Not only that, but it is also clear that the researchers have been heir to the personal disease-of-the-will notion, the origins of which can be traced back well beyond the start of the twentieth century. In fact, Cahalan and Room, '. . . sought to cover all major areas of content considered to be a part of alcoholism or problem drinking . . .' (p.5). These fell into three broad areas, one being the area of *consequences* of drinking which was used by them to define a 'drinking problem'. Of the others one concerned drinking *behaviour* itself. Three scales were employed to measure this component: heavy intake (the highest point on this scale being, 'twelve or more drinks at a time at least once a week, or eight or more drinks at least nearly every day'); binge drinking (the highest point being, 'stayed intoxicated several days at a time five or more times in the last three years'); and symptomatic drinking (the highest point being reached with five affirmatives from the following items—skipping regular meals while drinking, tossing down several drinks to get a quicker effect, having a quick drink when no one was looking, having a few quick drinks before a party to make sure he had enough, waking the next day unable to remember what he had done while drinking, often taking a drink first thing in the morning, shaking a lot after drinking, and sometimes getting high or tight drinking by himself) (pp.240–1).

The third area, psychological *involvement*, clearly has the greatest implications for a psychological model of excessive behaviour. Two scales were employed: psychological 'dependence' (a complex sum of points awarded for admitting to drinking in order to forget, to cheer up when in a bad mood, drinking when tense and nervous or depressed, etc.); and 'loss of control' (again a complex scale involving admitting that it was difficult to stop drinking once started, keeping on drinking after promising not to, trying to stop or cut down but failing, worrying about drinking, losing control over drinking, fearing becoming alcoholic, etc.).

Cartwright *et al.* (1975) considered three essentially similar elements which they termed excessive drinking, dependence on alcohol, and disturbance or interference (problems), pointing to the 1952 definition of alcoholism given by the World Health Organization which made reference to these three ingredients (see p.12 above). The similarity between the Cahalan and Room (1974) and Cartwright *et al.* (1975) concepts of 'alcoholism' is more apparent than real, however. First, Cartwright *et al.*'s assessment of excessive drinking was based simply on an estimate of a subject's mean daily intake of alcohol in centilitres and certainly took no account of binge drinking or other aspects of drinking pattern or style. Secondly, and more interestingly, Cartwright *et al.*'s measure of 'dependence' on alcohol corresponded partly to Cahalan and Room's symptomatic drinking and partly to their 'loss of control' (hands shaky in the morning after drinking, drinking first thing in the morning to steady nerves, and feeling on any occasion unable to stop drinking), and certainly did not involve any aspect of what Cahalan and Room termed 'psychological dependence'. Despite the apparent consensus of opinion between well-informed research workers about the concept of 'alcoholism' as a disease-of-the-will entity, it is clear that there is enormous confusion about what 'dependence' is, let alone about how it should be measured. Part, but only part, of the difficulty lies in the confusion, which Jellinek (1960) unsuccessfully tried to clear up, between 'dependence', which is thought to be purely 'psychological', and 'dependence', involving an altered physiological response to the substance involved. It will become clear later in the book that the distinction is difficult to maintain (see Chapter 10).

The list of factors taken into account by the epidemiologists faithfully reflects the modern concept of 'alcoholism' as a constellation consisting of abnormally heavy drinking, indulged in for abnormal reasons, resulting in abnormal behaviour, harmful short-term and long-term consequences, and abnormal difficulty in ceasing or reducing drinking. At the same time it poses many of the dilemmas with which this book attempts to deal. If harmful consequences are central, can 'problem drinking' be defined absolutely and independently of a person's social environment, his or her responsibilities and obligations, and the ways family and others respond? Are there cultures which promote drinking for reasons, and with a style, that are abnormal by the standards of others? Is someone who drinks heavily and regularly but who is unconcerned, more or less dependent than someone who drinks less, and less often, but who is more concerned? How can one distinguish between being unable to stop and not wanting to stop? These and other questions are relevant not only to excessive drinking but also to excessive behaviour of the kinds considered in the following four chapters.

They should not, however, stand in the way of our recognizing the facts of excessive alcohol drinking. These include the distress at being unable to control their drinking of which Lilian Roth and John Gardner wrote and of which countless others have complained; the needs to which Father Mathew and the temperance campaigners, not to mention the Prophet Muhammed, were responding when they used their influence to reduce or prohibit consumption; the preoccupation of governments past and present with the task of restraining excess; and the flourishing of self-help and professional forms of 'treatment' for 'alcoholism'. There may be disagreement about how best to construe excessive drinking, and about its causes and solutions, but of its existence there can be no doubt.

CHAPTER THREE

Excessive Gambling

> There is no doubt that the social conscience is as yet only very partially awakened to the widespread character of the gambling evil and to its grievous consequences. Like a cancer, the evil thing has spread its poisonous roots throughout the length and breadth of the land, carrying with them, where they strike, misery, poverty, weakened character, and crime. (B. Seebohm Rowntree in the Preface to *Betting and Gambling: a National Evil*, 1905.)

For some the explanation of excessive drinking as a form of drug 'addiction', as altered pharmacological response to the ingested substance, is sufficient. It is just because such an explanation is impossible in the case of excessive gambling, that the latter constitutes such an important example of excessive appetitive behaviour. If it can be demonstrated that excessive gambling is in most respects similar to excessive drinking or drug-taking, then it follows that an adequate explanation of excessive appetites in general must account for this non-drug form of 'addiction'. The main argument of this chapter will be that the parallels between excessive gambling and excessive drinking are, in fact, many and close.

The idea that the appetite for gambling could become excessive is no more a modern invention than is the notion of alcoholic excess. As Lindner (1950) put it, 'The fact that [it] . . . could assume a pathological form characterized by symptoms related to the various addictions . . . seems always to have been common knowledge among common folk everywhere' (cited by Herman, 1976). An article by Clemens France in the *American Journal of Psychology* for 1902 chronicles the many nations from ancient to modern which have been accused of fostering widespread gambling of a harmful kind. Since Roman Emperors and their wives have been charged with all manner of behavioural excesses, it is not surprising to find that this author, living himself in a relatively puritanical time and place, should quote good authority to the effect that several Emperors, including Augustus, Caligula, Claudius, and Nero, were themselves 'addicted' to gambling. Even Domitian, who so effectively demonstrated his concern over excessive drinking by having half the vineyards in the Empire destroyed (Glatt, 1958), is described as 'an inveterate gambler'. Under Constantine, '. . . every inhabitant of that city [Rome], down to the populace, was addicted to gambling' (Steinmetz, cited by France, p.366).

Many societies, according to France, had found it necessary to have legal controls on gambling behaviour. In France under Henry IV, 'incalculable social affliction' resulted from gambling despite stringent anti-gambling laws, and in the reign of Louis XIV:

> . . . men . . . left off tennis, billiards and other games of skill, and consequently became weaker and more sickly, more ignorant, less polished, more dissipated . . . The women, who till then had commanded respect, accustomed men to treat them with familiarity, by spending the whole night with them at play . . . (Steinmetz, cited by France, p.367).

As well as illustrating a prejudice against games of chance in favour of games of skill, a prejudice that is not infrequently betrayed by those who write on the subject of immoderate gambling, this quotation displays the extra opprobrium which often attaches to women when their behaviour is thought to go beyond the bounds of moderation.

In the England of Henry VIII legislation was passed prohibiting common people from playing cards except at Christmas (France, p.368), and Italy of the early sixteenth century was one of a number of countries which, from time to time, legislated for total prohibition of gambling but failed to suppress gambling behaviour (France, p.370).

Many of the descriptions of gambling which France unearthed from an earlier period are remarkably similar to current accounts of 'compulsive gambling'. For example, a book published in 1619 under the title, *The Nicker Nicked, or the Cheats of Gaming Discovered*, includes the following passage about gambling house activities of the period, which describes the phenomenon of escalation from moderation to excess that is such a recurring theme in both historical and modern accounts of excessive appetites:

> Most gamesters begin at small game; and, by degrees, if their money or estates hold out, they rise to great sums; some have played first of all their money, then their rings, coach and horses, even their wearing clothes and perukes; and then such a farm; and, at last, perhaps a lordship (Ashton, 1898, cited by France, p.368).

Amongst France's historical witnesses were the Englishman Cotton (1674) whose description of gaming as, '. . . an enchanting witchery . . . an itching disease . . .' is well known, and the Frenchman Barbeyrac. In the latter's three-volume work, *Traite du jeu*, published in 1737, Jean Barbeyrac had this to say:

> I do not know if there is any other passion which allows less of repose and which one has so much difficulty in reducing. . . . the passion of gambling gives no time for breathing; it is an enemy which gives neither quarter nor truce; it is a persecutor, furious and indefatigable. The more one plays the more one wishes to play; one never leaves it, and with difficulty one resolves to leave off a little while from dice and cards to satisfy the needs of nature . . . it seems that gambling had acquired the right to occupy all his thoughts. . . .

The idea that *it* takes over, becomes a preoccupation, and that the wish to reduce or leave off altogether is opposed by a stronger force that leaves the will powerless, is as clear here as in Lillian Roth's and John Gardner's modern-day accounts of 'alcoholism'.

The Russian novelist Dostoevsky is often referred to as the most famous of all 'compulsive gamblers'. Yet he can hardly be considered typical. There have been a number of case studies of the writer, mostly by psychoanalysts, one of the best known being that by Paul Squires published in the *Psychoanalytic Review* in 1937. He drew on about fifty sources, including Dostoevsky's own letters and his second wife's diary. Although there was mention of his 'gambling mania' and of dire financial troubles, it was his epileptic seizures and his restless, irritable, egotistical character that were to the forefront. Indeed, Squires made no mention of excessive gambling in the formal diagnosis with which he concluded:

> Our formal diagnosis runs as follows: Dostoevsky was an epileptic schizophrene, paranoid type, complicated by hysterical overlay. . . .

Not that an absence of reference to behavioural excess in a formal psychiatric diagnosis need imply that it was of no importance. For example, from Dostoevsky's wife's account of the year in which they married, Squires concluded that Dostoevsky was, 'Powerless in the clutches of his terrific gambling mania, which blunted his sense of moral responsibility as effectively as extreme alcohol addiction could' (p.372). Stripped of the glamour that surrounds the life of a world renowned artist struggling with his temperament and his appetites, Dostoevsky's life story contains moments that compare with the experiences of the most obscure man or woman who has struggled with an excessive appetite for gambling. There is, for example, the irrational conviction that some strategem or attitude to the game will bring certain gain. Writing to his first wife's sister from Wiesbaden, where he took up roulette *en route* for Paris to meet his mistress Suslova, he said:

> I really do know the secret: its terribly silly and simple and consists in restraining oneself at every moment, no matter what the phase

> of the game, and not becoming heated. This is the whole thing, and to lose with this is simply impossible (Minihan, 1967, p.237).

In his short novel, *The Gambler*, which he intended partly as, '. . . a firsthand and most detailed portrayal of roulette gambling . . .' (Minihan, pp.314–5), the hero, Aleksey Ivanovitch, describes the intense attraction of the sights and sounds of the gambling hall:

> With what trembling, with what faintness of heart I hear the croupier's cry . . . With what greed I look at the gambling table along which are strewn louis d'or, friedrichs d'or, and thalers, at the little columns of gold when they are scattered from the croupier's shovel into piles glowing like fire, or columns of silver a yard high lying stacked round the wheel. Even while approaching the gambling hall, two rooms away, as soon as I begin to hear the clinking of money being poured out, I almost go into convulsions (cited by Minihan, p.319).

His relationship with his second wife Anna seems to have contained episodes the recounting of which would be thoroughly in place at a meeting of Gamblers Anonymous or of Gam-Anon (for family members of compulsive gamblers) in Croydon or Exeter in 1985 (see Boyd and Bolen, 1970, for descriptions of the effects of 'compulsive gambling' on some present-day marriages). They were constantly in financial difficulties and Dostoevsky was for ever trying to relieve them by further gambling. His gambling was interspersed with protestations of regret and requests for forgiveness and more money with which to make good former losses. On one occasion Fyrdor and Anna travelled to Baden-Baden so that Dostoevsky could gamble. They stayed about a month, Anna spending the days waiting in their hotel room. The infuriating inconsistency in the behaviour of someone whose appetite is excessive is well portrayed in a passage in Minihan's biography which relates to a period just after the birth of Fyrdor and Anna's first daughter. The confinement had been expensive:

> Dostoevsky went a third time . . . He lost, pawned his rıng and begged his wife to send him the last hundred francs: '. . . Don't consider my request for a hundred francs mad. I'm not mad. And also don't consider it depraved; I won't act meanly, won't deceive, won't go to gamble . . .' On the same evening he wrote a second letter; he had lost the money received from pawning his ring . . . (Minihan, p.332).

Finally, much later, came a turning point, an occasion, similar to those that many lesser mortals have experienced, when Dostoevsky underwent some sort of experience, impressive, difficult to describe, but associated with a radical change in the formerly-excessive appetitive behaviour. It was during Anna's third pregnancy that Dostoevsky went to Wiesbaden to gamble, apparently, so Minihan would have it, at his wife's suggestion:

> Dostoevsky lost everything, and at night in despair ran in search of a Russian priest . . . At midnight he wrote to his wife 'Now this fantasy has ended for ever . . . Moreover, I have, as it were, been wholly reborn morally . . . A great thing has happened to me. The hideous fantasy that tormented me for almost ten years has vanished . . .' Actually, he underwent some sort of mystical experience. From that day Dostoevsky never gambled again in his life. 'The fantasy' had disappeared instantly and for good (Minihan, p.385).

There seems little doubt that those closest to Dostoevsky thought his gambling excessive, and possibly he thought so too from time to time. But was his gambling 'compulsive' or 'pathological'? As with drinking, so with gambling, the nature of 'true dependence', if such a thing exists, is elusive. Unnecessary controversy on this point has dogged discussions of behaviour in each of the areas considered in this book.

As is the case with *modern* commentary on the use of opiates, hallucinogens, and some other drugs, in older writings on the subject of gambling the distinction between gambling in moderation and gambling to excess is scarcely drawn at all. This is evident in the fourth revelation which Baasher (1981) mentions as part of the step-wise process towards prohibition of alcoholic drinks in the Muslim community. Here alcohol and gambling are clearly linked and total abstention from both is commanded: 'O ye who believe! Strong drink (khamr) and games of chance and idols and divining arrows are only an infamy of Satan's handiwork' (cited by Baasher, p.237). The failure to distinguish moderation and excess is also there in many of the sources cited by France in 1902 and in other writings of that period, such as those to be found in the book edited by Seebohm Rowntree at the suggestion of the York Anti-Gambling League in 1905. The Victorian moral view of gambling is well expressed in the latter work. Although reference was made to immoderate or excessive gambling, no form or degree of gambling is free from moral taint according to this view:

> Gambling involves the denial of all system in the apportionment of property: it plunges the mind in a world of anarchy, where things come upon one and pass from one miraculously . . . generates an emotional excitement that inhibits those checks which reason more or less contrives to place upon emotional extravagances. The essence of gambling consists in an abandonment of reason, an inhibition of the factors of human control. In the history of mankind, civilisation of the individual has chiefly consisted in and been measured by this increased capacity of rational control—a slow, gradual, imperfect taming of the animal instincts which made for emotional anarchy of conduct . . . The practice of gambling is thus exhibited as a deliberate reversion to those passions and that mental attitude which characterise the savage or pre-human man in his conduct and his outlook (Hobson, 1905, pp.5–6).

This view that gambling is itself undignified and appealing to the irrational and irresponsible parts of human mentality, still survives (Cornish, 1978; Herman, 1976). It offers 'something for nothing', involves 'unnecessary risk', offers gain at the expense of others' loss, and is contrary to the principle of reward for effort. Such a view was well represented in the report of the Royal Commission on Betting, Lotteries, and Gaming in 1951, and in recent publications of the Churches' Council on Gambling (e.g. 1960–1968, cited by Cornish, 1978).

Thus, although 'excessive' and 'immoderate' were adjectives often employed to qualify the term 'gambling', and hence the possibility of moderate use was acknowledged by implication, moderate and immoderate forms of gambling were not often clearly separated in the minds of writers on the subject. The idea that people can be more or less clearly separated into one group or another, or at least that we may talk and write on the subject as if they were, is a relatively recent invention. Stekel (1924) recognized gambling as one of the 'manias'—others, for example, being dipsomania, narcomania, and nymphomania—and psychoanalytic writers have recognized for some time that gambling, like sexual and other types of appetitive behaviour, could take on a compulsive form (e.g. Bergler, 1958). The creation of 'compulsive gambling' as an entity, and the possibility of 'treatment' for it, are new, however.

There are many recent accounts by psychiatrists and others of cases they have treated for 'compulsive gambling' (e.g. Barker and Miller, 1968; Goorney, 1968). The three case histories given by Barker and Miller illustrate the harm that can be associated with gambling, as well as demonstrating the range of personal reactions which this harm can evoke in the excessive gambler himself. They also hint at the possibility of inter-generational transmission of gambling problems which would provide yet another parallel with excessive drinking which does 'run in families' (Goodwin, 1976). Their Case I was a man in his early thirties, married with two children, who had recently been jailed for 18 months for obtaining money for gambling by fraud:

> He had been gambling excessively on 'fruit machines' almost continuously for the past 12 years. His 'addiction' began in Rhodesia shortly after marriage. A business client invited him to a club where a 'one-armed bandit' was installed. After a few initial wins he returned to the machine every night, claiming that he gambled 'to provide a house and furniture and decent standard of living for his wife'. Within 2½ years of marriage his gambling debts exceeded £500 which were settled by a relative. On returning to England, he continued to gamble furiously and several cheques drawn for money to feed 'fruit-machines' were not honoured.
>
> Recently he had spent all his wages (up to £15 per week) in a 'fruit-machine' in a public house every Friday night and invariably reinvested—and lost—all his winnings. Consequently his wife had to work throughout their marriage to support the family and repay

> his gambling debts. She vividly portrayed the situation thus: 'Over the last few years we have had a monster living with our family—a monster in the shape of a "fruit-machine". Practically every penny my husband earned went into that machine and while it consumed, we starved. He was obsessed by it. Frequently we were without food, fuel and light.' After 13 years of marriage they still lived in a rented apartment and possessed nothing but their personal effects. His wife repeatedly threatened to leave him if he did not stop gambling, and she eventually persuaded him to seek medical help (pp.287–8).

Case II impressed Barker and Miller as a very different personality whose reaction to his gambling was in marked contrast to that of Case I. He was a 50-year-old unmarried man, living with his sister and elderly father in their old family house. He had worked with the same firm for 20 years and had had no previous financial difficulties:

> He had placed a few shillings on horses and pennies on cards for years but had never shown any tendency to large scale gambling. For the past 8 months he had become 'addicted' to gambling on 'one-armed bandits'. During this time he lost more than £450 and accumulated debts and IOUs amounting to £50. As soon as he saw a 'fruit machine' he became totally immersed in gambling within seconds and spent every penny that he possessed in them. He gambled on two machines in a club and public house respectively but drank very little. His gambling followed a succession of wins on the first occasion and then he found he was unable to stop. It is significant that his wages increased considerably just before he started gambling so that for the time in his life he found he had money in excess of his needs. Finally, after spending £21 and £24 on successive nights, he became so concerned about his future that he sought psychiatric help (p.288).

Here, then, is a man, described by Barker and Miller as, '. . . somewhat shy, introverted . . . exhibiting some obsessional traits', who seeks help after a *relatively* short and harmless gambling history. Case I, by way of contrast, is persuaded to seek treatment after a much longer and troublesome history. Interestingly, Barker and Miller described Case I as, '. . . a co-operative and plausible man . . . showing marked psychopathic traits. He had an ebullient but unstable personality . . .'. The confusion between excessive appetitive behaviour and 'bad character' is a theme that recurs constantly in the literature on gambling, drinking, and other forms of excess.

Case III was similar to Case I in age, circumstances, family history of gambling, and the possession of, '. . . some psychopathic traits'. His particular problem, however, unlike the others, was 'the horses':

> He had gambled in 'betting shops' for more than 2 years and had lost over £1,200. Initially he ascribed his gambling mainly to boredom, but he had recently gambled to repay his debts, which exceeded £100. His usual practice was to spend all his salary (£15 to £30 per week) in a betting shop on Saturdays. He invariably reinvested his winnings on horses and returned home with nothing so that his wife and children went without food, clothes and fuel. He occasionally gambled on 'one-armed bandits' but this was not a major problem. Matters came to a head when he put his own money and the complete pay packet of a sick friend (who had asked him to collect his pay) on one horse and lost £40. This resulted in 18 months probation. His gambling had been causing serious marital difficulties and was affecting the health of his wife and his eldest son. He was referred for treatment by his doctor (pp.288–9).

As is the case with 'alcoholism', 'compulsive gambling' implies a number of things which are not necessarily implied by simply engaging in an activity with a greater frequency or at a greater intensity than others. 'Alcoholism' is said to be more than just heavy drinking; similarly, 'compulsive gambling' is said to be more than merely heavy gambling. The first implication is that excessive gambling is one of the most important things to be said about the person concerned. It becomes a vital piece of information; it needs to be known if a person's behaviour is to be understood. It explains much, particularly any harm that a person is experiencing or problems that have befallen him or her. The status of 'compulsive gambler' may become a kind of 'master status' which may then be taken to 'explain' a variety of ills such as neglect of family, incompetence at work, financial difficulties, even marital infidelity (Herman, 1976). Like Alcoholics Anonymous, upon which it is closely modelled, Gamblers Anonymous (GA), successfully started in America in 1957, has done much to foster this view of excessive gambling. To acknowledge 'I am a compulsive gambler', is a crucial step in the GA recovery programme.

The second implication of being a 'compulsive gambler' is the supposition that there exist hallmarks—one would be inclined to call them 'symptoms' if the view is taken that 'compulsive gambling' is an illness of some kind—which make the gambling experience qualitatively different from that of the moderate or normal gambler, and sets the 'compulsive gambler' apart from him. These assumptions, that people whose gambling is excessive have much in common and that all are in marked contrast to others whose gambling is not excessive, follow easily once an apparently scientific term such as 'compulsive gambling' is used, exactly as they do in the case of drinking and 'alcoholism'. Moran (1970, 1975) is a British psychiatrist who has taken a special interest in excessive gambling, which he prefers to call 'pathological gambling'. His reasons for preferring the latter term are interesting because they touch upon one of the central facets of the psychology of excessive appetitive behaviour, namely ambivalence and conflict. Following Lewis (1936) he argues that compulsions are the behavioural aspects of obsessional states in which a person finds his own behaviour alien and tries to resist it. It is the element of resistance which in his view defines compulsion, and the term compulsive should otherwise, '. . . not be used no matter how strong the urge to indulge in the activity' (Moran, 1975, p.417). In his view, although ambivalence about gambling is usually present to some extent, many excessive gamblers experience enjoyment of the activity and many do not wish to stop. This betrays the existence of a common misunderstanding, namely that enjoyment and compulsion are incompatible, and it is a central matter to which this book will return in a later chapter.

Moran referred to 'the syndrome of pathological gambling' and considered that it could be recognized by the presence of any of the following:

1 Concern on the part of the gambler and/or family about the amount of gambling, which is considered to be excessive.
2 An overpowering urge to gamble so that the individual may be intermittently or continuously preoccupied with thoughts of gambling; this is usually associated with the subjective experience of tension which is found to be relieved only by further gambling.
3 The subjective experience of the inability to control the amount once gambling has started . . .
4 Disturbances of economic, social and/or psychological functioning of the gambler and/or the family as a result of persistent gambling (p.418).

It is interesting to see the close parallels that exist between this list and the list of signs and symptoms of 'alcoholism' discussed in the previous chapter. The amount of the activity itself is mentioned, although it is concern about amount rather amount *per se* which is thought to be the criterion. So too are strength of desire and preoccupation, loss of control, and harm caused by gambling in economic, social, and psychological spheres. According to Moran the latter includes debt, loss of employment and friends, eviction, criminality, marital problems, family problems, depression, attempted suicide, and behaviour disorders in the children of compulsive gamblers. Only those aspects of 'alcoholism' which can be ascribed to alcohol being a drug (tolerance and withdrawal symptoms) are missing. Even then, Moran makes mention of tension, '. . . which is found to be relieved only by further gambling', and a recent article in the *British Journal of Addiction* reports that 30–50 per cent of a sample of GA members described disturbances of mood or behaviour on ceasing to bet which, if described by 'alcoholics', would be termed 'withdrawal symptoms' (Wray and Dickerson, 1981). Of those who completed a standard questionnaire (another group who responded in open-ended fashion reported almost as much disturbance) 40 per cent indicated five or more disturbances of mood or behaviour and 39 per cent listed at least one somatic disturbance. Amongst the results for individual 'symptoms', 32 per cent said they had felt anxious and 46 per cent said they had felt irritable. These percentages are remarkably similar, and in the case of irritability somewhat higher, than the comparable percentages from some studies of 'withdrawal symptoms' amongst excessive drinkers (Wray and Dickerson, 1981).

As disagreement over terms is the norm when excessive appetites are being discussed, it is no surprise to find not a little confusion in the literature on excessive gambling. This confusion, often borne of the view that someone with an excessive appetite is qualitatively different from other people, is exemplified by Bergler (1958) in his book *The Psychology of Gambling*, where he wrote, 'To avoid misunderstandings: not everyone who gambles is a gambler [*sic*]. There are millions of "harmless" gamblers who play for diversion or sociability' (p.viii). His view was that 'real' or 'pathologic' gamblers were, unlike other people, 'neurotics' with an unconscious wish to lose. Whatever one thinks of that view, he clearly recognized the possibility that gambling could constitute a very troublesome and excessive form of appetitive behaviour for some people, as his list of characteristics of the 'real gambler' shows:

> Gambling is habitual.
>
> Gambling absorbs and precludes all other interests.
>
> The gambler is always optimistic, never learning lessons from losing (he is, '. . . the last optimist . . . beyond the reach of all logical objection and argument', p.3).
>
> The gambler cannot stop when winning.
>
> The gambler may be cautious initially but eventually risks more than he can afford.
>
> The gambler seeks and enjoys an enigmatic 'thrill' ('pleasure–painful tension', to cite 'an observant patient' of Bergler's).

Moran would not recognize all these features as universal to 'pathological' gambling, however, since some of them, in his view, are only characteristic of certain sub-types. One of these sub-types of pathological gambling listed by Moran was 'impulsive' gambling—others being symptomatic gambling (associated with mental illness), psychopathic gambling, neurotic gambling, and subcultural gambling (arising from a social background of heavy gambling). Impulsive gambling, according to Moran, was characterized by loss of control and symptoms of craving. It is intriguing to find that these two 'symptoms' receive prominent mention in discussions of excessive gambling, as they have long been the *sine qua non* of 'alcoholism', and have come under serious attack in recent years for the way in which they have lent to the field of alcohol problems a spurious sense of precision and a medical aura (e.g. Pattison *et al.*, 1977).

Table 4 shows one of a number of questionnaires which are in existence, based upon these ideas of 'compulsive gambling' and particularly upon the tenets of Gamblers Anonymous, and which are designed for the self-detection of 'compulsive' or 'pathological' gambling.

The special entity or syndrome idea of excessive appetitive behaviour has come in for much the same kind of criticism when applied to gambling as it has when

Table 4 A typical questionnaire for the self-diagnosis of compulsive gambling

1	Have you ever lost time from work due to gambling?
2	Has gambling made your life unhappy?
3	Has gambling affected your reputation?
4	Have you ever felt remorse after gambling?
5	Have you ever gambled to get money to pay debts or to otherwise solve financial difficulties?
6	Did gambling ever cause a decrease in your ambition or efficiency?
7	After losing did you feel that you must return as soon as possible and win back your losses?
8	After a win have you had a strong urge to return and win more?
9	Have you often gambled until your last penny was gone?
10	Have you ever borrowed to finance your gambling?
11	Have you ever sold any real or personal property to finance your gambling?
12	Are you reluctant to use 'gambling money' for normal expenditures?
13	Has gambling ever made you careless of the welfare of your family?
14	Have you ever gambled longer than you had planned?
15	Have you ever gambled to escape worry or trouble?
16	Have you ever committed, or considered committing, an illegal act to finance your gambling?
17	Has gambling ever caused you to have difficulty in sleeping?
18	Did arguments, disappointments, or frustrations ever create within you an urge to gamble?
19	Have you ever had an urge to celebrate any good fortune by a few hours of gambling?
20	Have you ever considered self-destruction as results of your gambling?

applied to the drinking of alcohol. Indeed, just because gambling is not a pharmacological agent, anything resembling a disease concept of excessive gambling may lack the plausibility which the disease concept of 'alcoholism' possesses. Herman (1976), for example, clearly regarded the GA tendency to define all problems as stemming from 'compulsive gambling' as an over-simplification which is functional for its members rather than being an accurate statement of cause and effect. As he said, 'This kind of ''single cause'' theory may not satisfy the moralist, but it may be just the ticket for the relatively uncomplicated rehabilitation of the member' (p.101). He stated his view that there were no dividing lines between moderate gamblers, heavy gamblers, problem gamblers, addicted gamblers, compulsive gamblers, or pathological gamblers, and that creating a separate category of 'compulsive gambler' served no useful purpose. Indeed it, '. . . generates a set of new problems that would not otherwise exist' (p.103).

In his very comprehensive review on gambling in Britain carried out for the Home Office Research Unit, Cornish (1978) appeared to support the division into moderate and immoderate, although he used what the present writer considers to be the most accurate expression for the latter—namely 'excessive' gambling—and fully recognized the difficulty of separating the two. He avoided defining excessive gambling in terms of supposed hallmarks or symptoms such as craving or loss of control, but rather focused upon gambling which was a social problem. As we shall see later in this book, this tactic of considering only problematic or harmful appetitive behaviour is an attractive one, but it bypasses the central questions to which this book is addressed: What is the psychological nature of excessive appetitive behaviour? When and why does it occur, and under what circumstances does it disappear? Nor, as Cornish was aware, does it solve the problems of definition. He put the case for relativity as follows:

> First, the extent to which behaviour constitutes a social problem is a function not only of the behaviour itself but of its nuisance-value or its social and economic costs to the community in other ways; similar behaviours when manifested by different individuals or social groups may vary in their level of 'visibility' . . .
>
> Secondly, an individual is more likely, or likely more rapidly, to define his behaviour as constituting a problem in some circumstances than others. The heavy gambler with plenty of money and spare time, and few other commitments, will be considerably less likely to view his behaviour with anxiety than a similar person less fortunately placed in these respects (p.76).

This may be even more the case for gambling than for drinking, he suggests, for at least in the latter case the health hazards of drinking large quantities of alcohol impose some sort of upper limit above which relativity no longer applies.

Despite the difficulties, Cornish could at least conceive of an epidemiology of excessive gambling—the possibility of defining a case in quantitative terms, and of counting the number of those cases in a defined population. A body of epidemiological knowledge about excessive gambling does not exist to anything like the extent that it does in the case of excessive drinking, although estimates of the 'size of the problem' abound. The best that could be done in Cornish's view was to estimate the number of those 'at risk' on account of the regularity of their gambling. Based upon the results of the latest Gallup Poll (1976), Cornish estimated there to be two million regular (more often than weekly) gamblers on football pools aged 16 years or over in Britain, 1.3 million regularly engaging in off-course betting, one million in bingo gambling, 77,000 in gaming club gambling, and 24,000 in on-course betting. Employing the argument that those particularly at risk were those engaging regularly in forms of gambling which involved the possibility of continuous betting, and those who had relatively little personal disposable income (for both of which factors he found evidence), he estimated just over one million at risk of excessive off-course betting and just under one million at particular risk of excessive bingo gambling. The number of regular on-course betters and gaming club gamblers was comparatively very small, and the quite large number of regular football pools gamblers were not considered particularly at risk because of the non-continuous nature of the gambling activity involved.

Other estimates for Britain include Moody's (1972) estimate, prepared for the Churches' Council on Gambling, of the numbers of 'regular and committed' or 'thorough-going' gamblers. This estimate was 725,000, although no details were given of exactly how this figure was reached. Cornish considered this to be an example of the propaganda value for the anti-gambling lobby of maintaining estimates on the high side. The most carefully reasoned estimate is that of Dickerson (1974) based on his own close research on betting shops in the Birmingham area. He estimated 5.3 'gamblers' for each of about 15,000 betting shops in the country. 'Gamblers', according to Dickerson's definition, bet whenever there was an opportunity, stayed more than two hours in a betting shop, and bet until the end of racing. Of this group in Dickerson's study, 56 per cent thought they spent most of their own money on betting and had betting debts, 75 per cent regularly spent more than they intended, 45 per cent regularly lost all they had with them, and 36 per cent experienced some desire to cut back or to stop. He had thus identified a group who reported a high level of trouble related to their gambling and felt 'dissonance' regarding it.

A survey of gambling behaviour in the United States, carried out by the Institute for Social Research at the University of Michigan, demonstrated the extent of gambling activity but at the same time illustrated some of the difficulties and confusions involved in trying to define and enumerate 'compulsive gambling'. The survey report (Kallick *et al.*, 1979) estimated that a total of 22.4 billion dollars was ventured annually in the United States on some gambling activity or another (the equivalent figure for Britain in 1975/76 was £3.5 billion according to Cornish, 1978) and that 4.4 billion dollars, equivalent to 0.4 per cent of total personal income, was lost (or 'outlayed', i.e. amount bet minus winnings). The range of possible betting activities considered was wide, including betting with a bookmaker on various sporting events, playing commercially available 'games' such as 'jai alai', 'pickit', and 'numbers', and a whole host of ways of betting 'with friends', some of which Kallick *et al.* thought quite unusual:

> Almost one-sixth of the United States population said they bet whether some event would happen or where it would happen. For example, the hour of someone's birth, the first snowfall, whether someone would resign—or the date of that resignation—and similar events (p.18).

When it came to estimating the extent of excessive gambling, the authors of this report adopted two strategies, both of which are unsatisfactory but for different reasons. One was to propose the concept of 'level of gambling activity'. The lowest level was not gambling at all; the next gambling only with friends or on legal, commercial games; the third level, illegal but not heavy gambling; and the highest level, illegal, heavy gambling which they defined as spending at least 50 dollars on such betting in a year. Although they demonstrated that this scale correlated with rates of divorce or separation, with proportions of subjects having children with problems, with job dissatisfaction, and with amount of time off work, this scale clearly equates and confuses 'excess' with both amount of gambling activity and with illegality.

The second, and even less sound, method was based on the common confusion, which will be discussed further in Chapter 11, between excessive appetitive behaviour and character or personality. The method consisted of assembling a 'compulsive gambling scale' from items included in eight personality inventories (of self-acceptance, risk-taking, anomie, external control orientation, etc.) which best discriminated 120 'compulsive gamblers' and an equal number of church members. The scale was then used to estimate the number of 'probable compulsive gamblers' and 'potential compulsive gamblers' in the national survey sample. The fallacy of labelling people in this way on the basis of a scale that made no direct reference to gambling behaviour is obvious.

These difficulties and confusions notwithstanding, individuals *do* seek help on account of excessive gambling and this fact is illustrated by the growth of Gamblers Anonymous in Britain. By 1975 the *Journal of Gamblers Anonymous* advertised 47 groups throughout the country, and Dickerson (1974) estimated the rate of referral to GA to be of the order of 2,000 a year with an additional 300 referrals to psychiatrists specifically on account of excessive gambling. As with 'alcoholism', referral rates of this kind are usually assumed to represent only the tip of the iceberg—those for whom excessive behaviour has become chronic and intolerable—and the 'real' prevalence of the problem is assumed to be very much greater. Rates of excessive gambling amongst clients of probation officers, and particularly amongst prisoners, are considerably greater than for the population as a whole (Cornish, p.81)—a further similarity with excessive drinking. However, it should be clear that the problems of defining and counting the incidence of 'compulsive' or 'pathological' gambling are such that very little faith can be placed in differences between reported rates from different populations. An apparently high rate amongst prisoners may reflect a truly greater than normal rate of excessive gambling, or may be a reflection of a greater involvement in gambling by members of lower socio-economic status groups from which prisoners are disproportionately drawn. Alternatively, it may be a result of the sensitivity of prison or probation staff to the possibility of excessive gambling, or the greater readiness of prisoners to attribute their problems to gambling. The status 'compulsive gambler' may be a less stigmatizing one than that of 'criminal' on account of the former's connotations of sickness and reduced responsibility.

It is partly this implication of reduced responsibility for behaviour which lies behind criticisms of the concept of 'compulsive gambler', as it does behind criticisms of any designation implying that excessive appetitive behaviour is the result of a condition over which a person has only limited control. In the case of gambling this debate was nicely illustrated by a leading article which appeared in *The British Medical Journal* for 13 April 1968 which followed a report in *The Times* of 2 April describing how a 'compulsive gambler' had been referred to a medical specialist and treated by the use of brain surgery. The *BMJ* leader objected to the involvement of psychiatry in such cases: 'The gambler enjoys every bit of his "compulsion" . . . He may say "I cannot stop" but what he means is that he does not want to stop—the attractions are too great.' These statements go right to the heart of the dilemma presented by the phenomena of excessive appetitive behaviour. How is it possible to posit a 'disease of the will' when the object of a person's so-called compulsion is an activity which constitutes for most people a source of enjoyment? The leader went on to press the distinction between true compulsions and excess behaviours like gambling and drinking:

> . . . the rituals of the compulsive [i.e. the true compulsive] are uncontrollable because they arise outside consciousness. The gambler's behaviour is a source of pleasure . . . the compulsive's is a burden which makes him anxious and depressed . . . the excessive gambler lacks a sense of responsibility or of duty to society, but again this does not make him a psychiatric casualty. Every man in the street can imagine himself in his place. . . .

The distinction between true compulsions and excessive behaviours is the same distinction which convinced Moran (1975) that the expression 'pathological' was preferable in the case of gambling, although it did not convince him that excessive gambling was outside the realm of psychiatry or the other helping professions. Nor did it so convince a number of readers of *The British Medical Journal* who wrote protesting about the leader, and these letters were published in subsequent issues (e.g. Carstairs, 1968; Gunn, 1968).

These and other clinicians who have been asked for help by people in distress over their own or a family member's gambling are left in no doubt that it is an over-simplification to state that all gamblers enjoy their gambling and could control their behaviour if they wished. They are as impressed by the accounts which some people give of the difficulty of controlling an activity which has become greatly excessive and damaging as have others been by the accounts of those who wish to control their drinking, drug-taking, smoking, or eating but find they cannot. Words such as 'addiction' or 'dependence', or terms such as 'compulsive gambling', seem to serve the purpose of 'explaining' or at least of describing such apparent paradoxes.

Whatever the rights and wrongs on the issue of whether excessive gambling constitutes any sort of entity or condition, and if so what such an entity should be called, it remains a fact that the availability of opportunities for gambling represents for society the same sort of behavioural control problem which alcohol presents. The control of gambling activities is as perennial a concern for national governments as has been the control of alcohol consumption. The difficulty of getting legislation right is well illustrated for gambling in recent British history by the permissive Betting and Gaming Act of 1960 and the quickly following and relatively restrictive Betting, Gaming, and Lotteries Act of 1964 and Gaming Act of 1968. There is an interesting parallel here with the reversals of the Acts of 1729, 1736, and 1751 which were aimed at the control of the sale of alcohol.

The details of the social control of a nation's gambling behaviour are as much at issue as ever. A book published by the Churches' Council on Gambling advocated, for example, the setting up of a Betting Board to complement the existing Gaming Board, totalizator rather than bookmaker betting systems, a restriction on the licensing of horse race betting facilities at other sporting events such as tennis tournaments and cricket matches, and the abolition of certain features of betting shops, such as staggered times of races from different courses and the provision of continuous commentaries direct from the racetrack (Moody, 1974). It was one of the particular arguments of that publication, which was supported by Cornish (1978), that the licensed off-course betting office, with the almost continual opportunity which it provides during racing hours for betting, listening to commentary, and then betting again on the next race, creates an atmosphere which encourages continuous or uncontrolled betting in a way that was virtually impossible before 1960 when betting was limited to on-course or unlicensed off-course betting.

In Britain the Churches' Council on Gambling has generally campaigned to reduce opportunities for gambling, whilst at the same time lending support to the modern distinction between controlled and excessive forms of gambling behaviour. The Council has defended its campaign on the grounds that a high level of gambling turnover reflects public acceptance of gambling and a climate favourable to all forms of gambling, including those that are more dangerous; that it allows more opportunities for individuals to begin gambling; and that participation in less dangerous forms of gambling may lead by generalization to participation in more dangerous forms. The parallel which this last argument suggests with hypotheses about escalating use of drugs is made the more obvious by the use of the terms 'soft' and 'hard' by the Churches' Council and other writers on gambling when writing about forms of gambling such as football pools betting and horse race gambling, respectively.

Although there is persuasive evidence that the amount of excessive drinking in a population is directly related to the total amount of alcohol consumption in that population as a whole (Kendell, 1979), Cornish (1978), for one, doubted that the same relationship held in the case of gambling behaviour. He argued that whereas all alcoholic beverages contain the addictive ingredient alcohol, gambling activities were qualitatively different, for example in the degree to which they encouraged continuous play. His view on this would not be shared by many members of Gamblers Anonymous which advises its members to avoid even the casual playing of cards with no exchange of money, on the grounds that even such an apparently innocuous activity contains a measure of the active ingredients of tension and excitement.

The British Gaming Board has a double pronged policy for the control of gambling activities. It has argued, first, that new recruits to gambling can be limited by avoiding the artificial stimulation of demand. To this end it has succeeded in limiting the numbers and locations of gaming clubs. Secondly, it has argued for limiting the intensity of gambling by those recruited by preserving the 'essential nature' of gambling activities which are not in themselves dangerous. It has viewed Bingo, for example, as an essentially social activity and has resisted attempts to subvert this purpose by turning it into a relatively 'hard' form of gambling. Not that all bodies have shared the Gaming Board's charitable view that Bingo is a, 'neighbourly game played for modest stakes'. The Churches' Council on Gambling, for example, described it as a sterile and uncreative activity (CCG, 1960–1968, cited by Cornish, 1978).

Football pools betting is generally considered a fairly harmless form of gambling, but even in this case it is as well to remember that as recently as 1933 a Royal Commission recommended its abolition, and much more recently abolition of football pools has been advocated on the grounds that this type of betting takes place at home, thus placing young people at risk of involvement and of possible escalation to other forms of gambling.

As Cornish (1978) points out in the preface to his review, gambling occupies an equivocal position in our national life. Massive public participation, with over 80 per cent of adults taking part in one form of gambling or another, contrasts with continuing criticism of gambling on moral, social, and economic grounds, and continued awareness of the dangers of excess. Thus, gambling presents society with a problem very similar to that presented by the availability of alcohol: the problem of how to arrive at a balanced response which helps to minimize the dangers of immoderate use while at the same time detracting as little as possible from the enjoyment associated with the moderate use by the majority of citizens.

CHAPTER FOUR

Excessive Drug-taking

> . . . from this date the reader is to consider me as a regular and confirmed opium-eater, of whom to ask whether on any particular day he had or had not taken opium would be to ask whether his lungs had performed respiration, or the heart fulfilled its functions. (Thomas de Quincey, *Confessions of an Opium Eater* (Collected Writings, Vol. III, 1897, p.400).)

> . . . many in this kingdome have had such a continuall use of taking this onsavorie smoke, as now they are not able to forbeare the same, no more than an olde drunkard can abide to be long sober, without falling into an incurable weakness and evill constitution . . . (King James I, *A Counterblaste to Tobacco* (1604, cited by Jaffe, 1977, p.205).)

OPIATES

Because of events which are in very recent memory, drug-taking in the West is often taken to be virtually synonymous with heroin use. In many minds it conjures a picture of intravenous injection followed almost immediately by a total enslavement accompanied by moral and social decline. In the popular Western imagination of the 1960s, 1970s and 1980s 'drugs' are not in the same category as drink and gambling, and certainly not of the same kind as eating and sex, all of which, certainly the last two, are acceptable in moderation, although they carry the risk of excess for a minority. In fact, even a cursory examination of the literature on drug-taking demonstrates the variety of forms of drug and drug-taking in the present day, the variety of forms of use of the same drug at different historical periods, and differences in attitudes, reactions, and attempts to control drug-taking at different times and in different places. Many of the same questions about the nature of excessive behaviour, of definitions of 'dependence', and of the appropriateness of different forms of control and treatment which were raised in the cases of drinking and gambling, arise again with drug-taking. The study of drugs, in addition to the drug alcohol which has been given a chapter to itself, is vital in order to establish a psychological theory which does justice to the full range of excessive appetitive behaviours.

Whatever arguments there may be about the real physical or psychological nature of 'addiction', there can be no disputing troublesome opiate-taking as a social fact; something described by many who believe they have experienced it themselves and the existence of which is acknowledged by countless others. Kurland (1978) has provided a useful historical summary of the development of concern with individual opiate 'addiction' over the last 200–300 years. At the beginning of the eighteenth century a London physician, John Jones, was able to write his, *The Mysteries of Opium Revealed*, which included a section entitled, 'The effects of sudden leaving off the use of opium after a long and lavish use thereof'. These were:

> . . . great and even intolerable distress, anxieties and depression of the spirits, which in a few days commonly end in a miserable death, attended with strange agonies, unless men returned to the use of opium; which soon raises them again and certainly restores them (Sonnedecker, 1958, cited by Kurland, pp.1–2).

As has been the case with most troublesome drugs, opium was formerly used with approval as a medicine. It had been used in the relief of pain, to induce sleep and calm, and to control such common symptoms as cough and diarrhoea, and had been so used for hundreds of years. Laudanum, a mixture of opium and alcohol, was introduced by the English physician Thomas Sydenham late in the seventeenth century, and it was to laudanum that one of the most celebrated self-confessed drug-takers of all time, Thomas de Quincey, became 'enslaved'. His, *The Confessions of an English Opium Eater*, first published in the *London Magazine* in 1821, is thought to have been of much influence in the slow development of awareness during the nineteenth century that opium-taking might be extremely difficult to leave off. He first used opium, on the recommendation of a friend, to relieve unpleasant facial pain which had lasted for several weeks. In his confessions he sung the praises of opium not only for its ability to relieve his pain but also for the positive enjoyment which the drug brought him; so much so in fact that some have accused him since of being responsible for initiating many others into opiate use. It appears from his confessions that de Quincey took laudanum only occasionally, recreationally, and for pleasure, for a period of nearly ten years. For much of this time he confined his use to one or two occasions a week, and used it to enhance the pleasure of solitary walks around London or visits to the opera.

At this stage he extolled opium's advantages over alcohol. Alcohol's enjoyment was 'gross and mortal', opium's 'luxuries' were 'divine'; the pleasure from alcohol intoxication, quickly declining, was a 'flickering flame' compared to the 'steady and equable glow' from opium; wine 'disorders the mental faculties, . . . robs a man of his self-possession, . . . unsettles the judgement . . .'; opium, on the other hand, 'communicates serenity and equipose to all the faculties . . .' (pp.213, 383).

Only later, after these years of intermittent and moderate use, did de Quincey become, '. . . a regular and confirmed opium-eater' (p.398). Following a recurrence of stomach pain which he had had as a youth, he started to take opium daily and increased his dose eventually to 8,000 drops of laudanum a day. It was only then that he became aware of the 'addicting' properties of the mixture which he had formerly seen in such a favourable light. He wrote of, '. . . the morbid growth upon the opium-eater of his peculiar habit' (p.417), and of, '. . . the accursed chain which fettered me' (p.211). The conflict which he described puts his experience on a par with that of Lillian Roth, John Gardner, Dostoevsky, and others who have struggled to control excessive appetites.

It has been pointed out that laudanum contained 45 per cent alcohol, and that de Quincey was also a, 'generous partaker of wines and cordials' (Terry and Pellens, 1928, cited by Kurland, p.23). Hence, he may have been consuming more than the equivalent of a pint of whisky a day when his laudanum-taking was at its greatest, and his case should therefore be considered, not as one of pure opium 'addiction', but rather as one of 'multiple drug abuse'.

Enormous changes have taken place in society's reactions to opiate use since the early nineteenth century and it is of the utmost importance to appreciate that the social context surrounding opiate use is utterly different for a modern street addict than it was for de Quincey partaking of his laudanum. De Quincey lived at a time when opium-taking was tolerated and quite unrestricted, a state of affairs diametrically opposite to that which exists now. Great detail has recently been added to our knowledge of opium use and reactions to it in the nineteenth century by the historical research of Berridge at the Addiction Research Unit in London. She comments that, prior to the Pharmacy Act of 1868:

> Imported opium, mostly Turkish in origin, could be bought almost anywhere—not just from chemists, druggists, or pharmacists, but in village shops, from grocers, general stores, and corner shops in the back streets of the growing industrial cities (Berridge, 1977a, p.78).

For example, it was accepted that, '. . . large numbers of people of all ages and classes . . .', living in the fenland area of Lincolnshire, Huntingdonshire, Cambridgeshire, and Norfolk, were regular takers of opium (Berridge, 1977b). The *Morning Chronicle* in 1850 referred to Ely as the 'opium-eating city'. Many commentators of the time attributed this local predilection to rheumatism, neuralgia, and the ague, which were known to be particularly common in this low-lying and poorly drained part of the country. Although opium use may have been less widespread than in areas such as the Fens, less tolerance was shown towards the habit in urban areas, and increasing concern was expressed about working-class opium use in particular (Berridge, 1978).

Berridge and Rawson (1979) have presented trade figures from the time showing that consumption in England and Wales at least doubled between the 1820s and the late 1850s. It is of interest to note that this was a time of free trade policy, and that duty on imported opium fell during this time. It stood at four shillings a pound between 1828 and 1836, was reduced to one shilling a pound in 1836, and was finally abolished altogether in 1860 (Berridge and Rawson, p.353). Use by women was as much cause for concern as use by men. Even those who were not prepared to accept that regular opium use was widespread amongst adults, were concerned about the dosing of infants with opium-containing preparations such as Godfrey's Cordial, Daffy's Elixir, Dalby's Carminative, and other 'children's draughts'.

Consistent reports of violent deaths from opium poisoning were kept by the Registrar General from 1863 onwards, and Berridge and Rawson (1979) reveal that they show a rate of around five deaths per million of the population during the 1860s, that the rate was only very slightly higher for males than for females, and was much the highest in the age group 0—4 years with the over-30s showing a higher rate than adults below 30. Thus, the sex, and particularly age distribution of opiate-related deaths was very different from recent modern experience.

The tolerance with which opium was viewed in Britain in quite recent history is illustrated by the literature which Berridge (1977c) has collected on the cultivation of the opium poppy in this country between 1740 and 1823. There was much debate about the type of poppy—the garden or white varieties—best cultivated, methods of sowing and harvesting, and ways of keeping down costs. Quite considerable prizes were offered by such bodies as the Society of Arts and the Caledonian Horticultural Society. One major grower in the 1820s recommended interspersing plants of papaver somniferum with potatoes, the latter to be planted in February and the poppies in April. Harvesting opium juice from poppy heads has always been a labour-intensive operation and, not surprisingly, the use of child labour was recommended at this time. Thomas Jones recommended employing boys between eight and twelve years, and, 'To the youngest I gave three pence per day, and, if tractable and well-disposed, an additional penny for every additional year' (cited by Berridge, 1977c, p.93).

Of particular relevance to the theme of this book is Berridge's (1979) attempt to trace the development of concepts of 'addiction' in the nineteenth and early twentieth centuries. She pointed out that although the early part of the nineteenth century was characterized by increasing concern about the consumption of opium and the harm it might be causing, there was a general lack of medical conceptualizations, and certainly very little formal use of the notion of 'addiction':

> Addiction existed, yet often unrecognized even by the addicts themselves. Where it was recognized, it was seen as a vice, or just a bad habit, not an illness requiring medical attention. Isaac Milner, Dean of Carlisle, and himself dependent on opium after a nervous breakdown, advised William Wilberforce who was taking opium regularly for ulcerative colitis: 'be not afraid of the habit of such medicine, the habit of growling guts is infinitely worse. There is nothing injurious to the constitution in the medicines, and if you use them all your life there is no great harm. But paroxysms of laxity or pain leave permanent evil' (Berridge, 1979, p.69).

Although de Quincey's confessions, and particularly the comments which they contained on opium-eating by Manchester cotton workers, were important in bringing the subject to public attention, they were not much discussed in medical circles until late in the nineteenth century when the medical concept of 'addiction' was developing. Early medical involvement in fact was prompted much more by concern about infant mortality, about the open sale and availability of poisons, and about the question of opium-taking and longevity. The latter first arose on account of a disputed insurance case. The Earl of Mar died in 1828 of jaundice and dropsy and his insurance company refused to pay, arguing that opium-taking was a habit which shortened life and that his daily use of both solid opium and laudanum, which he admitted to his house-keeper, should have been admitted to the company when taking out the policy. In the event the case was settled against the company on a technical point, but it led to considerable medical debate and analysis of case series. De Quincey, incidentally, who did declare his habit was, a few years earlier, refused life insurance on these grounds by fourteen offices in succession.

This stage in the development of medical thinking gradually gave way to the emergence of a concept of 'addiction' that was given great impetus by the increasing use of the hypodermic, allowing for the accurate and rapid administration of a narcotic, in the later part of the century and awareness of the existence of 'morphinism', particularly amongst doctors themselves. Morphine, the active ingredient of opium, had been isolated in 1803 and became available in pure form towards the end of the century (Kurland, 1978). Amongst the more eminent 'morphinists', according to Brecher (1972), was Dr William Halstead, a New York surgeon and co-founder of the Johns Hopkins Medical School. Formerly a regular user of cocaine as a result of his experiments on anaesthesia, he later switched to morphine and remained 'addicted' for most of his distinguished working life. Although his efforts to come off morphine altogether were unsuccessful, he is reported to have been successful in reducing his dosage. Interestingly, it was at first thought that morphine administered by hypodermic would not be 'addicting'. Because the stomach was bypassed, it was argued, administration would not give rise to an appetite for continued drug-taking.

Berridge cited a famous article by Allbutt in *The Practitioner* in 1870:

> Gradually the connection began to force itself upon my notice, that injections of morphia, though free from the ordinary evils of opium-eating, might, nevertheless, create the same artificial want and gain credit for assuaging a restlessness and depression of which it was itself the cause (cited by Berridge, 1979, p.73).

Nevertheless, as Berridge noted, the new concept of 'addiction' was a hybrid theory incorporating both medical and moral ideas. For one thing, it had close links with both temperance and anti-opium agitation. The two were linked in the concept of 'inebriety'. According to Kerr, then President of the Society for the Study of Inebriety, there was a disease of inebriety allied to insanity and characterized by an overpowering impulse or craving for the oblivion associated with 'narcotism'. The disease took various forms depending upon the drug employed: alcoholomania, opiomania, morphinomania, chloralomania, and chlorodynomania (Kerr, 1889, cited by Berridge, 1979, p.76).

The new 'addiction' view incorporated much of the moral perspective of the temperance movement and in many ways the new approach was harsher, combining as it did moral and medical condemnation. The Society for the Suppression of the Opium Trade, founded in 1874, was campaigning against Britain's involvement in supplying opium to China, but its propaganda influenced British medical opinion about the problem at home. The Chinese Opium Wars provide a fascinating nineteenth-century example of the dynamics of national and international control of a substance that readily gives rise to excess. As Inglis (1976) stated in his account:

> Opium had the effect, invaluable for traders, of making hungry where most it satisfied. Those consumers who became addicted to it maintained a rate of demand which seemed proof against price increases (p.16).

Opium-smoking in China, as opposed to opium-eating or opium-drinking which were the customs in India and elsewhere, spread to such an extent as a result of the East India Company's operations that in 1729 the Imperial Court in Peking banned the importation of opium except under licence for medical use. Penalties for dealing in the drug were to include the wearing of a large wooden collar, known as a cangue, and the receipt of up to a hundred strokes of the bamboo. Just as in Europe and America two hundred years later, however, this edict did not prevent continued trading and the entry into China of large quantities of opium from British India, mainly through Canton. By the 1830s a member of the Imperial Court, Hsü Nai-Chi, who had lived in Canton, was recommending legalization on familiar pragmatic grounds:

> The law as it stood, Hsü argued, had demonstrably failed. It was no good saying that this was because it was unenforceable. As the ban had failed to prevent the drug from entering the country, it could

> not be said to do any good; but demonstrably it did immense harm, breeding crime, banditry, extortion and blackmail (p.111).

The newly appointed Commissioner for Canton, however, favoured a twin-pronged attack, equally familiar to us now, of tightening of controls on illegal imports plus prevention particularly directed at the young:

> To facilitate detection of opium-smoking among the young, who were most in need of protection, schoolmasters were to report any student who to their knowledge took the drug; and also to form the students into groups of five, each being responsible for the good behaviour of the other four (Lin's reasoning being that as no group would wittingly include anybody known to smoke, it would be easier to discover who the smokers were). Members of the public who in their own interest admitted their addiction would be helped to give up the drug (p.117).

Commissioner Lin's views would not have been out of place as evidence to the New York Academy of Medicine Committee which reported in 1955 and proposed a similar combined approach of reducing availability by controlling the drug traffic plus early detection and rehabilitation of those who needed it (Kurland, 1978).

In pursuit of his first aim, Lin blockaded the headquarters of the foreign merchants in Canton who were obliged to hand over around 2.5 million pounds of opium. There followed the symbolic act, which the Commissioner supervised personally, of mixing the drug with salt, lime, and water and pouring it ceremoniously into the Canton river. No doubt this act gave the same sort of uneasy satisfaction which the pouring down the sink of a bottle of whisky gives to the distraught wife or husband of an excessive drinker in London or New York.

In England, Gladstone referred to, '. . . an infamous contraband traffic . . .', and the fact that, '. . . we, the enlightened and civilised Christians, are pursuing objects at variance with justice and with religion' (cited by Inglis, pp.140, 145). Palmerston, on the other hand used arguments, also familiar to us, in favour of the continuation of the trade legally:

> The plenipotentiaries must not be given the impression that they were under any compulsion to legalise it; they were simply to be told that they would be wise to, as the British could not put down the opium traffic, 'because even if none were grown in any part of the British territories, plenty of it would be produced in other countries, and would then be sent to China'. In addition, the Chinese should be reminded of the revenue which they could expect to get from licensing the drug (p.153).

Medical writings in Europe were using such expressions as 'disease of the will', 'a form of moral insanity', 'evidence of a mental failure', 'moral orthopaedics', and 'the re-education of the will'. Levinstein's *Die Morphiumsucht*, translated into English in 1878 as *Morbid Craving for Morphia*, distinguished between 'morphinists', who wished to be cured, and 'morphinomaniacs', who were irredeemably enslaved. Many English doctors preserved this distinction in their own writings (Berridge, 1979, p.73). Whether later, twentieth-century, concepts of 'addiction' and 'dependence' have succeeded in unravelling the moral and medical strands is a debatable question. As we shall see below there are many who believe that they have not.

One of the effects of the medicalizing of ideas on opiate-taking which is highly relevant to present-day debate about concepts of 'alcoholism' and drug 'dependence', was the tendency to obscure the distinction that some would make between regular but moderate users of a drug and those whose use is excessive or uncontrolled. When the question of opium use was discussed earlier in the nineteenth century, prominence was given to moderate consumption and the stable opium-taker, the person who could take a limited dose of the drug and function adequately for many years. Berridge commented that the moderate, stable addict may have been a casualty of the new 'disease-of-the-will' formulation. Allbutt had a patient who took a grain of opium every morning and evening for fifteen years and who was, 'never so presumptious as to endeavour to suppress', this habit. But he concluded that, 'the familiar use of opium in any form is to play with fire, and probably to catch fire' (Allbutt, 1897, cited by Berridge, 1979, p.79). The possibility of 'controlled illicit drug use' (Zinberg *et al.*, 1977) is one to which this book will return in Chapter 10.

Heroin was first synthesized in 1874 and interestingly, in view of the present-day use of methadone in the treatment of heroin-users, it was itself used for a while in the treatment of 'morphinism'. Indeed, for a few years heroin was welcomed as a useful medication for a wide range of conditions. However, the medical use of heroin naturally gave rise to cases of 'heroinism' much as morphine had resulted in cases of 'morphinism' before it.

The history of Western reaction to heroin in the twentieth century illustrates a number of points. It shows the intense concern of law-makers with the control of a drug believed to be highly dangerous, but also illustrates how divergent may be the responses in different countries. Furthermore, by comparing twentieth-century reaction to heroin in the United States with reaction in Britain, and, providing an even greater contrast, with the picture in the nineteenth century, evidence is provided which is readily interpretable as illustrating the effect of legal reaction upon the problems associated with the use of a particular drug. The following brief account of the development of legal controls in the United States is based upon accounts given by Brecher (1972) and by Kurland (1978, Ch.1).

The first local statutes regulating the formerly unrestricted use of opiates in the United States were passed in San Francisco in 1875 and New York in 1904. The first Federal regulation was the Pure Food and Drug Act of 1906 which required that medicines containing opiates had to declare this on their labels. The Act was later amended to require also that the quantity of opiates contained be stated. The real turning point, according to most later writers, was the Harrison Narcotic Act of 1914. The Act required the registering and taxing of all producers, importers, and sellers of opiates, but was not intended as a prohibition law and was not to apply to a, '. . . physician . . . in the course of his professional practice . . .'. The latter, however, was interpreted by law enforcement agents to mean the treatment of disease, and 'addiction' did not qualify as such. There had in fact been a number of clinics, more than forty in number and mainly private, set up for the treatment and legal dispensing of opiates to 'addicts'. These had come under criticism for their lack of treatment orientation and what was seen as their maintenance of 'morbid appetites'. Many doctors were prosecuted under the new Act, all the clinics had closed within ten years of the Act being passed, and hence the Act became a *de facto* Act of prohibition. Many medical commentators were immediately aware of what would now be called the 'deviance amplifying' effects of the Act upon opiate users.

An editorial in *American Medicine* for 1915 reported:

> Instead of improving conditions the laws recently passed have made the problem more complex. Honest medical men have found such hardships and dangers to themselves and their reputations in these laws . . . that they have simply decided to have as little to do as possible with drug addicts or their needs . . . The druggists are in the same position . . . Abuses in the name of narcotic drugs are increasing . . . A particular sinister sequence . . . is the character of the places to which [addicts] are forced to go to get their drugs and the type of people with whom they are obliged to mix (November 1915, pp.799–800, cited by Brecher, 1972, p.50).

The U.S. clinics of the early part of the century were, arguably, ahead of their time having adopted a basically maintenance approach similar to the methadone maintenance system popular in the United States in the 1960s and 1970s and to the British system which allows the medical prescribing of heroin to addicts. The basis of this latter system, with its ideas of 'addiction' as a disease and as 'addicts' as suitable subjects for treatment, was laid by the report of the Departmental Committee on Morphine and Heroin Addiction (The Rolleston Report) in 1926, in very similar terms to parallel statements about 'alcoholism' and recent statements about 'compulsive gambling' discussed in the previous two chapters:

> . . . there was general agreement that in most well-established cases, the condition must be regarded as a manifestation of disease and not as a mere form of vicious indulgence. In other words, the drug is taken in such cases not for the purpose of obtaining positive pleasure, but in order to relieve a morbid and overpowering craving. The actual need for the drug in extreme cases is in fact so great that,

> if it be not administered, great physical distress, culminating in actual collapse and even death, may result, unless special precautions are taken such as can only be carried out under close medical supervision, and with careful nursing (cited by Berridge, 1979, pp.67–8).

Even from such a short, and third-hand, glimpse at the recent history of opiate use, it can be seen that the injecting of heroin by young, post-Second World War 'junkies' is only a part of the reality of opiate use in just one culture. As Berridge observed, 'History invites that we distance ourselves a little from preconceptions which otherwise coerce us' (1977a, p.80). Certainly, nineteenth-century use of opium and its various preparations and derivatives poses many of the same questions about the nature and definition of excessive appetitive behaviour as are raised by a consideration of present-day alcohol use and gambling activities, and these are questions which can go unasked if attention is confined to modern 'hard' drug use. These questions are pressing, however, and have had to be asked when the 'softer' or non-opiate drugs are discussed.

TOBACCO

Along with opium, alcohol, and hemp and its derivatives, tobacco must be rated as one of the most ubiquitous and socially significant of all drugs. Yet current attitudes towards tobacco could scarcely provide a bigger contrast to attitudes towards the opiates. As van Lancker (1977) puts it, '. . . smokers almost all over the world can now enjoy their habit with the tacit approval of their government, vigorous encouragement of the tobacco industry, absolution of their church, and the resigned silence of their physicians'. Indeed, acceptance has been so great, the licit involvement of governments and commerce so strong, and until very recently the dangers of the drug so ignored, that tobacco has scarcely been recognized as a 'drug' at all. Jarvik (1970), Russell (1971), Jaffe (1977), and van Lancker (1977) are amongst those who have commented on the history of nicotine and pointed out how attitudes and practices have varied and changed.

Official reactions to tobacco have run the gamut from total condemnation and persecution to permissive licence in a way that we should now expect of responses to appetitive behaviour generally—judging from the historical and cultural variations to be found in reactions to alcohol, gambling, and the opiates. For instance, in the seventeenth century tobacco-smoking was at one time or another punishable by death in Turkey, Russia, Persia, and Germany. At other times in Turkey the nose of a convicted tobacco-user would be pierced, the stem of a pipe passed through it, and the user ridden through the streets on a donkey. Van Lancker (1977) lists a number of religious groups and sects which have more recently banished tobacco altogether: Mormons, Seventh Day Adventists, and Parsees and Sikhs in India, for example.

According to Corti (1932, cited by Jaffe, 1977) one of the first Europeans to note the addicting properties of tobacco was a Spanish missionary Bishop who, upon questioning Spanish settlers about their 'disgusting habit' of tobacco-smoking, was told that they found it impossible to give it up. Soon after its introduction to Europe from the New World, King James I organized in Oxford in 1605 the first public debate on the effects of tobacco, producing black brains and viscera supposedly obtained from the dead bodies of inveterate smokers (van Lancker, p.235), an interesting forerunner of modern health education campaigns of the fear-arousing type. And in his famous, *A Counterblaste to Tobacco*, in 1604, King James compared tobacco's black smelly smoke to the horrible vapours that 'exhale from hell'.

On the other hand, it should not surprise us that van Lancker is able to list a number of publications from the sixteenth and seventeenth centuries praising tobacco on medical grounds. One writer claimed to have cured headaches, coughs, asthma, gout, stomach pains, constipation, renal stones, flatulence, rheumatism, toothache, and hemoptysis with tobacco syrups, enemas, or inhalation of tobacco smoke. He even recommended that hot tobacco leaves be applied to the navel to reduce pains associated with delivery or pregnancy.

In the nineteenth century, physicians of temperance persuasion were, by contrast, strong in their condemnation. One such believed that to 'break the chains' of tobacco enslavement, 'requires the sternest efforts of reason, conscience and the will' (Harris, 1853, cited by Jaffe, 1977, p.206).

Jaffe drew attention to what he believed to have been a reaction to such moralistic attacks between the First and Second World Wars. He cited Brill, a pioneer of the psychoanalytic movement, who believed that, 'most of the fanatical opponents of tobacco that I have known were all bad neurotics', and a German pharmacologist, Lewin, who expressed the common belief of the time that smoking did not lead to 'suffering of the body or morbid desire for the drug' when given up. Indeed, the latter believed it to be:

> . . . an enjoyment which man is free to renounce and when he indulges in it he experiences its benevolent effects on his spiritual life . . . [unlike wine] . . . it adjusts the working condition of the mind and the disposition of many mentally active persons to a kind of serenity or 'quietism' during which the activity of thought is in no way disturbed . . . (Lewin, 1924, cited by Jaffe, p.207).

Of particular interest is his quotation from Sir Humphrey Rolleston whose report on opiates was to be of such importance in the history of drug-taking in Britain in the twentieth century. On tobacco, he is quoted as saying:

> This question turns on the meaning attached to the word 'addiction' . . . That smoking produces a craving for more when an attempt is made to give it up . . . is undoubted, but it can seldom be accurately described as overpowering, and the effects of its withdrawal, though there may be definite restlessness and instability, cannot be compared with the physical distress caused by withdrawal in morphine addicts.

> To regard tobacco as a drug of addiction is all very well in a humorous sense, but it is hardly accurate (Rolleston, 1926a, quoted by Jaffe, pp.207–8).

Even Seevers, described by Jaffe as 'one of the giants in the field of pharmacological research on drug dependence', was of the view that, 'By no stretch of the imagination can either nicotine or caffeine conform to any accepted definition of addiction' (Seevers, 1962, quoted by Jaffe, p.208).

The last twenty years have seen renewed concern, principally in the form of a vastly increased rate of research into the medical effects of regular tobacco-smoking, and a consequent increase in awareness of the medical dangers of smoking (Bernstein, 1970). Most modern commentators now accept the evidence for a link between habitual cigarette-smoking and the development of cardiovascular disease, chronic bronchitis, emphysema, cancer of the lung and bladder, and other diseases (Bernstein and McAllister, 1976). This evidence has been publicized in Britain by reports from the Royal College of Physicians (e.g. 1977) and in the United States by the Advisory Committee to the Surgeon General (1964). The United States remains, according to Eckholm (1977), the world's topmost cigarette-smoking country nevertheless, with Japan a close second. Eckholm also reported tobacco-smoking spreading rapidly to developing countries, in some cases with the connivance of governments of the 'developed' nations. He cited, for example, the United States Public Law 480 'Food for Peace' programme of concessional agricultural sales to developing countries, under which large amounts of tobacco have been shipped overseas on favourable terms. Like the Spaniards introducing hard liquor in large quantities to Latin American Indians (Bunzel, 1940) and the British trading in Indian opium to China, this seems to be yet another example of a powerful nation creating economic dependence by pushing an 'addictive' substance upon a native population and creating a demand which turns out, in economic terms, to be remarkably 'inelastic'.

Rather like medical awareness of opiate use in the nineteenth century, modern concern with tobacco focused first on tobacco-related medical damage—morbidity and mortality—rather than 'addiction'. Concepts of 'addiction' and 'dependence' are now sufficiently familiar, however, that the idea of tobacco or nicotine 'dependence' is readily to hand and is not seen as particularly alien. With publicity given to the damaging effects of cigarette-smoking, the mounting of anti-smoking health campaigns on a large scale, and even the setting up of clinics to help people give up smoking—itself a sign that giving up is difficult for some people—has come the realization that many people who may wish to give up smoking are unable to do so. One American survey carried out in Chicago in the early 1960s reported only 24 per cent of smokers ever having tried to quit and only a third of those having been successful. The author of the survey described continuing smokers as either 'uninformed', 'unbelieving', 'unmotivated', or 'unable' (Straits, 1965, cited by Bernstein, 1970)! Russell has argued that cigarette-smoking is a 'dependence disorder':

> We can no longer afford to regard cigarette smoking as a 'minor vice'. It is neither minor nor a vice, but a psychological disorder of a particularly refractory nature and all the evidence places it fair and square in the category of dependence disorders (Russell, 1971, p.1).

Difficulties in defining 'dependence' have already been met in the context of excessive alcohol use and excessive gambling, and the difficulties are the same in the context of tobacco use. At one time the World Health Organization wished to distinguish between 'addiction' and 'habituation', defining the former as:

> A state of periodic or chronic intoxication, detrimental to the individual and society, produced by the repeated administration of a drug; its characteristics are a compulsion to take the drug and to increase the dose, with the development of psychic and sometimes physical dependence on the effects of the drug, so that the development of compulsion to continue the administration of the drug becomes an important motive in the addict's existence.

'Habituation', on the other hand, was defined as:

> A condition resulting from the repeated consumption of a drug. Its characteristics include: a desire (but not a compulsion) to continue taking the drug for the sense of improved well-being which it engenders; little or no tendency to increase the dose; some degree of psychic dependence on the effect of the drug, but absence of physical dependence and hence of an abstinence syndrome; detrimental effects, if any, primarily on the individual (World Health Organization, 1964a).

Quite apart from the evident difficulties in deciding whether a desire is sufficiently strong to be rated as a compulsion, and whether society is or is not harmed, the difference hinged upon the questions of the development of tolerance (and hence the likelihood of increasing the dose) and the presence of a syndrome of effects upon withdrawal or abstinence. Although it is clear that adolescents increase their daily intake in the course of developing a tobacco habit (McKennell and Thomas, 1967), and that smokers describe 'withdrawal symptoms' such as gastric disorders, dry mouth, irritability, sleeplessness, headaches, weight gain, tremors, nausea, impaired concentration, and restlessness, as well as a strong desire for cigarettes (Bernstein, 1970), it is by no means an easy matter to establish whether these effects constitute increased tolerance and an abstinence syndrome in a strict psychopharmacological sense. Bernstein (1970) is among those who believed that the evidence was, strictly speaking, lacking, whilst Russell (1971) believed the case to be proven in the form of experimental evidence of withdrawal effects such as sleep disturbance, sweating, gastro-intestinal changes, a drop in pulse rate and blood pressure, disturbed time perception, and impaired performance of simulated driving tasks, as well as EEG changes (p.3). He pointed out that, unlike the case of alcohol or the barbiturate drugs, intermittent or occasional use of tobacco is a rarity. Most people who smoke go on to become regular smokers, he argued, citing McKennell and Thomas's results (1967) in his support. We should not be surprised that this is the case, he wrote, since the absorption of nicotine through the lungs during smoking is about as rapid and efficient as an intravenous 'fix' of morphine or heroin (p.3). There was many a smoker who would, '. . . reach for a cigarette first thing on waking, will seldom go more than an hour without a cigarette, and, should his supply run out, will go to great lengths to obtain more' (p.4). In this way the heavy smoker maintains a certain level of nicotine more or less continuously throughout the waking day.

Russell strengthened his case by reference to continued 'dependence' on a national level since the sixteenth century, and in recent years the inelasticity of demand for tobacco. On the first point he noted that although tobacco use was unknown in Europe, as in Asia and Africa, before the discovery of the New World, once introduced the form of tobacco consumption may change, but a country seems never to rid itself entirely of its use. Table 5, reprinted by Jarvik from a U.S. Government report of 1964, which shows changes in the form of tobacco use in the United States between 1900 and 1960, supports Russell's argument.

Table 5 Changing consumption of tobacco products, U.S.A. 1900–1960 (from Jarvik, 1970)

Year	All tobacco (pounds)	Cigarettes (number)	Cigars (number)	Pipe tobacco (pounds)	Chewing tobacco (pounds)	Snuff (pounds)
1900	7.42	49	111	1.63	4.10	0.32
1910	8.50	138	113	2.58	3.99	.50
1920	8.66	611	117	1.96	3.06	.50
1930	8.88	1,365	72	1.87	1.90	.46
1940	8.91	1,828	56	2.05	1.00	.38
1950	11.59	3,322	50	.94	.78	.36
1960	10.97	3,888	57	.59	.51	.29

On the second point, Russell's own analysis of changes in cigarette price and changes in level of consumption by males in Britain between 1946 and 1971 showed that, although price increases regularly resulted in a small reduction of consumption, and reductions in real price were followed by increases in consumption, demand was inelastic in the sense that for every 1 per cent change in real price, consumption changed by only approximately 0.6 per cent (Russell, 1973).

In his interesting paper entitled, *Tobacco Use as a Mental Disorder*, Jaffe (1977) also asked why modern psychiatry had been so indifferent to the question of tobacco use and 'dependence'. He pointed out that psychiatric textbooks tended to devote more room to glue-sniffing than they did to tobacco, that the International Classification of Diseases (ICD) made no mention of 'dependence' on tobacco although 'dependence' on cannabis and even on caffeine were listed, and that the second version of the American Psychiatric Association's *Diagnostic and Statistical Manual* (*DSM*) had no separate section on tobacco 'dependence' (unlike alcohol) although it was mentioned as an example of 'dependence'.

Jaffe then outlined recent developments which gave evidence of cautious, and ambivalent, inclusion of tobacco as a 'dependence producing substance'. In 1975 a draft version of the ninth edition of the *ICD* did not include tobacco under 'drug dependence', even though this was defined in such a way that withdrawal and tolerance (the original hallmarks of 'addiction') were not considered necessary conditions. Where it was included was in a special section on 'non-dependent abuse of drugs' defined as follows:

> . . . cases where a person for whom no other diagnosis is possible, has come under medical care because of the maladaptive effect of a drug on which he is not dependent and that he has taken on his own initiative to the detriment of his health or social functioning.

Strangely, the subsection on tobacco, under this heading of abuse, specifically included the possibility that 'tobacco dependence' might be present, but defended the decision not to include it in the section on 'drug dependence', '. . . because tobacco differs from other drugs of dependence in its psychotoxic effects' (quoted by Jaffe, p.210).

At the same time the American Psychiatric Association were reviewing their *DSM* with a view to bringing out a third edition and Jaffe reported that this would include Tobacco Use Disorder to be defined as follows:

> 1) The patient experiences distress at the need to repeatedly use tobacco; or
> 2) Both (a) and (b):
>   (a) In the judgement of the diagnostician the individual manifests a serious medical disorder in which tobacco smoking is a significant etiological or exacerbating factor; and
>   (b) There is evidence of current physiological dependence on tobacco or nicotine either by the presence of the tobacco withdrawal syndrome or by the daily intake of nicotine of sufficient magnitude that the diagnostician judges that the withdrawal syndrome would ensue if the intake of tobacco stopped for more than 24 hours
>
> (quoted by Jaffe, p.213).

Such a tortuous definition, as Jaffe admitted, leads to certain obvious inconsistencies. Paragraph 2(b) makes quite explicit the belief in the possibility of 'addiction' in the sense of altered physiological response but makes no mention of 'psychic dependence'. Furthermore, if this is absent, and if the individual concerned does not experience distress, then tobacco-use disorder is said not to exist, whilst distress alone is sufficient for 'diagnosis' even in the absence of medical harm and 'addiction'. Such an effort at definition demonstrates all the problems of attempting to make a definable disorder out of a problem of excessive habitual behaviour. The problem is almost exactly parallel to problems incurred in trying to define 'alcoholism', 'compulsive gambling', 'compulsive eating', or 'hypersexuality'.

Not only are there these difficulties in pinning down 'addiction', 'dependence', or 'disorder', but furthermore not everyone agrees on the criteria to be employed. The lay notion of 'addiction' probably incorporates notions of need, and of difficulty in quitting, but almost certainly is not specific about tolerance and withdrawal. Authorities on the subject frequently define 'addiction' in a manner closer to the lay definition than to that of the World Health Organization in 1964. For example, Bernstein cites Tomkins' (1965) criteria: the absence of the addicting substance is always noted by the addict; awareness of this absence produces intense negative feelings for which there is also awareness; and the addict expects that only the addicting substance can reduce these feelings (cited by Bernstein, 1970, p.6). Jarvik prefers the even more straightforward definition: 'Drug addiction is a behavioural pattern characterised by a tendency to obtain and introduce into the body quantities of the drug to achieve pleasurable effects' (Jarvik, 1970, p.183). Hence, neither physical adaptation nor tolerance are necessary for 'addiction' according to this definition. Finding the distinction between 'addiction' and 'habituation' unworkable, the World Health Organization subsequently recommended dropping both terms, substituting the single concept of 'dependence', arguing that each drug produced its own brand of 'dependence' (dependence of alcohol type, dependence of morphine type, etc.), and that increased tolerance and an abstinence syndrome would be more or less a feature of the picture in different cases and with different drugs. The 'alcohol dependence syndrome', discussed in Chapter 2, is a development of this thinking.

Whatever the ins and outs of such wrangles over definitions, the evidence that many people are 'addicted' to tobacco-smoking, in the lay sense of that word, is overwhelming. There is no better evidence for this than the results of the study of adults' and adolescents' smoking habits and attitudes, carried out for the Government Social Survey by McKennell and Thomas (1967). In the Summer of 1964 they interviewed a representative national sample of 854 16–20-year-olds and 984 adults. 'Addiction' was defined by four items:

> Frequently when I haven't got any cigarettes on me I feel a craving for one (craving).
>
> The respondent thought he/she would find it, 'Fairly or very difficult to go without smoking for as long as one week (difficulty anticipated).

If the respondent had tried to give up he/she had found it, 'Fairly or very difficult to do so' (difficulty experienced).

The respondent thought he/she would find it, 'Very difficult to give up altogether' (difficulty altogether).

McKennell and Thomas's report is particularly noteworthy for their introduction of the concept of 'dissonant smoking', a simple and straightforward concept which may go some way towards clearing a great deal of the confusion that surrounds such terms as 'addiction' and 'dependence'. A 'dissonant' smoker is simply one who would like to behave otherwise than he or she does: someone who feels he or she smokes when non-smoking would be ideal or who smokes more than an amount considered ideal. As McKennell and Thomas wrote, 'One of the most remarkable findings that emerges from social surveys of smokers' habits and attitudes is the very large number who either express a wish to give up smoking or else have tried to do so' (p.96). Dissonance was operationally defined by them in terms of just two questions: 'Would you like to give up smoking if you could do so easily?'; and 'Have you ever tried to give up smoking altogether?' Table 6 shows the percentages of respondents defined by them as dissonant or consonant in their smoking on the basis of answers to the above two questions. They commented: 'Dissonant smokers appear to be people who are trapped by the smoking habit, somewhat against their will. The majority of them have in fact tried several times to give up smoking . . .' (p.90). They presented a great deal of evidence on the development of smoking, particularly during the teenage years, and they pointed out how the majority of respondents who had smoked at all reported escalating to regular and often 'addicted' or 'dissonant' smoking within an average of two to three years. They commented on the relative rarity of 'true' or 'genuine' long-term occasional smoking, and indeed Russell (1971) leant heavily on this finding in arguing that tobacco was one of the most highly 'dependence-producing' drugs of all. In fact this point may have been overstated: their figures show as many as 18 per cent of adolescents and 11 per cent of adults reported smoking only once, 13 per cent and 9 per cent reported smoking more than once but never as frequently as once a week for as long as a month, and 8 per cent and 2 per cent reported smoking at least once a week for as long as a month but never regularly.

Table 6 Percentage of dissonant smokers (McKennell and Thomas, 1967)

	Adolescents (%)	Adults (%)
Dissonant:		
Wish and tried—highly dissonant	38	30
Wish but not tried—dissonant	11	15
Consonant:		
No wish but tried in the past—consonant	22	22
Neither wish nor tried—highly consonant	29	33

Debate about the nature and prevalence of 'addiction' aside, there can be no denying widespread present-day concern. One estimate (Luce and Schweitzer, 1977) put the economic cost of smoking in the United States at $41.5 billion, or 2.5 per cent of the country's gross national product. Of this, $7.5 billion was estimated to be direct health care cost, $18 billion lost earnings due to death and disease, $15.5 billion retail cost of tobacco products to the consumer, and $167 million costs due to fire damage to property.

Health education campaigns consisting of some combination of lectures, films, pamphlets, posters, and exhibits have been mounted in large numbers in the United States in recent years (Bernstein, 1970) and the same is true in Britain. Numerous self-help smoking cessation books have also appeared on the market. A more personal and individual approach is offered by the 'smoking withdrawal clinics', the first of which was opened in Sweden in 1955 (Bernstein, 1970). A whole range of individual and group psychological treatments has been employed in these clinics, some of which will be considered in more detail in a later chapter. Of particular interest, because of the major role played by drug substitution therapy in the management of opiate use, is the use of medication in smoking clinics. Various drugs, including caffeine and nicotine itself, have been used from time to time, probably the most popular having been lobeline, normally used in the form of lobeline sulphate, which mimics to some degree the effect of nicotine (Bernstein, 1970). The drug is used with or without other preparations, one example being a cherry flavoured lozenge branded Smokurb.

Despite all this activity, overall trends in consumption do not show the dramatic reduction in smoking consumption that some had hoped for. Schuman (1977), summarizing material collected by the American National Clearing House for Smoking and Health which was set up shortly after the Surgeon General's Advisory Committee Report in 1964, noted a reduction in the proportion of adult males currently smoking from 53 to 39 per cent between 1964 and 1975. However, the change for adult women had been far less dramatic, from 31.5 per cent to 29 per cent, and there is evidence that new recruits to smoking are starting at an earlier age, and that girls and young women are starting to smoke in larger numbers than had previously been the case. This latter trend was already apparent in Britain by 1964 when McKennell and Thomas carried out their survey. They noted in their report that whilst males were still tending to smoke earlier and in greater numbers than females, as they had previously done, nevertheless, 'The pattern of female smoking had in fact been transformed over the past 20 years so as to resemble that which has long been established amongst males' (p.14). It should be noted here again that a particular concern with the behaviour of young people, and with women, has always been a notable characteristic of the debate about the dangers of potentially 'addicting' substances and activities. All the excesses considered in this book, with the possible exception of over-eating, have commonly been thought to be habits mainly indulged in by adult males, and particular worry is expressed when either women or young people appear to be adopting them in larger numbers.

OTHER DRUGS

Tobacco is of course not the only non-opiate drug substance which can cause problems of excess and give rise to difficult questions about the existence or nature of drug 'dependence' or 'addiction'. The full list of mind-altering drugs, both naturally occurring and synthetic, would be huge, and only some of the main categories will be discussed here. Of these, the so-called sedative hypnotics have a good case for being given pride of place, in particular the barbiturates. In the 1960s there was increasing evidence of the use of both oral and injected barbiturates as ancillary or alternative drugs for heroin users (e.g. Mitcheson *et al.*, 1970), although there is now evidence that they may be in the process of being ousted by the benzodiazepines (Jauhar, 1981). Recent studies of drug-related problems dealt with by casualty departments of London hospitals showed barbiturates, sometimes obtained from a general practitioner or a hospital treatment centre but most often obtained illegally, to be the commonest drugs involved in incidents of overdose (Ghodse, 1977). In the United States the Drug Abuse Warning Network (DAWN) set up by the National Institute on Drug Abuse to monitor the type and extent of drug-related incidents occurring in emergency rooms, crisis intervention centres, hospitals, and surgeries in 29 cities across the country, has reported a similarly high rate of barbiturate overdoses and medical complications (Wesson and Smith, 1977, pp.53–4).

There is another side to barbiturate use, however, which bears closer resemblance to middle-class opium-taking in the nineteenth century than to deviant or illicit abuse or overdose. In 1975, according to Williams (1981), no less than 47.5 million prescriptions for psychotropic drugs were dispensed at retail pharmacies in England. The scale of licit, medically prescribed 'drug-taking' is thus huge. Furthermore, Balint *et al.* (1970) found that 40 per cent of patients in a general practice setting were given *repeat* prescriptions of psychotropic drugs. Of those receiving barbiturates or amphetamines at least once, 50 per cent were still receiving the same medication four years later, 25 per cent eight years later, and 9 per cent 16 years later. With the number of medical prescriptions for barbiturates running in the region of 20 million annually, in England and Wales, at that time, it is not surprising that estimates of the number of long-term users of barbiturates, most medically prescribed and with continual medical knowledge, are high. Swinson and Eaves (1978) cite a 1966 estimate of the number of 'barbiturate dependants' in the United Kingdom to be in the region of 100,000 with 500,000 other 'regular users without dependence'. Barbiturates are fairly widely regarded as having high 'dependence potential' and their use as leading to increasing tolerance and withdrawal effects. Wesson and Smith (1977), for example, rate the barbiturate drugs as similar to alcohol but less potent than heroin in terms of the speed with which they can produce both 'psychological' and 'physical dependence', but rate them stronger than alcohol (weaker than heroin) in their capacity to bring about increased tolerance. Thus, the barbiturates have now acquired a bad reputation in medical circles, and voluntary restraint by doctors in

Britain reduced the number of prescriptions markedly after the mid-1960s (Bennett, 1981).

Because of the widely differing circumstances under which barbiturates have been taken there is ample room for differences of opinion about the use of such terms such as 'misuse' and 'abuse', both terms widely but loosely used in connection with drug-taking of many types. As Wesson and Smith (1977) have pointed out, the term 'abuse', '. .. is likely to be applied to individuals living on the fringes of the dominant culture rather than to those living within it who use similar amounts of barbiturates. The latter group's behaviour is more likely to be labelled "misuse" or "overuse" ' (p.55). They cited a number of attempts to define the term 'drug abuse'. Whilst the Committee on Alcohol and Addiction of the American Medical Association (1965) attempted precision by defining barbiturate abuse as the, '. . . self-administration of excessive quantities of barbiturates leading to tolerance, physical and psychological dependence, mental confusion and other symptoms of abnormal behaviour', Einstein and Geritano (1972) emphasized cultural relativity by defining abuse as:

> . . . behaviour, so designated by professionals and other community representatives, describing the use of particular drugs in particular ways for particular reasons which are contrary to the agreed upon rituals in a given community at a given point in time (cited by Wesson and Smith, p.56).

If, as Wesson and Smith argued, use of the word 'abuse' involves a judgement of one person upon another, depending upon the age, social position, and occupation of both, the quantities of drug taken, the reasons for which it is taken, whether it is taken orally or by injection, and the source from which it is obtained, a parallel with other substances and activities is again readily apparent. Gambling, drinking, sexual behaviour, and opiate use have more commonly been criticized discriminatively rather than wholesale, and have been judged on the basis of who is indulging in what form of the activity and why. Nineteenth-century concern with the motivations for opiate use constitute one of the best examples. Quotations from the period show that discriminations were frequently made between medicinal use, or use as a pick-me-up by the under-privileged poor, on the one hand, and use as a 'stimulant' or a 'luxury' (hedonistic use) on the other. The former was frequently condoned, the latter was not (Berridge, 1979). In present-day Islamic countries, according to Baasher (1981), the problem of controlling the use of the many, new, manufactured drugs has added to the long-standing problems of controlling opium, cannabis, and khat. Although Islamic law has proscribed any substance having the properties of Khamr (wine), which causes clouding of the mind and interferes with rational thinking, the fact that, unlike alcohol, they recieve no mention in the *Qur'ān*, can be an impediment to control. Baasher referred to a number of attempts adopted in different countries in the Islamic world to control the use of different drugs, including the attempt to inculcate discriminate khat-chewing in

Democratic Yemen by restricting consumption to weekends and official holidays. As we shall see below, the breakdown of discrimination in the use of a drug or activity is central to the process of becoming excessive.

Amongst the great range of relatively new synthetic drugs now available in many parts of the world there are, not surprisingly, many which when first developed were unknown quantities. Chemically they do not sit neatly into any one of the well-known major categories and it takes time before their potential is known. Amongst these are a number, the effects and potential for 'dependence' of which, are said to closely resemble the barbiturates. Meprobamate is one and glutethimide is another. An interesting further example discussed by Schecter (1978, Ch.11) is methaqualone. The story of this drug's promotion in the United States and United Kingdom could be repeated for many recent drugs and bears a striking similarity to the much earlier history of morphine and heroin and to the much more drawn-out process that occurred during the nineteenth century as the harmful potential of opium slowly became apparent. Despite widespread 'abuse' of methaqualone in Japan when it was available there over the counter in the early 1960s, and evidence from the same country that individuals could become 'addicted' to the point of experiencing withdrawal convulsions and delirium symptoms, methaqualone was introduced to the American medical market in 1965 for the treatment of insomnia and anxiety with the claim that it was a non-barbiturate hypnotic with no potential for 'abuse' and 'dependence'. Schecter has related how the drug rapidly developed a reputation for producing a particularly pleasant state of intoxication, earning the tag 'heroin for lovers'. Conflicting views as to whether methaqualone could or could not produce 'physical dependence' appeared at that time. Schecter's view would probably now be widely accepted by the experts, namely that methaqualone is very similar to most barbiturates in producing tolerance, and in carrying particular dangers of 'dependence' and death by overdose. He referred to the practice, known as 'luding out', of taking methaqualone with wine, a particularly hazardous habit because of the compounding effect of the drug with alcohol. At one time methaqualone gained special favour with former heroin addicts maintained on methadone because methaqualone was not looked for in the routine urine samples required of participants in methadone maintenance programmes.

The drug scene is further complicated by the marketing of preparations which combine different drugs. A well-known example in Britain, the subject of much concern about 'abuse' in the 1960s, was Mandrax, a combination of methaqualone and an amphetamine, diphenhydramine (Swinson and Eaves, 1978, p.151).

A particularly important class of drug, because of the enormous numbers now prescribed (over 30 million prescriptions in England and Wales in 1978 (Bennett, 1981)), is that of the benzodiazepines or, as they are sometimes called, 'minor' tranquillizers. The group includes diazepam (Valium) and chlordiazepoxide (Librium). The benzodiazepines are sometimes classed with barbiturates as sedative-hypnotics, although they are generally thought to be of much lower 'dependence potential' and to be much safer than the barbiturates. This is the conclusion reached, for example, by Marks (1978) in his review. From the evidence from animal experiments, which he reviewed, he concluded that 'dependence' could be produced when animals self-administered large doses of the drug intravenously over a long period of time. Indeed, he concluded that all drugs which have a sedative or depressant effect on the central nervous system had some potential for 'dependence', but that this varied greatly from drug to drug, and was low in the case of benzodiazepines. Marks critically reviewed the human literature in great detail and stated that it confirmed the animal studies. He pointed out that the study by Hollister *et al.* (1961) in which hospitalized psychiatric patients were made 'dependent' upon chlordiazepoxide, in fact involved dosages very much in excess of the normal therapeutic level, administered for several months. Marks found 42 documented cases where there was, 'reasonable evidence', for 'dependence' within the framework of medical therapeutic use, and 151 cases within the framework of, 'multiple drug abuse (polytoxicomania) or alcoholism'. In addition he found 15 and 250 cases in those two categories, respectively, where he considered the evidence for 'dependence' to be 'poor'. In a high proportion of the cases with 'reasonable evidence', he considered there to be evidence of 'physical dependence' in the form of abstinence symptoms similar to those observed in cases of alcohol or barbiturate 'dependence', but normally less severe and occurring later after withdrawal—usually on the third to sixth day.

On the basis of these published cases, plus a number of unpublished reports based upon records held by the monitoring system of Hoffmann–La Roche and Company, the drug manufacturers for whom Marks had previously worked, and using a reasonable estimate of the number of 'patient months at risk' in the United Kingdom (150,000,000 for the period 1960 to mid-1977), he calculated the incidence of recorded cases of benzodiazepine 'dependence' to be extremely low (one recorded case for every 5.3 million patient months of use in the United Kingdom, excluding recorded cases from other countries, mostly the United States and Germany).

Lader (1981) was less sanguine in his review, however. There had been many reports of tension, trembling, dizziness, insomnia, anxiety, and even fits and psychoses upon discontinuing therapeutic use abruptly, and he reported similar experiences for 20 patients known to him who complained of difficulty stopping benzodiazepine use and who underwent withdrawal in hospital. About half of this group had escalated the dose to several times the usual and he attributed the 'symptoms' they experienced on cessation to 'withdrawal' on the grounds that they were often untypical of the kind of anxiety for which the drug was probably prescribed in the first place, and that they subsided over a period of two to four weeks. Note here that Lader's concept of 'dependence' relied heavily upon medical evidence of 'withdrawal symptoms' and took little account of the psychological complexities introduced by those who have pondered the nature of 'addiction' in the context of such appetitive behaviours as drinking, tobacco use, or gambling.

The incidence of recorded cases is in any case a poor basis for estimating real incidence, even assuming that such a notion as 'real incidence' in the case of something as ill-defined as 'dependence' is conceivable at all. This is quite clear in the context of alcohol, as discussed in Chapter 2, and would certainly be accepted by most commentators in the field of gambling. Recorded cases of 'dependence' on minor tranquillizers establish at least that such a phenomenon is reported. The rate with which such a phenomenon occurs can only be established by studies which draw samples from the general population or from the population of users of these drugs. Marks was able to find only five large-scale studies of patients. Of these, four appear to have been superficial studies involving records of several thousands of users of tranquillizers. Two reported no case of 'dependence', the other two studies reporting one and two doubtful cases, respectively. These studies probably prove little other than the obvious fact that 'dependence' will not be found unless it is looked for. The fifth study, by Maletzky and Klotter (1976), was dismissed by Marks on the grounds of inadequate data although, '. . . taken at its face value this appears to show that a high proportion of the patients taking diazepam presented some evidence of dependence' (p.34).

In fact, the Maletzky and Klotter report represents a fascinating and detailed look at the attribution of 'dependence' on the part of medical practitioners and patients. Of the 50 patients of a military psychiatric clinic who were the subjects of Maletzky and Klotter's study, half had increased the dose of diazepam used, many without asking their doctors, and most had not subsequently returned to the original level. There was considerable evidence of 'dissonance', to use the term that McKennell and Thomas employed in the context of smoking. Twenty-four patients had attempted to stop, all but 2 unsuccessfully, and 30 rated themselves as 'dependent' to some degree (14 'slightly', 8 'moderately', 4 'greatly', and 4 'severely'). Of those who had attempted to stop, 79 per cent experienced, '. . . withdrawal symptoms of moderate to extreme severity . . .' (p.106). The most common symptoms were anxiety, agitation, insomnia, and tremor and almost all complained of some symptoms not present before taking the drug.

A particularly valuable and intriguing part of their study concerned the effect upon the attribution process of knowing whether the drug described was a minor tranquillizer or not. When a panel of general practitioners, general surgeons, internists, and orthopaedic surgeons judged the degree of patients' 'addiction' from their replies to the standard interview which had elicited this information, *without* knowing the name of the drug involved, 31 were rated as having some degree of 'addiction' (20 at least 'moderately' so, and 9 of these 'greatly' or 'severely'). When the panel was asked to re-rate the degree of 'addiction' having been told that the drug concerned was diazepam, only 14 were rated as showing any 'addiction' (only 5 'moderate' and none 'great' or 'severe').

Maletzky and Klotter add, 'Often physicians commented, with relief, that "it was only Valium", thus could not be dangerous' (p.111). This, '. . . over-acceptance of diazepam's safety . . . may be falsely based upon a narrow concept of addiction: [that] unless withdrawal symptoms mimic those of heroin or alcohol, a drug cannot be addicting . . .' (pp.96–7).

The amphetamines constitute a further major category which raises salient questions about the psychological nature of excessive drug use. They have been in medical use for over 30 years for many conditions, latterly particularly for depression and for weight control in cases of obesity—yet a further example of the substitution of one appetitive behaviour for another (Swinson and Eaves, 1978, p.37). Reactions to them have followed the familiar pattern of medical enthusiasm followed by growing awareness of their dangers, followed, in the case of the amphetamines, by the introduction of legal and voluntary controls on prescriptions and availability in many countries. In Japan amphetamines were freely available without prescription, and by 1954 it was estimated that 2 per cent of the total population was 'addicted' (Swinson and Eaves, p.38), since when the problem has been brought under control with the help of legal restrictions and the spread of information about their dangers. In England, Connell (1958) reported cases of psychotic reactions due to excessive intake of amphetamines, and a study by Kiloh and Brandon (1962) suggested that 1 per cent of the population was receiving amphetamines and that one in five of users showed signs of some 'dependence'.

Amphetamines and mixtures containing amphetamines (for example Mandrax and Drinamyl or 'purple hearts') were popular recreational drugs in the 1960s, and for a short period, before restrictions on the prescribing of the drug were instituted, the intravenous injecting of methylamphetamine by numbers of young, often multiple, drug users was reported (e.g. Hawks *et al.*, 1969). Sweden was just one of many other countries that legislated to restrict the availability of stimulants in the 1960s, in this case only two years after their prescribing had been legalized (Swinson and Eaves, p.40).

Cocaine, classed like the amphetamines as a stimulant, is of particular interest because it occurs naturally in the leaves of the coca plant and was introduced to Europe at about the same time as tobacco. This was yet another drug that met with medical enthusiasm in the nineteenth century, on the part of Freud amongst others, and was tried as a cure for both opiate and alcohol excess. It too emerged as a recreational drug amongst young adults in the 1960s (Schecter, 1978). Although it may be injected intravenously, either alone or in combination with other drugs including heroin (when the mixture is known as a 'speedball'), the commonest method of use in the United States was, according to Schecter, absorption through the mucus membranes of the nose, a method popularly known as 'snorting'. It can also be rubbed on the gums and absorbed, blown from a straw on to the mucosal surface at the back of the throat, or absorbed through the mucosa of the vagina or the glans of the penis (Schecter, p.142). Like other stimulants, cocaine is often used alternately with a sedative-hypnotic drug in an 'upper–downer cycle'. On the question of 'dependence', Schecter's view was that 'psychological dependence' did occur, but that true physical dependence was controversial.

Chronic oral use of cocaine occurs in the form of coca leaf chewing in South

America, particularly in Peru. The problems such use poses for definitions of 'dependence', 'abuse', and excess are quite similar to those posed by nineteenth-century English opium-eating. According to Negrete's (1980) review, South American coca-chewing is so widespread that it is, '. . . among the larger if not the most extensive narcotic problem in the world' (p.285). 'Cocaism', he wrote, is culturally accepted and there is considerable controversy over the use of coca and its effects. It seems that its use is 'utilitarian' as opposed to 'hedonistic'. Ostensibly it is used to help concentrate at work, to withstand the climate and harsh life often lived at high altitude. Coca leaves are still given in some places as part of wages. There is little evidence of obvious 'dependence': 'Coca chewing is a case of orderly moderate and social use of narcotics. It cannot be equated with the usually individualistic, anarchic and more symptomatic problem of cocaine abuse' (p.286). The social and cultural setting, the user's motivation and other characteristics, the dose, and the route of administration of the drug are, if Negrete was right, as different from illicit cocaine injecting in urban America as fenland opium-eating in England was from the later junkie subculture. Negrete considered there was evidence for the suggestion that chronic coca leaf chewing produced long-term cognitive changes in the direction of lowered abstract thinking ability, but admitted that the problems of testing such an hypothesis thoroughly, ideally involving the use of controls and the partialling out of factors such as education and age, had not properly been overcome.

A further category of drug use which should be considered, because it illustrates the capacity of many readily available substances to be used to excess, is that of glue- or solvent-'sniffing' (or 'huffing', i.e. inhaling through the mouth, Cohen, 1979). Many industrial solvents and other commercial products, including fuels, cements, glues, and cleaners, contain chemicals which act as depressants or anaesthetics and can produce the experience of intoxication. The recent growth of aerosol sprays has added greatly to the list of products which can be used for this purpose. Window cleaners, deodorants and air fresheners, furniture polishes, insecticides, disinfectants, non-stick frying pan sprays, and, particularly popular among 'sniffers' according to Schecter, pressurized refrigerants such as cocktail glass chillers, all contain CNS-acting drugs if not as part of the active ingredient of the product, at least in the propellant (Schecter, 1978, p.186; Edwards and Holgate, 1979). Glue- or solvent-sniffing, often experimental but sometimes regular and in large quantity (referred to by Cohen, 1979, as 'solventism'), usually but not exclusively by boys in the age range 7–17, has worried the guardians of health, welfare, and the law in a number of countries, including Britain, the United States, Canada, Japan, Mexico, and countries in Africa and South America. Schecter reported that between one and two thousand adolescents were seen yearly in the New York City Juvenile Court system between 1963 and 1965 in connection with glue-sniffing, and Campbell and Watson (1978) reported on a sample of 18 boys, taken from a larger group, and known to the police, an assessment centre, or a psychiatric centre, in Glasgow in 1975. All had been sniffing for at least six months. One boy, described in greater detail, had been using as much as half a pint of adhesive per day, often with alcohol, and a second had been using glue almost daily for a year and had been hospitalized unconscious on one occasion. Physical 'withdrawal symptoms' were reported for one case and 'habituation' (an interesting reintroduction of a term long-since abandoned in the case of tobacco) was thought to have occurred in the remaining cases: 'Despite protestations by the sniffers that they could "kick the habit" tomorrow, most showed little inclination to do so' (p.209). Some deaths associated with glue or solvent 'abuse' have been reported and there is fear that it may lead to some degree of brain damage (Cohen, 1979). Cohen has reported an increasing number of older people (in the age range 18–29) counted amongst 'solvent abusers', more women, and more students than previously.

Of the many other drugs which could be added to the list, mention should finally be made of cannabis because of its long history and widespread current use, and because of the controversy which surrounds its use in present-day Britain, North America, and elsewhere. There is general agreement that cannabis preparations, made either from the resin (hashish) or from the flowers or leaf (marijuana), produce no very obvious phenomena of increased tolerance or physical effects upon withdrawal. Hence, cannabis is yet another drug which gives rise to confusion and controversy about the nature of excess and 'dependence'. There is in fact some evidence that one of the drug's active components, delta-9-tetrahydrocannabinol, gives rise to a degree of tolerance and to a mild 'withdrawal syndrome', but only when administered in dosages very much larger than those used by most human consumers (Schecter, 1978, Ch.14).

Even so, the use of cannabis has often provoked extreme negative reaction. For example, the medical director of a Cairo mental hospital wrote in 1903:

> The term cannabinomania may be employed to describe the mental condition of many hasheesh users. The individual is a good-for-nothing lazy fellow, who lives by begging and stealing, and pesters his relations for money to buy hasheesh . . . emotional outbreaks when refused their demands, garrulity, abusive threats, alternating with servility, are all marks of this state (Warnock, 1903, cited by Edwards, 1976).

An American pamphlet of 1936 included the following:

> While the marijuana habit leads to physical wreckage and to mental decay, its effects upon character and morality are even more devastating. The victim frequently undergoes such degeneracy that he will lie and steal without scruple; he becomes utterly untrustworthy and often drifts into the underworld where, with his degenerate companions, he commits high crimes and misdemeanours (International Narcotic Education Association, 1936, cited by Edwards, 1968).

Edwards (1976) has reviewed evidence for and against the proposition that cannabis use can produce harm of various kinds. He concluded that the assertion that cannabis can cause acute mental disturbance is irrefutable, but that there is little solid evidence for asserting that cannabis use produces a state of chronic lethargy, and the case for cannabis causing brain damage is even weaker. Interestingly, he made no mention of the possibility of cannabis 'dependence'. Surveys of cannabis use by university students (e.g. Kosviner *et al.*, 1973; Kosviner and Hawks, 1977) and the important participant observation study by Plant (1975) of drug-takers in one English provincial town, make no mention of cannabis 'dependence' either. Kosviner and Hawks referred to 'heavy use' by 7 per cent of cannabis-using university students, and defined this as use at least four times per week. Plant wrote that many of his subjects disapproved of 'excessive' cannabis use, although no definition of excessive in this context was offered.

Brecher and the editors of *Consumer Reports* (1972), in making their conclusions, drew particularly upon the interim report of the Canadian Government's Le Dain Commission (1970, the final report was published in 1972). The report concluded that 'physical dependence' on cannabis had not been demonstrated but that it might in some cases produce 'psychological dependence'. Unfortunately, the report went on to beg most of the questions which this book considers, by adding:

> Psychological dependence may be said to exist with respect to anything which is part of one's preferred way of life. In our society, this kind of dependency occurs regularly with respect to such things as television, music, books, religion, sex, money, favourite foods, certain drugs, hobbies, sports or games and, often, other persons. Some degree of psychological dependence is, in this sense, a general normal psychological condition (p.26, cited by Brecher, 1972, p.460).

Nevertheless, the World Health Organization has described 'drug dependence of cannabis type' (World Health Organization, 1964b), and 'dependence' on cannabis has been included in the International Classification of Diseases (Jaffe, 1977).

In conclusion of this chapter, then, it can be stated with some conviction that the varied forms taken by 'drug addiction' pose as much of a challenge in themselves to the development of a psychological understanding of excessive appetitive behaviour, as does a consideration of the similarities and contrasts found between excessive alcohol use and excessive gambling. Our theorizing must embrace de Quincey's experience as well as the modern experiences of the middle-aged 'physician addict' and the so-called 'street junkie' (Kurland, 1978, pp.179–96). It must account for the young 'glue-sniffer', and for those who take to excess over-the-counter analgesics or 'cough medicines' such as Colles-Brown's, an opium-based mixture (Murray, 1981), as well as those 'dependent' on medically controlled or illicit drugs. The major recreational drugs around the world, including tobacco, derivatives of hemp, coca, and khat, must figure also, and the historical perspective must be there too (Edwards, 1971). Only a few generations separate us from a time when 'spontaneous combustion' was one of the feared consequences of excessive alcohol or other drug use, and when excessive coffee or tea drinking were thought to give rise to a state of 'addiction' quite as horrifying as our more recent image of heroin 'addiction'. Allbutt and Dixon, British pharmacologists writing in the late nineteenth century, wrote of the excessive coffee drinker:

> The sufferer is tremulous and loses his self-command; he is subject to fits of agitation and depression. He has a haggard appearance . . . As with other such agents, a renewed dose of the poison gives temporary relief, but at the cost of future misery (cited in Peele, 1977, p.105).

And of tea:

> An hour or two after breakfast at which tea has been taken . . . a grievous sinking feeling . . . may seize upon a sufferer . . . so that to speak is an effort . . . The speech may become weak and vague . . . By miseries such as these, the best years of life may be spoilt (*ibid.*).

Our theories must account for these observations as for the observations that individuals may find it difficult to desist from an apparently compulsive expression of the normal biological acts of eating and copulating, the subjects of the following two chapters.

CHAPTER FIVE

Excessive Eating

> Sudden death is more common in those who are naturally fat than those who are lean (Hippocrates, aphorism number 44, cited by Mayer, 1968).
>
> In all maladies, those who are fat about the belly do best. It is bad to be very thin and wasted there (Hippocrates, aphorism number 34, cited by Mayer, 1968).
>
> Obesity . . . is usually taken to be a self-induced condition which can be easily remedied by a modest exercise of will. It is attributed to one of the easiest forms of self-indulgence in a prosperous culture. . . . Over-eating where food is in abundance requires neither courage nor skill, neither learning nor guile. Gluttony demands less energy than lust, less industry than avarice. The fat human being, accordingly, is taken to be both physically and morally absurd, and to constitute a living testimony to the reality and the vapidity of his sins (from Mayer, 1968, p.85).

The excessive appetites introduced up to this point have had as their objects drugs or activities none of which is essential to human survival. One way of coping with the risk of excess with such objects of behaviour is to abjure them totally. A large part of the purpose of these introductory chapters, however, is to draw parallels whilst at the same time pointing to contrasts which have to be accommodated in any satisfactory psychological model of excessive appetitive behaviour. Amongst the appetites considered so far have been those directed at ingestable substances and those such as gambling which are quite different; those which involve presently licit behaviour and those involving illicit activity; those which are more common amongst men and those which are more common amongst women. The diversity of appetites which can become excessive is the point.

The point is underlined in the present chapter, where we turn to eating—unlike those considered so far, a biological necessity, at least in moderation. Another point of comparison is the nature of the initial concern over excess. In the case of eating, it has often not been excess itself which has occasioned concern but, rather like tobacco-smoking, bodily damage or the risk of it. In particular, it was over-weight or obesity which first gave rise to interest in over-eating as a possibly 'addictive behaviour', although, as this chapter will attempt to make clear, obesity is not necessarily the most appropriate starting point for the student of excessive appetite.

Most authorities have seemed satisfied that there was an association between over-weight and increased mortality (Kaplan and Kaplan, 1957; Mayer, 1968; James, 1976; Bray, 1978) even though most of the data upon which this conclusion has been based consists of actuarial tables drawn up for life insurance companies. Although there is a possibility that people who apply and are accepted for life insurance are not wholly representative (James, 1976), this has not been considered by most to alter the basic conclusion. Bray (1978), for example, showed an impressive graph demonstrating a much increased mortality ratio once 'body mass index' (weight in kilograms/height in metres squared) rose above about 30. James (1976) included a table based on a study of Provident Mutual policy-holders. This table not only shows increased mortality with over-weight, but also shows the importance of age at the time of issue of the policy. For those aged 50–65 at issue, the mortality ratio (100 representing average mortality) was 118 for those weighing 23 lb or more above 'standard weight', whilst the corresponding ratios were 130 and 146 for those with similar degrees of over-weight in the age-groups 35–49 and 14–34, respectively.

Those who have examined the evidence in detail, however, warn that correlation need not imply *cause*. The results of two major large-scale studies are contradictory on the question of whether obesity predicts heart disease, for example, independently of other factors such as age, blood pressure, serum cholesterol, and smoking (James, 1976).

Mayer (1968) was in fact particularly critical of the assumption that over-weight is a bad thing *per se*, and that it causes a very wide range of unpleasant and sometimes fatal conditions. He pointed out that proponents of this position, in their efforts to persuade others of the damaging consequences of obesity, go back as far as Hippocrates in their search for suitable sources. Whilst Hippocrates' aphorism number 44 linking mortality and over-weight is much quoted, number 34, suggesting the opposite, is rarely quoted. Nor, he added, was it so frequently remarked upon that insurance company mortality tables such as those from Metropolitan Life showed a *reduced* mortality ratio for the over-weight for certain forms of cancer (cancer of the stomach, and breast cancer in women, for example), rates of death by suicide (ratios of 78 and 73 for men and women, respectively), and particularly for tuberculosis (21 and 35). In his review, Ley (1980) also pointed out that studies of obese people in the general population, as opposed to those who seek help, have sometimes found over-weight people to be *less* anxious and depressed than the non-obese (Crisp and McGuiness, 1976, cited by Ley).

There have been a number of attempts to estimate the prevalence of obesity. The results of the main studies in the United States and Britain have been summarized by Ley (1980). Several of these studies show over-weight to be more prevalent amongst women and to be more strongly associated with age for women than for men, and this trend was also evident in the results of Silverstone's study conducted amongst patients of two general practices, one in a relatively high status North West London suburb, the other in a lower status East End practice. The same study also found an association with social class, the proportions at least 'markedly' obese (more than 30 per cent over-weight) being increased in social classes IV and V in comparison with social classes I–III (Silverstone, 1968, 1969). Ley concludes from his review that the same association has been found in a number of studies, including those from the United States. For example, the Midtown Manhattan Study (Srole *et al.*, 1962), which involved a very large normal sample of New York adults, found a quite striking relationship between socio-economic status and obesity: in this case the prevalence of obesity being seven times higher amongst women reared in the lowest socio-economic status group in comparison with those belonging to the highest group.

Most of these authors who have considered the prevalence of obesity have, like those who have attempted to count excessive drinkers, gamblers, or drug users, commented upon difficulties and inconsistencies in definitions. It is often pointed out, for one thing, that being over-weight by some standard or another is not the same thing as being obese (Kaplan and Kaplan, 1957; Mayer, 1968). The different ways to assess one or the other have been reviewed by James (1976), the U.S. Department of Health, Education and Welfare, Public Health Service (1977) and by Ley (1980). The commonest method is to compare actual weight with a population average for the appropriate age group, or with some 'ideal weight' which is often that given by the Metropolitan Life Company. It is difficult to gauge the validity of these 'ideals', and although a range of weights is given for small-, medium-, and large-framed men and women, the determination of frame size is subjective. The body mass index, already referred to, is a favoured index because it overcomes such problems and can be compared with norms independently of height.

There is an even greater area of uncertainty, however, and one which is of greater importance for the present account, and that concerns the relationship between obesity or over-weight on the one hand and excessive food consumption on the other. It is often assumed that people who are obese or over-weight are so because they eat excessively. Indeed, most psychological theories of obesity attempt to explain why some people eat more than others (Ley, 1980). Quite apart from the truth or falsity of that assumption, it could be said to be illogical in any case to attempt a psychological account of over-weight or obesity which are, in themselves, not psychological phenomena. To confuse obesity with an excessive appetite for food is rather like equating liver cirrhosis with excessive drinking, forgery with excessive gambling, or venereal disease with excessive sexual behaviour. The confusion is instructive nevertheless. The history of ideas in the field of excessive appetitive behaviour is partly the history of looking for psychological phenomena behind the appearance of troublesome physical or social events. The extent to which the underlying psychology is 'recognized' depends upon the epoch and upon the activity. 'Alcoholism' or excessive drinking as a construct to explain certain events is currently popular, difficulty in giving up tobacco-smoking is becoming more available as an explanation for lung cancer, whilst immoral but not necessarily 'dissonant' sexual behaviour has long been popular as an explanation for venereal infection.

In the case of eating and obesity the link may well have been exaggerated. It is now often stressed that obesity is by no means a unitary entity (e.g. James, 1976; Leon and Roth, 1977). For one thing, it can be caused by a variety of different physical conditions, including hypothalamic lesions, hypothyroidism, hyperinsulinism, and ovariectomy, as well as sometimes being genetically transmitted (Bray, 1978). The distinction between endogenous, metabolic, or endocrine obesity on the one hand and exogenous, or simple, common obesity caused by over-eating, was favoured at one time (Kaplan and Kaplan, 1957), but it is now recognized that the distinction is not an easy one to draw. Indeed there is now more than a little evidence that obese or considerably over-weight people eat no more (and some studies have found *less*) than people of normal weight (Ley, 1980; James, 1976). James drew attention to one explanation for this, namely the differentiation, long favoured by French scientists, between 'dynamic' and 'static' forms of obesity. In the first there is an energy imbalance with fat progressively accumulated, whilst in the latter form the energy balance has been restored, and the person may eat normally, or even less than normally in accordance with reduced exercise, but remains fat. According to this reasoning it is not necessary to assume that the obese are currently over-eaters, only that they have at some time eaten more than they needed (James, p.34).

One of the difficulties in reaching consensus about the relationship between over-weight and excessive eating lies in the very different populations which have been studied and to which the term obese has been applied (Leon and Roth, 1977). The same problem is evident here as in the study of drug use or of any one of the other forms of appetitive behaviour: it is necessary to study a wide range of people, varying at least by sex, age, and socio-economic status, before a comprehensive account of over-weight and excessive eating can be given. As is the case with the other forms of behaviour considered here, generalizations about forms of eating behaviour become less and less tenable the further the matter is looked into. Stunkard (1959, cited by Leon and Roth), for example, described a number of eating patterns of obese individuals which he considered to be fairly distinct. One of these was the 'night eating syndrome' characterized by excessive eating in the evening, insomnia, and avoidance of eating altogether in the morning. A second pattern he described was that of 'binge eating' in which large quantities of food would be consumed in a short period of time, these periods being interspersed with longer periods of normal or restrained eating. A third pattern he described, which he called 'eating without satiation', where the individual found it difficult to stop eating once intake had started, he felt might be related to central nervous system damage.

Particular attention has been focused recently on the pattern which Stunkard called 'binge eating' and which has been variously referred to by others as 'compulsive eating', 'bulimia nervosa', 'bulimarexia', the 'dietary chaos syndrome', or simply the 'stuffing syndrome' (Wardle and Beinart, 1981). A number of authors have described people who show extreme preoccupation with food and weight, who episodically consume enormous amounts of food in short periods of time in an 'orgiastic' manner (episodes varying in frequency from more than once a day to once every few weeks), and who experience guilt, shame, depression, and self-condemnation following 'binges'. The parallel with apparently 'compulsive' patterns of gambling or drinking is immediately striking. Indeed, it is this eating pattern that most readily invites the label 'addictive' (Hamburger, 1951). Further parallels are suggested by the clinical reports that the two most common 'triggers' for binges are emotional stress and the ingestion of small amounts of 'forbidden' food (Loro and Orleans, 1981; Wardle and Beinart, 1981).

Loro and Orleans (1981) have made a special study of binge eating amongst 280 obese and over-weight adults attending a dietary rehabilitation clinic in the United States and have found the phenomenon much more common than has sometimes been supposed. Just over half the sample reported, 'consuming large or enormous quantities of food in short periods of time', at least once a week, and only 20 per cent stated that this never happened. It was more common amongst those who reported already being over-weight in childhood or adolescence. The latter were more likely to have had some psychological treatment for weight loss, which lead Loro and Orleans to suggest that those who manifest binge eating may require more intensive treatment. They did not consider the possibility that binge eating might at least partly be a *consequence* of treatment or at least a consequence of efforts at self-control which had failed (Wardle and Beinart, 1981). They did, however, raise the possibility later in their paper that adhering to an overly strict and unrealistic diet could itself lead to a pattern of oscillating between self-denial, rigid dieting and fasting at the one extreme, and binge eating at the other.

Their clients reported that binges usually lasted between 15 and 60 minutes, rarely lasting more than 4 hours, and that the number of calories consumed was usually within the range 1,000 to 10,000. In addition to stress-related precipitants, another similarity with excessive drinking was that binge eaters preferred privacy and isolation and an element of secrecy prior to and during a binge. A further parallel lay in the loss of self-respect which this pattern of behaviour entailed and which was experienced most acutely following a binge.

Wardle and Beinart (1981), reviewing what has been written about this pattern of eating, showed that although it has been reported to occur amongst obese people, it occurs also amongst people of normal weight, and amongst those who are below normal weight including those who are anorexic. Bruch (1974) was one of the first to describe a pattern of alternating bingeing and starving. These 'thin fat people', as she called them, often had a history of over-weight. This and later reports described frequent self-induced vomitting and purging as well as fasting by people with this pattern, plus the sense of despair, shame, and experience of preoccupation with eating or resisting eating felt by the 'victims' of this 'condition'. Patients with anorexia nervosa have been noted sometimes to have periods of over-weight in their previous or subsequent histories, and those who use vomitting and purging as well as dieting as ways of keeping weight down are recognized as a sub-type within the category of anorexia (Wardle and Beinart, 1981).

Nor, it seems, are experiences of uncontrolled binges preceded and followed by stringent attempts at self-control and the use of deliberate weight control methods include fasting and self-induced vomitting, limited to clinical populations. Wardle (1980) found that a group of women medical students reported an average of nearly five eating binges per month, and men two. As always, history helps us to see that this is not a new phenomenon. According to Bruch (1974) Roman women had to suffer, literally by starving, in order to keep slim, and the Romans are known for the invention of the 'vomitorium' which, '. . . enabled them to indulge in exessive eating and then to relieve themselves, a method reinvented by modern college girls' (Bruch, p.17).

The recognition that apparently 'addictive' forms of eating are not confined to the over-weight and that many obese people may in fact eat quite normally are amongst the factors that have produced a shift in attention from the variable over-weight versus normal weight to a new variable, restrained versus unrestrained eating. It has been pointed out that many people diet or 'watch their weight' closely, and that these vigilant or 'restrained' eaters differ from unrestrained eaters in theoretically predictable ways. For example, Herman and Polivy (1975), using their Restraint Questionnaire which has been much used in research since, found that unrestrained eaters ate significantly less when made anxious, whilst restrained eaters tended to eat *more*. Coates (1977) summarized research by Herman, Polivy, and others showing that whilst unrestrained eaters tend to eat less after a milk shake 'preload', restrained eaters tend to eat *more*. Polivy (1976) found that restrained subjects, after a preload which they perceived to be of high calorie content, ate *more* of a standard meal than did those who thought the preload to be of low calorie content, whilst unrestrained subjects did the reverse.

Rodin (1978) has also presented results suggesting that over-weight or obesity itself may not be the most important criterion upon which to focus from a psychological perspective. In one of his experiments the insulin responses of over-weight and normal weight subjects on being shown a grilling steak after 18 hours of food deprivation differed markedly, with the insulin levels of over-weight subjects rising to a much higher peak. With a further division of obese subjects into those who appeared highly responsive to food-relevant cues (whom Rodin called 'external'), and those who did not, and with the addition of a group of people who were formerly, but were no longer, obese but who were nevertheless still 'external', the picture became even more complicated. The formerly fat, external, subjects showed a relatively extreme insulin response (but not as extreme as the currently obese externals), whilst the non-external obese showed a much lower level of response (although not as low as non-external normal weight subjects). It is not clear that 'externality' as Rodin defined it is to be equated with 'restraint' as Polivy and others have used that term, but Rodin's results certainly suggest that some aspect of psychological response to food cues may be more significant than the fact of over-weight itself.

Findings of this kind have been seen as consistent with the theory proposed by Nisbett (1972) that individuals are biologically determined to be of a certain degree of fatness. Amongst the main determinants of this 'set point', or 'ponderostat', may be the number and composition of adipose or fat cells, which may in turn be the result of genetic determinants or early feeding experiences (Coates, 1977; Ley, 1980). Ley reviewed findings consistent with this view: for example that heavy-weight subjects who reduced weight by stringent dieting returned easily to their former weight despite maintaining a normal or even lower than normal diet, whilst relatively light-weight people might have difficulty putting on weight even when they ate excessively. Others, such as Coates (1977), have cautioned that the biological set-point theory should not be accepted uncritically. He found it equally plausible to suppose that such individual differences could be accounted for in terms of social learning history.

The matter is complicated further if it is considered that food intake constitutes just one part of the 'energy balance equation'. A certain amount of energy is required to maintain the body even in an inactive state (the basic metabolic rate (BMR)), and additional muscular exercise necessitates the use of further energy. Hence, amount of exercise is considered by many to be a crucial part of the equation and the control of energy output may be as important in accounting for over-weight as is the control of appetite (James, 1976, Ch.5). The control of energy balance in man is, however, a highly complex and as yet little understood process (James, 1976; Garrow, 1978). For example, there is ample evidence, reviewed by Garrow, that BMR falls with underfeeding. This represents a rudimentary control system such that when energy supply is reduced expenditure falls, tending to protect energy stores from excessive depletion—a source of frustration to the obese person trying to lose weight. There is, in addition, much speculation and dispute over the effects of diet and weight upon processes of thermogenesis. Is there a cumulative 'dietery-induced thermogenesis' effect of a series of large meals so that in the chronically over-fed person more energy than usual is used both at rest and also during exercise, for example? Do obese people require less thermogenesis under conditions of cold because of fat insulation, or do they even choose warmer conditions, thereby reducing their energy requirements compared with leaner people (Garrow, 1978)?

All these complications aside, it is undeniable that there are many individuals who experience an appetite for food which they or others judge to be excessive and which leads to self-initiated attempts at behavioural control or to recommendations for restraint from others. A low carbohydrate diet, modifications of which have been popular ever since, was recommended to William Banting by a Dr Harvey in 1862. So impressed was he that, after years of trying and failing, his weight had declined on this diet form 202 lb to 156 lb a year later, that he published a pamphlet entitled, *A letter on Corpulence Addressed to the Public* (1863), in which he stated, 'Of all the parasites that affect humanity, I do not know of, nor can I imagine any more distressing than that of obesity' (p.7, cited by Bray, 1978).

With increased interest in the treatment of obesity in recent years, practitioners have published numerous short case histories to illustrate the fact of difficult-to-control eating behaviour and the motivation to seek help on its account. Morganstern (1977) cited, for example, the case of an extremely obese 24-year-old graduate student whom he called Miss C:

> In addition to eating three regular meals a day, the client reported that she ate candy and 'junk' all day long, completely unable to control herself despite countless attempts at dieting and medically prescribed appetite suppressants. Miss C also stated that she had been in some sort of psychotherapy for six, nearly continuous, years. This previous treatment had included two instances of hospitalization of very short duration and contact with five separate therapists whose techniques, reportedly, ran the gamut from psychoanalysis to desensitization . . .
>
> A preliminary analysis of Miss C's eating habits reavealed an enormous consumption of five principal types of food: candy, cookies, doughnuts, ice cream, and pizza. Base-rate data for three weeks indicated that the client ate close to 200 pieces of candy and dozens of cookies and doughnuts per week. In addition, she indulged in pizza and ice cream at least once a day, and often as many as three times in the same day (p.106).

Crisp and Stonehill (1970) described seven people who were severely obese and who between them illustrated a range of underlying psychological and family problems. Amongst them was a 58-year-old housewife, Mrs E. H., referred to a psychiatric department on account of arthritic complications of 'massive obesity' which had proved unresponsive to attempts at dietary control. Her excessive eating appears to have commenced at the time of her first pregnancy:

> When she became pregnant with this child she and her husband accused each other of infidelity. At this time she became depressed and began to overeat and her weight increased from 12 or 13 stones to about 18 stones at which level it remained. She grew into the image of the jolly fat woman and was no longer overtly depressed although she had a multitude of somatic complaints. . . . She was admitted three times to the psychiatric unit. On her first admission . . . she was treated by dietary control and aversion therapy. Her weight

> dropped to 16½ stones but she became increasingly irritable and hostile on the diet and was discharged . . . For the next two years her weight remained at 16–17 stones but in 1965 it increased up to 20 stones and she sought further treatment . . . Treatment consisted of dietary control, weekly supportive psychotherapy, group therapy, anorectic aversion therapy . . . On discharge from hospital she weighed just over 15 stones. Since this time her weight has increased but has fluctuated (pp.332–3).

A description of the same woman elsewhere (Meyer and Crisp, 1977) makes reference to secret eating in hospital. Hamburger (1951) also refers to cases where excessive eating has apparently led individuals to steal food or money to buy food, to hide and hoard food, and to lie about their eating activities:

> These patients crave food like an alcoholic addict craves drink. Over and over [one patient] . . . spontaneously compared her compulsive eating jags to the behaviour of an alcoholic. She said she could no more eat one piece of food than an alcoholic can take one drink. On an eating spree she would go from drug store to restaurant 'like an alcoholic making his rounds'. She was afraid to take a cocktail for fear her compulsion would switch from food to alcohol. In this connection, it may be more than chance that two patients in this series were known alcoholics at one time or another (pp.491–2).

Such accounts make it clear that there are closer parallels with the more readily acknowledged 'addictions' than might at first be supposed. Those who have written from a psychoanalytical viewpoint, such as Fenichel (1945), Bruch (1974), and Wise and Wise (1979), have recognized an 'addictive' or 'neurotic' need for food. Bruch quoted 'typical' expressions used by some of her clients: ' "I get 'mad' in my stomach", or "I get this gnawing feeling and nothing can change it but a luscious meal", or "It is my mouth that wants it; I know that I have had enough" ' (Bruch, p.127). The familiar 'addiction' elements of an appetitive drive alien or in opposition to the conscious will or real self is found here as in accounts of excessive drinking, gambling, or drug-taking, and the drive in this case is felt to be located in the stomach or the mouth, anywhere in fact but in the seat of reason or will.

Bruch also quoted a woman whose pattern of eating corresponded to Stunkard's night eating syndrome:

> She was one of the many fat people who succeeded in showing a fairly complacent attitude towards the world during the daytime. She was quite efficient in her work, although her severe obesity became increasingly a handicap. When she was alone at night, the tension and anxiety became unbearable. 'I think then that I am ravenously hungry and do my utmost not to eat. My body becomes

> stiff in my effort to control my hunger. If I want to have any rest at all, I've to get up and eat. Then I go to sleep like a newborn baby (Bruch, 1974, p.129).

Bruch considered that an inability to stabilize at any one particular weight was more serious than stability at a relatively high weight, and she provided in her book several case descriptions of women and men who alternated between excessive eating and dieting or fasting, and between fat and thin states. In a chapter entitled 'Thin Fat People', she appears to have anticipated the later discovery of 'restrained eating'. She wrote of '. . . eternal vigilance and conscientious semi-starvation dieting . . . (p.196), of those who make, '. . . a fetish of being thin and follow reducing diets without awareness of or regard for the fact that they do so only at the price of continuous strain and tension and some degree of ill health' (p.197). A patient described by Wijesinghe (1977) is of particular interest in the light of earlier discussion on the relationship between over-weight and excessive eating: she illustrates the now commonly recognized complaint of periodic excessive eating without obesity. The patient was a 37-year-old woman referred with a six-year history of compulsive eating which had become progressively worse in the previous two years:

> It had started after her husband had left her, but even before that when she was depressed or frustrated she used to find solace in eating biscuits or chocolates. . . . There was a regular pattern of 'binges' two or three times a week. At the beginning of an episode she would have sensations which she described as 'feverish excitement' which would compel her to go to the nearest baker's shop and buy large quantities of sweet, starchy foods—cakes, biscuits, chocolates—and either drive out in her car to some secluded place or take the food home. She would then set about consuming this food in a voracious manner 'making a pig of myself' as she put it. This would continue for an hour or two, by which time she would feel 'bloated, tired and sick'. This would usually be followed by loss of appetite for a day or two, whilst she would feel extremely guilty. The abstinence from food after a compulsive eating episode kept her weight within bounds. Nevertheless it seriously disrupted her work . . . and also her social life (p.86).

In all these clinical cases eating behaviour had become a major issue and target for modification and in some cases over-weight had become a chief complaint. Quite apart from these clinical cases, however, concern about over-weight and often over-eating is widespread in countries like Britain and the United States. National opinion polls carried out in America in 1950, 1956, and 1966 showed that 21, 23, and 36 per cent of men at the three polls, and 44, 45, and 42 percent of women considered that they were over-weight (Dwyer and Mayer, 1970, cited by James, 1976, p.57). In their survey in the London borough of Richmond,

Ashwell and Etchell (1974) found that half of the women and a third of the men considered themselves to be over-weight. There was a strong but imperfect relationship between believing oneself to be over-weight and Ashwell and Etchell's objective assessment of over-weight arrived at by comparing actual weight with ideal weight for a person of 'medium frame' according to the Metropolitan Life Tables. Of women and men who were actually over-weight by this index, 89 and 69 per cent, respectively, considered themselves to be over-weight. Even of those considered objectively to be of 'suitable weight' (within 10 per cent either side of the ideal weight), 36 per cent of women and 17 per cent of men thought themselves to be over-weight. Silverstone (1968, 1969) found much the same thing in his survey in two London general practices, but he remarked upon the number of obese people (i.e. 30 per cent or more above ideal weight) who did not consider themselves over-weight and who did not consider it to be a problem. He cited results for 20 obese men, 14 of whom considered themselves over-weight and 7 of whom considered their weight to be a problem; and for 30 obese women, 24 of whom considered themselves over-weight and 20 of whom considered their weight to be a problem. Of particular interest, only 5 and 4, respectively, considered that they over-ate. Six obese men though food was 'very important' to them, and only 1 said that he ate more when anxious (both figures being identical to those obtained from the sample of 20 *non*-obese men), whilst 11 of the obese women considered food to be very important to them, and 17 claimed to eat more when anxious (versus 6 and 7 out of 30 non-obese women).

This picture of widespread 'dissonance' regarding weight, even though over-weight may not always be attributed to over-eating, is matched by a high level of interest in controlling eating and a high prevalence of attempts at dieting, particularly for women. Of Silverstone's 30 obese women, 25 wanted to lose weight, but so did 10 of the 30 control non-obese women. Corresponding figures for men were 15/20 obese and 2/20 non-obese wanting to lose weight. Ashwell and Etchell (1974) reported that two-fifths of their total sample (half of the women and a quarter of the men) had tried to lose weight at some time. James (1976) remarked that only 7 per cent of men and 14 per cent of women in the U.S. national opinion polls were actually dieting despite the very much higher percentages who considered that they were over-weight. Nevertheless these percentages represent an enormous number of people attempting to gain control over appetitive behaviour, and in any case they leave out of account those who have attempted dieting in the past but who are no longer doing so.

It is interesting to note the differences between the sexes which recur in these studies. Unlike excessive consumption of alcohol, excessive gambling, and *some* forms of disapproved or excessive drug use, we are dealing here with a form of concern about behaviour which is decidedly more prevalent amongst women than men. There are various possible explanations for the difference—biological, psychological, and sociological—but the fact of the difference in levels of concern remains and provides a striking contrast with some other forms of excessive appetitive behaviour. The sex difference, and the comparison with other forms of appetitive behaviour, are instructive also concerning the difference between 'objective' and 'subjective' indices. Although surveys in Western and particularly in developing societies nearly all show a higher prevalence of 'objective' over-weight amongst women than men (Ley, 1980), there are studies that have found very similar percentages of men and women over-weight (e.g. Ashwell and Etchell, 1974, and the National Health Examination Survey in the United States, 1964, cited by Ley) and it is 'subjective' *concern* about weight and eating which most clearly distinguishes men and women (Dwyer *et al.*, 1970). Over-eating, or eating at times of stress, may be a female sex-typed behaviour, but there is more substantial evidence for the supposition that concern about perceived over-weight, and interest in dieting as a means of reducing weight, are quite strongly sex-typed behaviours. In the following chapter, which deals with excessive sexual behaviour, we come to an even more dramatic example of the same thing: a form of appetitive behaviour for which the evidence suggests men are objectively more 'excessive', but where the majority of cases that have come to clinical attention are women.

Several of those who have written about the psychology of over-weight have remarked upon the prejudice which exists towards the obese (Mayer, 1968; Dwyer *et al.*, 1970; Ley, 1980). Mayer drew upon a wide range of historical and fictional references to support his conclusion that, 'People who are not fat have attitudes, mostly hostile, toward those who are. People who are fat have attitudes, mostly self-deprecatory, towards themselves' (p.91). Ley (1980) also cited a number of recent studies showing that people hold negative stereotypes of fat people or those with endomorphic physiques; that fatness elicits a higher frequency of negative descriptions such as 'lazy', 'sloppy', and 'stupid'; that the obese are discriminated against, for example in obtaining university places—this being especially true of women; and that the over-weight themselves tend to share these prejudices. Here again, then, as with other excessive appetites, there is evidence that obesity, itself the subject of serious medical and scientific interest, carries for many people strong moral connotations. There is probably more than a grain of truth in Mayer's eloquent statement, quoted at the beginning of this chapter, to the effect that over-weight is often viewed as a sign of weakness and moral depravity.

Ley (1980) believes such prejudices may be partly responsible for pressure upon women in particular, and especially young women, to reduce weight, and an increase in anxiety about weight and eating, and Mayer (1968) has stated his belief that the inverse relationship between socio-economic status and over-weight referred to above might partly be brought about as a result of social attitudes. As he pointed out, however, it would be wrong to conclude that social factors necessarily *cause* over-weight. Rather, the association may partly be explained as a result of obesity reducing chances of social advancement.

It is also important to bear in mind, and here again eating joins company with other forms of appetitive behaviour, that social attitudes are not constant but vary and have varied from place to place and from time to time. Crisp (1978) and Ley (1980) both remind us that other ages and other cultures than our own have preferred women to be of a weight which might well qualify as obese by some modern standards, and that fatness has been viewed sometimes as a sign of health, wealth, and success, or as escape from a culture of poverty and malnutrition (Bruch, 1974). Paradoxically, when viewed from the present-day perspective, several human societies have had 'fatting sheds' instead of slimming clinics (Ley, 1980).

Nevertheless there can be little dispute over the central point of the present chapter; that many people find it difficult to control their eating which they view as excessive. Nothing attests more clearly to this fact of serious concern about excessive eating and over-weight than the range of remedies that have been attempted, the generally disappointing results produced by different forms of treatment, and the absence of clear indications that one treatment is better than another, either overall or for different types of people or problem. Once again, this state of affairs is reminiscent of that to be found in the fields of treatment for other forms of excess.

In the case of food, the seriousness of the concern which is evoked and the lack of response to more 'conservative' approaches is displayed by the existence, and apparently growing popularity, of a number of quite radical treatments. Foremost amongst these are various forms of operation in which, by surgical means, a length of the intestine is bypassed. According to James (1976), early attempts to bypass the absorptive area of the intestine, which involved joining the upper jejunum to the colon, met with frequent complications, and the most favoured operation more recently has been the jejunum–ileal bypass with retention of 14 inches of jejunum and four inches of ileum. The results of such surgery are quite dramatic (Ley, 1980). Not only are large weight losses (by comparison with the results of other treatments) produced for many of those who undergo this operation, but weight loss for 18 months or more has been reported in at least one study cited by Ley, and patients in the same study more frequently reported being less irritable, less often depressed, less insecure and lonely, and to be experiencing a more normal and contented sex life at follow-up than did members of a control unoperated sample (Quaade, 1978). Naturally there are complications associated with so drastic an operation: James (1976) cited operative mortality as lying between 2 and 7 per cent, and post-operative complications include troublesome diahorrea and a comparatively high frequency of complaints of abdominal pain, rumbling, and flatulence (James, 1976; Quaade, 1978). Clearly, it is likely to be only the very obese who will be considered for this type of treatment (Ley, 1980).

Even psychosurgery is not unknown in the treatment of obesity, having been used in an attempt to destroy feeding centres in the hypothalamic area of the brain, either by irradiation or by stereotactic surgery. However, few cases have been reported and, because of the dangers, the method is not in general use (James, 1976).

A further physical method, which nicely demonstrates both the 'dissonance' which some people feel about their eating and the behavioural conflict which their behaviour poses for them, consists of fitting a 'dental splint' or 'jaw wiring' to prevent the person taking in other than liquid sustenance. Since some people are willing to put up with this restraint for several weeks or months at a time, and since it produces, not surprisingly, dramatic weight reductions, this method has a number of medical advocates. There has been relatively much less work evaluating this method, in comparison with work on bypass surgery, and it is not known what are the long-term effects upon weight and quality of life (James, 1976; Bray, 1978). The method is not without risk, for example of permanent damage to teeth or asphyxiation if vomitting occurs (Bray, 1978).

A range of medications have been prescribed to control excessive eating, as they have for all forms of excessive appetitive behaviour. The most popular in the case of excessive eating have been the amphetamine-like stimulants used to suppress appetite—an example of the tendency to treat one form of excessive appetite with a procedure that puts the person at risk of developing another. There appears to be general agreement that amphetamines are moderately effective in controlling appetite (Bray, 1978; Ley, 1980) although they are often employed in conjunction with dietary advice and, like most treatments, their long-term efficacy is doubtful (James, 1976). In addition, a largish component of their short-term effectiveness may be attributable to placebo response (Ley, 1980). Bray (1978) recommended the use of agents such as fenfluramine and phentermine, with lower 'potential for drug abuse' than some others such as methamphetamine and amphetamine, but in practice the prescribing of all appetite-suppressant drugs has become less popular as recognition of the possibilities for excessive drug use has grown. Thyroid hormone is another agent that has been used for many years, not to reduce appetite, but rather to increase energy expenditure. Other drug remedies have been tried from time to time, including injections of human chorionic gonadotropin, an extract of pregnant human urine, although according to Bray there is no evidence even of the short-term effectiveness of this. Bruch (1974) was particularly scathing about drug treatments which have been fashionable and often lucrative to the manufacturers and suppliers, and have continued to be popular with physicians long after the theoretical rationale for their use had been repudiated and, in the case of the amphetamines, long after the possible dangers had been exposed. The worst abuse, according to Bruch, was the fashion for 'treating' obesity with 'rainbow pills', which consisted of various combinations of drugs offered in different colours, to be used at different times of day (Bruch, p.317).

Starvation routines of one kind or another have also been used to try to bring about rapid decreases in weight and to 'break the habit' of over-eating. Short-term fasting, of a few days only, appears to be ineffective (Swanson and Dinello, 1969; James, 1976), but there have been a number of published accounts of prolonged starvation, up to a hundred days or more, in hospital. Such regimes, not surprisingly, have dramatic effects upon weight, but once again the long-term effects are not so clear. There are also risks, with prolonged starvation, of adverse psychological reactions such as irritability, depression, and even psychotic reactions, and there have been several deaths reported (Bray, 1978; James, 1976). Hence, compromises between short- and long-term fasting regimes have been used including in-patient fasting for one or two weeks followed by one or two days of fast each week as an out-patient, or protein-supplemented out-patient fasting (Swanson and Dinello, 1969; Bray, 1978).

These therapeutic experiments are revealing about the nature of eating as a possible 'addiction', and there are intriguing parallels with other forms of excessive behaviour. The willingness to undergo drastic regimes, often involving total abstinence from the difficult-to-control behaviour, is reminiscent of the 'alcoholic', the 'compulsive gambler', the 'drug addict', and the person 'driven to distraction' by sexual temptation. Swanson and Dinello also commented that hunger was virtually absent during such in-patient fasts. There is a clear parallel here with the case of a person who finds it difficult to control alcohol or other drug use in the natural environment, but who experiences little or no desire when in the protective institutional environment of hospital or prison.

Varieties of other treatments have been used, including acupuncture (Bray, 1978) and hypnosis (Erikson, 1960), but the most popular forms of treatment have consisted of dietary advice. By 1886, when the Congress of Internal Medicine in the United States discussed the pros and cons of various diets, a number had already become extremely popular (Bruch, 1974). These included the Harvey–Banting diet of high protein content, Epstein's diet which was high in fat content, and the Dencel–Oertel Cure which involved fluid restriction and systematic exercise. To this day numerous varying diets have been proposed, all in Bruch's view fraudulently put over in a way that quite erroneously suggests that their use will be easy. Many are based either on 'counting calories' to reduce energy intake, or upon reducing carbohydrate intake, but others include those involving protein only with vitamin supplements, amino acids and minerals with varied small quantities of carbohydrates, high egg diets, high grapefruit diets, chicken only diets, and many others (James, 1976).

In comparison with the large number of techniques aimed at reducing eating, increasing energy output through exercise has been surprisingly neglected (James, 1976), perhaps partly because of the assumption that it will be even more difficult to change this aspect of people's life-styles than to change eating habits, and perhaps partly due to the expectation that increased activity would merely be compensated for by increased consumption of food. Nevertheless, there has been renewed interest in exercise as an approach for the obese (e.g. Harris and Hallbauer, 1973; Bray, 1978).

In recent years there has been a veritable explosion of techniques of 'behaviour modification' aimed at the control of over-eating. It is not surprising to find, for a start, that aversion techniques have been applied to eating as they have to virtually all forms of appetitive behaviour which can get out of control. Leon (1976) and Ley (1980) have each reviewed the range of aversion and other behaviour modification methods. Aversive stimuli have included electric shock, foul-smelling substances such as butyric acid, acetimide, and pure skunk oil, cigarette smoke, and pictures of the person who wishes to reduce weight clothed in scanty underwear or swimwear. The connection between eating-related and aversive stimuli can be made in imagination, as in the procedure known as 'covert sensitization', and other imaginal procedures have been used such as 'coverant control', whereby negative thoughts about eating are immediately followed by positive thoughts about being slim, followed by some 'high probability behaviour' such as answering the door or opening a magazine. Clients have been rewarded with tokens or social approval by the therapist, by repayment in instalments of deposits put down at the beginning of treatment, or by 'self-reward' of various kinds. However, the greatest recent developments in behavioural treatments have taken the form of varieties of 'self-control' procedure, or what Bray (1978) calls 'behavioural engineering'. Following pioneering work by Ferster *et al.* (1973) and Stuart (1967), these techniques usually involve close 'self-monitoring' of food intake and weight; they aim to modify eating style, for example by encouraging eating only at meals laid in one place, pausing between bites, chewing food well and leaving some food at the end of a meal; and involve controlling the environment in such a way as to reduce temptation, for example by avoiding exposure to unsuitably tempting foods, shopping after eating rather than before, and asking other members of the family to prepare their own late night snacks.

The list of contents in a book on *Behavioural Treatments of Obesity*, edited by Foreyt (1977), illustrates the variety of behavioural approaches currently being used. They include, 'massed electrical aversion treatment', 'aversion-relief therapy', 'self-managed aversion therapy', 'assisted covert sensitization', 'coverant control and breath-holding', 'self-management application of the Premack principle', 'social reinforcement', 'successive contracts', 'contingency contracting', 'bibliotherapy', 'self-directed program', and 'self-reward, self-punishment, and self-monitoring'.

The appeal of self-help and commercially run weight-reduction groups, documented for example by Sagarin (1969) and Ashwell (1978), is further testimony, if any more were required, to the fact of widespread 'dissonance' over eating behaviour. Weight Watchers, started in the United States in 1961 and in Britain in 1967, is the largest of these groups with over 800 weekly classes in the United Kingdom according to Ashwell (1978) and a million members all told according to Bray (1978). TOPS (Take Off Pounds Sensibly) could claim 345,000 members, according to Ashwell, in over 12,000 Chapters throughout the world, with Chapters delighting in names such as Taperettes, Shrinking Violets, Pound Pushers, and Tummy Tuckers. Silhouette Slimming Clubs and Slimming Magazine Slimming Clubs were other British variants with over 1,000 and over 400 classes throughout the country, respectively, in 1977. U.S. varieties included Over-eaters Anonymous, Diet Kitchen, and Diet Workshop.

The evidence for including over-eating as an excessive appetite or an 'addiction' in the popular meaning of that term, is overwhelming. Although the link between over-eating and over-weight or obesity is by no means clear, the fact remains that millions of people feel that their eating is excessive, would like to be able to control it better than they do, but find great difficulty in so doing. As a result, people join, in their hundreds of thousands, organizations devoted to helping their members control their eating behaviour, and an enormous amount of clinical service and research time and effort has been devoted to devising ways of helping people achieve this aim. That many people who try to control their eating are battling against an appetite of considerable strength is suggested by the modest success achieved by even the most promising treatment approaches. All who report upon evaluation of their own or others' treatments conclude that the long-term results are unknown or disappointing. There is a pervasive therapeutic pessimism in much of the literature which is nicely captured by Stunkard's often-quoted statement: 'Most obese persons will not stay in treatment for obesity. Of those who stay in treatment, most will not lose weight, and of those who do lose weight, most will regain it' (1958, p.79, cited by Foreyt and Frohwirth, 1977).

CHAPTER SIX

*Excessive Sexuality**

. . . too much frequency of embraces, dulls the sight, decays the memory, induces gout, palsies, enervates and renders effeminate the whole body, and shortens life (John Evelyn).

[Sexual excess leads to] . . . palsies and epilepsies, falling sickness, trembling of the joints, pale dejected aspects, leanness, and at least rottenness and other filthy and loathsome distempers (Daniel Defoe, cited by Stone, 1979, p.313).

Terms commonly used to describe excessive appetitive behaviour—such as 'addiction' and 'dependence'—as well as theoretical debate around this area, have been particularly informed by a consideration of the excessive use of drugs having a direct effect on the central nervous system. It has been the argument of these opening chapters that this narrow focus has constrained our understanding and prevented the emergence of a complete theory of the 'manias', as excessive appetities would have been termed a hundred years ago. The debate must be widened, to include at least excessive gambling behaviour and excessive eating. The purpose of the last of these scene-setting chapters is to contribute further to the widening of discussion about the nature of excessive appetitive behaviour by considering a further example, namely sexual behaviour which is excessive.

It is important to make clear from the outset that this discussion is not concerned with sexual problems of a 'dysfunctional' kind such as difficulties in attaining erection or orgasm or with minority sexual appetites. As with excessive alcohol use and excessive gambling, for example, the focus is upon a type of behaviour which in moderation is considered in our culture to be normal (heterosexual behaviour with an adult partner) but which has become

*This chapter has been adapted, with permission of the editor, from an article by the author that appeared in the *British Journal of Addiction*, volume 73, 1978, pages 299–310.

immoderate or excessive. This topic rarely receives serious scientific attention at the present time, and theorists see little need to account for it. This is partly because such behaviour rarely presents itself in a clinical setting, and partly because it is unfashionable to speak of immoderate sexual behaviour, particularly when speaking of the behaviour of women, who have suffered from the application of the double standard in the past.

Neither feature is confined to sexual behaviour, however. A resistance to seeking help on particular account of an appetite that has become excessive is a feature of all types of such behaviour and there are good psychological reasons for this, as later chapters will attempt to make clear. The question is rather whether sexual behaviour can become the object of an appetite that is experienced by the individuals concerned to be, and observed by others to be, excessive? The tentative answer on the basis of the evidence adduced in this chapter, is yes, and hence the psychological model to be presented later in the book must embrace these experiences and observations. Nor is excessive sexual behaviour peculiar amongst the excessive appetites because it is unfashionable or apparently anti-feminist to suggest its existence. Precisely the same can be said of over-eating (Orbach, 1978): that women experience far greater social pressure to be moderate or restrained and therefore are much more likely to be labelled, or to label themselves, as immoderate or excessive. This in no way diminishes the argument that excess exists as a personal experience or as an observation by others. Indeed, it will be one of the cornerstones of the model to be presented in Part II of this book that excessive or 'addictive' behaviour is in the last analysis a *social* phenomenon, whether the object of the perceived excess is the opposite sex, gambling activity, food, or a drug.

In the case of excessive sexuality it is more than usually difficult to sort out truth from fiction amongst professional, quasi-professional, and lay contributions to the 'literature' on the subject. For example, the rulers of Rome are cited frequently as instances of excessive sexual behaviour, as they are as instances of excessive appetitive behaviour of other kinds. In their book, *Nymphomania: A Study of the Oversexed Woman* (1965), Ellis and Sagarin (both men) discussed Tiberius's wife Julia, Justinian's wife Theodora, and Claudius's wife Messalina (whose name is occasionally used to describe excessive sexuality in women—the Messalina complex) as possible 'cases' of 'nymphomania'. Amongst other historical figures discussed, George Sand, the French writer, was rejected as a 'true case' and Catherine the Great of Russia was considered doubtful. Readers of 'men's magazines' will be familiar with modern journalistic embellishments of the sex lives of such historical figures.

Krafft-Ebbing, in his notorious collection of sexual monstrosities and expressions of repressive sexual prejudice, *Psychopathia Sexualis* (1965, first edition, 1886), wrote of what he called 'hyperaesthesia' in which sexual desire was abnormally increased:

> . . . to such an extent that it permeates all his thoughts and feelings allowing of no other aims in life, tumultuously, and in a rut-like

> fashion demanding gratification without granting the possibility of moral and righteous counter-presentations, and resolving itself into an impulsive insatiable succession of sexual enjoyment . . . This pathological sexuality is a dreadful scourge for its victim, for he is in constant danger of violating the laws of the state and of morality, of losing his honour, his freedom, and even his life (pp.46–7).

Amongst the cases he cited was a married man of 53, a caretaker, who had nauseated his wife by being, 'insatiable in his marital relations'. Amongst other misdemeanours was his seduction of his sister-in-law and of a 16-year-old girl who was his ward:

> His excuse was hypersexuality. He acknowledged the wrongfulness of his actions, but said he could not help himself . . . There was no disturbance of his mental faculties, but the ethical elements were utterly wanting (p.48).

This one quotation alone illustrates two general and related features of excessive appetitive behaviour. One is the function of the construction placed upon behaviour: in this case the construction 'hypersexuality' or something similar serves to explain if not excuse the behaviour. Second is the attribution of immorality or lack of 'ethical elements', particularly if the offered 'excuse' of a condition that renders behaviour difficult to control is not accepted. These features have an important role to play in a social psychology of excessive appetites and they will be discussed further in later chapters.

In a much later section of his influential work, Krafft-Ebbing cited case reports of 'nymphomania' and 'satyriasis' (the female and male variants, respectively), although the distinction between these and 'hyperaesthesia' was not made clear. Most of these reports cited had been previously published elsewhere. Indeed, the rumour-like spread of information about the wildest extremes of behavioural excess is abundantly obvious here and elsewhere in the literature; the same 'cases' are to be found repeatedly as evidence of the existence of certain 'conditions'.

A very wide variety of terms have been employed at one time or another to describe excessive heterosexual behaviour. Sometimes subtle distinctions are drawn between the conditions to which they are supposed to refer, but mostly they are used synonymously. The list includes: the Casanova type, compulsive promiscuity, compulsive sexuality, Don Juanism or the Don Juan syndrome or complex, Don Juanitaism, erotomania, hyperaesthesia, hypereroticism, hyperlibido, hypersensuality, hypersexuality, idiopathic sexual precocity, libertinism, the Messalina complex, nymphomania, oversexuality, pansexual promiscuity, pathologic multipartnerism, pathologic promiscuity, satyriasis, sexual hyperversion, and urethromania. This list is certainly not exhaustive.

Not very long ago, in the 1930s, 'nymphomaniacs' were referred to by doctors as women '. . . who exceed the bounds of decent behaviour', as 'morally insane' driven by 'some moral poison' to carry out a 'disgraceful sacrifice of feminine honour' (cited by Levitt, 1973). Although the language has been moderated somewhat, books and articles in supposedly respectable journals such as *Medical Aspects of Human Sexuality*, and *Sexology*, still regularly testify to the fact that individuals do sometimes complain of an inability to control their own excessive sexual appetite. Morse (1963) provided a 'case history' typical of many:

> 'I developed these tremendous urges', she explained . . . 'I couldn't think about anything but sex. It was on my mind constantly . . . my desires were just too strong for me . . . I thought maybe I should see a psychiatrist . . . I was . . . all set to be a good wife [but] I would go out and find a man. Any man . . . There was one magical cure for depression, something a lot better than tranquillisers. Sex' (pp.40–2).

Despite Morse's statement that the histories he provided were, '. . . real histories of real individuals' (p.12), it is difficult to know how reliable are the quotations he provided. Nevertheless, this story has the ingredients of the subjective experience of uncontrollable desire, behaviour felt to be inappropriately excessive by the individual concerned given her life circumstances, the use of behaviour to control unpleasant affects, and guilt about behaviour—all frequent ingredients of excessive appetitive behaviour of other kinds. Other similar descriptions of excessive heterosexuality, in males as well as females, are provided by Auerback (1968), Chesser (1974), Ellis and Sagarin (1965), Golden (1968), Levitt (1973), Lewis (1971), McCary (1972), Miller (1969), Radin (1972), Robbins (1956), and Shiff (1961). In one of the more thoughtful articles on the subject of female excessive sexuality, Levitt (1973) described a person suffering from 'nymphomania' (a term he recommended abandoning) as, '. . . an emotionally disordered woman whose major symptom is an abnormally high frequency of sexual behaviour involving multiple persons, apparently without regard to their personal characteristics, or to other aspects of reality' (p.14). Radin (1972) has described Don Juanism in the male as, '. . . a driving need to have sexual relations with a great number of women' (p.4).

Another source of clinical material on excessive sexuality are the writings of clinicians concerned with marriage and the family (e.g. Eisenstein, 1956; Slater and Woodside, 1951; Dicks, 1967). Eisenstein listed 'hypersexuality' as one of six types of sexual problem affecting marriage, although he believed it was not a clinical entity in itself but rather a manifestation of neurosis. Sex became in such instances 'an addiction'. In his book *Marital Tensions*, Dicks wrote of the 'compulsive promiscuity pattern' of adultery. Eisenstein and Dicks agreed that such behaviour patterns were rarely described to clinicians unless the behaviour was known and objected to by the marital partner who insisted on help being sought. Students of 'alcoholism' and 'compulsive gambling', 'drug addiction' and over-eating would probably agree that these conditions are also unlikely to come to clinicians' attentions unless they occasion harm, or the perceived risk of it, either to the individual or to others.

A further source of clinical material comes from reports of the therapeutic use of antiandrogenic drugs such as cyproterone acetate for sex offenders or would-be offenders (e.g. Cooper *et al.*, 1972; Laschet, 1973; Money, 1970). Although most people treated with such drugs have displayed unlawful minority sexual behaviour such as pedophilia or exhibitionism, over half of the series of 120 patients reported by Laschet (1973) were non-delinquent and 17 were described as suffering 'hypersexuality' with or without excessive masturbation. Other 'anaphrodisiacs' include benperidol, a 'major tranquillizer', and oestrogen. Other treatments for excessive heterosexual behaviour include castration, used in cases of 'hypersexual delinquency' in countries such as Denmark in quite recent times (Cooper *et al.*, 1972), and the occasional use of aversion and other behavioural therapies for 'compulsive masturbation' (Hodgson and Rachman, 1976) and even for infatuation and adultery with a next door neighbour (Barker and Miller, 1968).

The whole idea of 'hypersexuality' as something that warrants a special name of this kind has been much criticized and the arguments are remarkably reminiscent of those that have been used to challenge concepts such as 'alcoholism' or 'compulsive gambling'. Criticisms of the concept of 'hypersexuality' fall under a number of related headings, and most of them apply equally whatever terms are employed to describe the supposedly abnormal sexual behaviour. One of the strongest arguments is that it is impossible to separate normal and abnormal sexual behaviour in other than an arbitrary way, and that there is no evidence of a separate sub-population of people whose behaviour is excessive and qualitatively different from that of others (Lewis, 1972; Levitt, 1973). The following quotation from Kinsey *et al.* (1948) is a good summary of this particular criticism:

> Even the scientific discussions of sex show little understanding of the range of variation in human behaviour . . . such designations as . . . excessively active, over-developed, over-sexed, hypersexual, or sexually over-active, and the attempts to recognise such states as nymphomania and satyriasis as discrete entities, can, in any objective analysis, refer to nothing more than a position on a curve which is continuous . . . Such a continuous and widely spread series raises a question as to whether the terms 'normal' and 'abnormal' belong in a scientific vocabulary (p.199).

The continuum is artificially split into abnormal and normal parts by the fact of a very small number of people complaining of excessive sexuality who have come the way of clinicians over the years. The special problems of this small minority have created a biased and generalized view (Golden, 1968; Lewis, 1972). This bias is displayed, for example, by Auerback (1968):

> Habitually promiscuous persons . . . come from disturbed homes where there were inconsistencies in training and discipline . . . Often

> [promiscuous] women have never accepted their femininity and they may have a large degree of unconscious homosexual colouring in their personality . . . they are often neurotic and immature, using sex in a manner comparable to a child who masturbates . . . Frigidity is common in the nymphomaniac . . . (pp.39,44).

Such 'explanations', attributing excessive behaviour to underlying deficiencies of personality or character, are of course common in certain types of clinical account, and in the context of excessive sexual behaviour they illustrate again the very different perspectives taken by those who approach the subject from acquaintance with a small number of individuals who have sought help and those, such as epidemiologists, who approach it from a study of normal populations. The difference in orientation between Auerback and Kinsey is much the same as that separating Jellinek and Cahalan in the case of alcohol, or Moran and Cornish for gambling.

The popular idea that 'nymphomaniacs' are unable to achieve orgasm is in fact rejected by many writers on the subject, even on the basis of their knowledge of highly unrepresentative clinical samples (e.g. Ellis and Sagarin, 1965, p.25). Notions which propose underlying motives opposite to those which are supposed to underlie 'normal' behaviour (e.g. people who indulge in a great deal of heterosexual behaviour really hate the opposite sex, or are really homosexual, or really find such behaviour very unsatisfying; people who gamble excessively really have a wish to *lose* not to win) support the division into normal and abnormal types but are clearly extremely difficult to prove or disprove. As with 'alcoholism', however, the commonest concept underpinning the notion of abnormal hypersexuality is that of 'uncontrol' or 'loss of control'. Numerous writers have criticized the loose application of such terms in this context as others have for 'alcoholism'. For example:

> Words like 'uncontrolled' when they are used as trait names, have an all-or-nothing flavour. They sound like dichotomies; the person is either uncontrolled on every occasion or controlled on every occasion. But certainly it is possible that an individual who has good self-control may become uncontrollable on a few special occasions. Or a person who is generally poorly controlled may nonetheless clamp down on his impulses occasionally. Once we allow that control—uncontrol is a continuum rather than a dichotomy, theory is again beset by the aggravating need to establish cut off points (Levitt, 1973, p.16).

It is hardly surprising that precise definitions of terms have been even less forthcoming than in the cases of excessive drinking, gambling, drug-taking, and eating. Particular writers may have a clear idea of the concept but can convey it only in the most indefinite terms. For example, Ellis and Sagarin (1965) considered the chief characteristics of 'nymphomania' to be lack of control, continuous need, compulsivity, and self-contempt (pp.26–7). As Levitt has pointed out, 'The key words that have repeatedly appeared in definitions of nymphomania are unusually relative and ambiguous' (1973, p.15). Under these circumstances it is not surprising to find that the experts are at pains to define 'true' or 'real' cases. For example, to Auerback (1968) the 'real nymphomaniac' is not just someone with an unusually large number of sexual contacts and partners, but is also someone, '. . . with no positive feelings emotionally' (p.210). Terminology can become quite confusing. Ellis and Sagarin (1965), despite making a serious and lengthy attempt to be clear thinking on the subject, created confusion by referring to the rarity of 'true' or 'endogenous' 'nymphomania' which Ellis claimed not to have seen, '. . . in my many years of clinical practice' (p.29). They distinguished 'true nymphomania' from 'compulsive promiscuity' and in the remainder of their book appear to be referring to the latter whilst using the former term. Elsewhere they refer to 'controlled promiscuity' and 'genuine nymphomania' amongst other terms, without clear exposition of the differences.

One familiar strategy for survival in such a conceptual jungle is to divide people up into types. This appears to deal with the frequent criticism that a single concept of 'hypersexuality' ignores the evident heterogeneity of people so defined, but such attempts are as open to criticism on grounds of arbitrary labelling and imprecision of definitions as is the single global concept. Lewis (1971), for example, described no less than nine types, including 'the frigid nymph', 'the promiscuous teenager', 'the sexual compensator', and 'the latent lesbian'. Oliven (1974) distinguished 'sociocultural deviance' from 'pathologic promiscuity' in women, and amongst males drew a subtle distinction between the emotional distance of the Don Juan, motivated purely by the incentive of sexual conquest, and the Casanova who wreaked still greater havoc by his repeated entanglements both sexual *and* affectionate (pp.423–5).

A further, major short-coming of a concept such as 'hypersexuality' which implies a pathological or illness-like entity is that it relegates differences in social habits and customs, and reactions to deviance, to a position of relative unimportance. This is particular folly when discussing sexual behaviour, and understandably concepts such as 'hypersexuality' and 'nymphomania' have been frequently criticized on these grounds.

Even within a relatively homogeneous culture there are sub-cultural and individual differences in what counts as 'normal' sexual behaviour. For example, Kinsey *et al.* (1948) were at pains to point out that differences between high frequency and low frequency sexual behaviour found amongst American males were of unusually large magnitude as judged by biological standards, and that discussions of what is right and proper in sexual behaviour are bound to be biased by the position of the discussants on this dimension (pp.198–9). On the basis of his British survey, Eysenck (1971a) has argued for the importance of the *reaction* of different personality types to their own sexual behaviour. A person high on the extraversion scale of his inventory typically described relatively 'promiscuous' behaviour but was not dissatisfied. Eysenck described such a person as 'a happy philanderer'. In contrast, the high neuroticism scorer reported relatively much guilt and low satisfaction. Interestingly, the high psychoticism scorer preferred impersonal sex, according to Eysenck, and believed in taking his pleasure where he could find it. However, this, '. . . has clearly not brought him much happiness; the libertinism is marred by a pathological streak . . .' (p.600).

Overlying great individual variation in sexual behaviour and attitudes are large differences in the formal and informal rules governing sexual behaviour to be found in different social and cultural groups (Ford and Beach, 1952). In the volume edited by Marshall and Suggs (1971) different cultural attitudes were described, varying from the highly permissive (by our standards) sexual culture of Mangaia in the South Pacific, to the highly repressive sexual atmosphere of the west coast of Ireland. Marshall's (1971) observations in Mangaia, the most southerly of the Cook Islands, led him to believe not only that adults assisted youths in early sexual behaviour and that there was great freedom and encouragement for pre-marital sexual intercourse, but also that the system of beliefs that upheld this pattern of conduct was in many respects quite contrary to our own. There was the belief, for example, that avoidance of continuous or regular intercourse with the same partner prevented pregnancy: a view quite opposite to the majority view held in the West which has certainly become more tolerant of pre-marital sex but only provided there is some regularity of partner. Indeed, number of sexual partners is central to the Western concept of 'hypersexuality'. In Mangaia, 'Personal affection may or may not result from acts of sexual intimacy, but the latter are requisite to the former—exactly the reverse of the ideals of Western society' (p.119).

By contrast, Messenger (1971) described Inis Beag, as he called the island off the West coast of Ireland which he studied, as '. . . one of the most sexually naive of the world's societies' (pp.14–15). He observed that discussion of matters even slightly sexual was avoided, that boys and girls, and to a large extent men and women, in their social lives were separated, that nudity was abhorred, and that there was even an absence of a 'dirty joke' tradition on the island. The roots of this attitude were, Messenger explained, intertwined with the complex roots of the Irish character, but they owed much to the influence of ascetic monasticism, Augustinianism, and Jansenism, the latter being a particularly, '. . . rigid and gloomy doctrine', introduced to Ireland in the late eighteenth and early nineteenth centuries. In Inis Beag, according to Messenger, normal, informal, social control in which the fear of embarrassment played a major part, was aided by 'clerical social control' in the form of the repressive activities of the local priests and the occasional visit to the island of week-long missions conducted by Redemptorist priests who had commonly taken 'controlling one's passions' as their theme (abstaining from intoxicating drink being another favourite). Clearly, what counts as 'hyper' or 'excessive' sexuality is not the same in two such divergent cultures as Inis Beag and Mangaia.

A most persistent criticism that notions such as 'hypersexuality' ignore social relativism concerns the 'double standard'. As Golden (1968) has put it: 'Perhaps the most apparent influence on our attitudes about human promiscuity relates to gender differences. People tend to view women as being 'promiscuous' and do not attach the same label to men . . .' (p.48). Many writers on the subject (e.g. Ellis and Sagarin, 1965) have commented on the apparent greater clinical incidence of 'nymphomania' than of male variants (satyriasis, Don Juanism, etc.), despite evidence from surveys that males indulge in a greater amount of pre- and extra-marital sexual behaviour with a larger number of partners. Thus, the social reaction is different, and the individual herself as a recipient of society's attitude reflects this in her own reaction to her own behaviour:

> . . . when a male in our society is highly promiscuous, nothing is done about it. In fact, his peers usually look up to him, they envy him: when a female behaves in a similar fashion, she is scorned, and if young, often taken in hand by the authorities. Every effort is made to have her *condemn* herself . . . (Ellis and Sagarin, 1965, p.177, their emphasis).

Thus, many who have considered the matter carefully are of the opinion that the problems resulting from excessive heterosexuality are the result of personal or social *reactions* to behaviour rather than the result of anything intrinsic to the behaviour itself. As Golden (1968) puts it, 'it doesn't make so much difference what one does as how one feels about it' (p.53). Kinsey *et al.*'s (1948) view was that:

> Most of the complications which are observeable in sexual histories are the result of society's reactions when it obtained knowledge of an individual's behaviour, or the individual's fear of how society would react if he were discovered (p.202).

The great importance of both individual and wider societal reactions to appetitive behaviour has arisen with each of the excesses considered here, and this will be one of the themes of later chapters. Suffice it to say at this point that the choice of the word 'excessive' to describe the forms of behaviour of interest in this book was made for the very purpose of underlining the relativity of reaction to behaviour.

Indeed, in the case of excessive sexuality, it has been argued by the critics of 'hypersexuality' that the notion rests squarely upon moralistic injunctions in American and like societies against non-marital sexual behaviour, sexual behaviour with more than a very small number of partners, and particularly sexual behaviour which is 'impersonal' or outside the approved context of a deep emotional relationship (Levitt, 1973, p.16). Fascinating reflections of American ambivalence over sex are to be found in content analyses of the media and popular literature (Ellis, 1951) and of confession magazines (Nunnally, 1961). The notion of 'hypersexuality' is likely to be viewed even more critically now as a result of the general relaxation of sexual inhibitions, the emergence of middle-class sub-cultures giving approval to practices such as co-marital and group sex which might otherwise be considered deviant (e.g. Smith and Smith, 1970; Ramey, 1972; Cole and Spanier, 1973), and particularly challenges to the assumption that women have naturally a lesser capacity to be sexually aroused than men (e.g. Schmidt and Sigusch, 1973). Terms such as 'varietist sex' and 'multi-partnerism' are in vogue whilst 'nymphomania' and 'satyriasis' are decidedly not.

Nevertheless, it is difficult to deny that some individuals have expressed distress and concern over their difficulty in controlling heterosexual behaviour that has become, in their terms, excessive. One outstanding work of undoubted relevance to the theme of this chapter is the anonymous 11 volume autobiographical sexual history, *My Secret Life*, written by a Victorian who called himself merely Walter (anonymous, 1966). We are fortunate in having two published and quite extensive analyses of *My Secret Life* and it is upon these that the following discussion is based. The first consists of two lengthy chapters in a book on sexuality and pornography in mid-Victorian England written by Stephen Marcus (1966) and based on material in the archives of the Institute for Sex Research (The 'Kinsey' Institute) at Bloomington, Indiana. The second analysis, itself in two volumes, is by two American psychologists, Eberhard and Phyllis Kronhausen (1967), and which quotes extensively from Walter's original. The two analyses take contrasting views of Walter's sex life and a comparison of them reveals many of the uncertainties and contradictions over the definition of excess in the area of sexual behaviour, and hence about the nature of excessive habitual behaviour in general.

Marcus and the Kronhausens agreed, first of all, that the work is probably authentic; that despite the seemingly incredible number of sexual partners whom Walter claims to have had, and the way the work concentrates exclusively upon matters sexual from the beginning of the first volume to the end of the last, the 11 volumes do largely represent the carefully recorded facts of the sexual life history of one man. Indeed, the Kronhausens were inclined to think that *My Secret Life*'s preoccupation with sex makes the work more credible; they argued that Walter developed an almost scientific interest in the subject. Certainly he reported developing the habit of recording his sexual behaviour in minute detail as soon as possible, usually within a day or two of the relevant events taking place; the work contains a questionnaire which he 'administered' orally and discreetly to as many of his partners as he was able; and one volume contains three essays which he hoped might impart useful knowledge to the young on matters, '. . . which owing to a false morality is a subject put aside as improper' (Marcus, 1966, p.165). Marcus believed the writing of this work, basically factual though it might be, served psychopathological needs in the writer. Even the Kronhausens, who took the more liberal, sympathetic, view, conceded that, '. . . the scabrous terms and frankly pornographic manner of expression are the least genuine . . .', and were perhaps, '. . . thrown in for the author's own retrospective benefit or . . . for the benefit of a prospective readership which demanded this kind of presentation' (Kronhausen and Kronhausen, 1967, p.326).

My Secret Life certainly portrays a man who was, to use the Kronhausens' preferred term, 'sexually active'. Despite, or perhaps because of, a childhood and adolescence characterized by the sort of ambivalence towards sex which we have come to associate with Victorian England—a mixture of dire warnings against masturbation from his uncle and intensely exciting partial sexual experiences with servants—and despite a lengthy, though unhappy, marriage, he acquired a large appetite for heterosexual variety which he pursued vigorously. His partners were legion and ranged from the high class to the low, from the courtesan to the 'park doxie', from the lengthy affair to the most casual of commercial arrangements, from the mature to the quite immature. In later life he seems to have acquired particular 'taste' (a metaphor, no doubt ugly to some, which makes the appetitive nature of much sexual behaviour quite explicit) for very young virgins—a taste perhaps shared by many of his contemporaries (Pearson, 1972).

The two analyses took contrasting views. To Stephen Marcus, *My Secret Life*, '. . . revealed to us the workings and broodings of a mind that had for an entire life-time been possessed by a single subject of interest' (pp.86–7). He referred to Walter's 'compulsive promiscuity', his 'compulsive need for variety, for having many different women all the time' (pp.172–3), and his 'obsessional state, his hypersexuality . . .' (p. 176). 'The need for variety . . .', he wrote, '. . . is itself monotonous . . .' (p.181). The author could not be thought of, he suggested, as an ordinary or normal person; his appetite was, '. . . strong, unreflecting, unconscious and unmanageable' (p.178), it turned women into 'commodities', 'objects', and its outcome was frequently 'brutal and disgusting' (pp.157, 160).

The Kronhausens were less blunt and straightforward. They admitted that, 'compulsive sexuality' is '. . . exemplified by the author of *My Secret Life* (p.x) although they disclaimed the use of the term themselves by attributing its use to Marcus. Later they wrote:

> The only thing about Walter's sexuality which we do consider pathological or neurotic, and here we agree with Prof. Marcus, lay in its obsessive–compulsive nature, which drove him literally from one sexual experience to another, with little time or interest for anything else, and which makes everything about him seem so grotesquely overdone and out of proportion (p.xix).

They noted that early on in his life Walter, '. . . gave up a job in the War Ministry and assured promotion in order to devote himself more fully to his erotic interests' (p.4). They agreed with Marcus, too, that Walter's behaviour with women was usually, '. . . clearly unromantic and unequivocally self-motivated . . . never anything like the kind of attitude that one, rightly or wrongly, describes as "love" in sexual relations' (p.126).

Although Walter had on the whole, '. . . emancipated himself from the prevailing scruples and conventions of his time' (Kronhausens, p.183) and,

'. . . felt little need to change and modify his style of life' (p.xxi) nevertheless he was by no means free of guilt and conflict. For instance:

> Yet, many a time, after such pleasure, I have been *disgusted with myself* for my weakness and have tried to atone for it—without the object of my solicitations ever having been aware of the reasons for my ultra-kindness (quoted by the Kronhausens, p.183, their emphasis).

At one period, conflict was particularly evident. Walter had a relatively long-term liaison with one particular partner at this time (indeed Marcus believed Walter made her his second wife, although the Kronhausens thought Marcus was mistaken) and aspired to be faithful to her:

> . . . Yet, such is my sensuous temperament . . . that no matter how much I struggle against it, I find it impossible to be faithful to her . . . I have wept over this weakness, I have punished myself by self-imposed fines, giving heavily to charities, thus disposing of the money which I would have paid for other women [a strategy now recommended by some behaviour therapy self-control therapists!]. More than that—I have masturbated to avoid having a woman whose beauty has tempted my lust . . . I have made love at home with fury and repetition so that no strength should be left . . . Always useless; the desire for change seemed invincible . . . My life is almost unbearable from unsatisfied lust . . . It is constantly on me, depresses me, and urges me to yield (quoted by the Kronhausens, p.184).

Further relevant historical case material is provided by Stone (1979) in his book, *The Family, Sex and Marriage in England 1500–1800*. Stone described in some detail the sexual exploits of two diarists, Pepys and Boswell, who experienced 'dissonance' on account of their own sexual behaviour. According to Stone, Pepys had some physical contact with no fewer than fifty-odd women in the last nine years before his young wife's death. He was restrained by fear of venereal disease and of pregnancy, and unlike Walter was not so absorbed in his pursuit of sexual pleasure that he allowed this to interfere with his work in the Navy Office.

This was the period of the Restoration when the monarch, Charles II, set a standard of sexual permissiveness in his court which others followed. Nevertheless, Pepys was perhaps too close to the Puritan period of anti-hedonistic restraint to be free of a guilty conscience. Stone stated:

> Finally, he was constantly torn between his nagging puritanical conscience and his irrepressible sensuality and love of pleasure. Forever making good resolutions, and forever breaking them, he lacked a strong moral centre to hold him together. Meticulous to

> a degree in his business affairs at the Navy Office, his private life was something of a mess, simply because he pursued women as a form of relief from the tensions in the office . . . Pepys was a naturally prudent cautious man, at the mercy of a growing sexual obsession . . . He recorded what he regarded as his failings as an aid to his reformation and at the New Year he would make futile good resolutions to be more chaste in the future. Pepys was a man at war with himself, and as such was an epitome of his time and his class (pp.344, 349, 350).

A hundred years later, when James Boswell was writing his diaries and letters, sexual permissiveness had become more the norm. The Puritan period was well gone, and the Victorian age was yet to come. Nevertheless, Boswell, brought up by a Calvinist mother, was not free of sexual guilt. He was, '. . . blessed or burdened with an overwhelmingly powerful sexual drive . . .' (p.352) which, as with Walter, caused him to pursue women irrespective of social class or marital status. In his twenties, before his marriage, he had numerous mistresses and liaisons and had sexual relations with well over sixty different prostitutes in many countries in Europe as well as in England and his native Scotland. He suffered from at least ten outbreaks of gonorrhoea before his marriage and seven after, and certainly appears to have obtained no lasting benefit from remedies such as 'Leake's Genuine Pills', 'The Specific', 'Lisbon Diet Drink', 'Doctor Solander's Vegetable Juice', or 'Doctor Keyser's Pills', advertised in fashionable newspapers of the time.

Nevertheless he was continually worried about the rights and wrongs of his sexual behaviour and on one occasion tried to increase his self-control by writing, '. . . a discourse against fornication along the hell-fire and brimstone lines of his early education by his mother' (p.353). Later he confided in his new friend Dr Johnson whom he greatly admired and who gave him stern advice on the subject. He drew up an 'Inviolable Plan' of moral reform and regeneration and was able to report that he had been chaste for almost a year after. After his marriage to Margaret Montgomerie he wrote no diary for three years until he went on a trip to London which revived his old temptations and made him resolve, '. . . never again to come to London without bringing my wife along with me' (p.363). He failed to keep that resolution, was soon back to his old ways, and after only a few years of marriage was thrown into moral indecision:

> . . . I told her I must have a concubine. She said I might go to whom I pleased . . . but I was not clear, for though our Saviour did not prohibit concubinage, yet the strain of the New Testament seems to be against it, and the Church has understood it so. My passion, or appetite rather, was so strong that I was inclined to a laxity of interpretation, and as the Christian religion was not express upon the subject, thought that I might be like a patriarch; or rather I thought that I might enjoy some of my former female acquaintances

> in London . . . the patriarchs, and even the Old Testament men who went to harlots, were devout. I considered indulgence with women to be like any other indulgence of nature. I was unsettled (p.365).

The remaining years of his marriage were characterized by the kind of conflict and vascillation that have been described in connection with other forms of excessive appetite. He was, 'Always confessing to his long-suffering wife, always repenting, always relapsing . . .' (p.367). Glimpses of his wife's reactions are almost as interesting as Stone's account of Boswell's behaviour itself. She was forgiving of his dalliance with prostitutes: on one occasion, when Boswell returned home and confessed, he wrote, 'She was good humoured and gave me excellent beef-soup, which lubricated me and made me feel well' (p.370). She was less forgiving, however, of his affection for other women, and was cooler in her reaction if she thought that Boswell had been sober at the time of an infidelity.

It is clear from Stone's account that Boswell could equally well have figured in the chapter on excessive drinking. Within three years of his marriage, there is talk of frequent all-night drinking bouts, of decreasing control over drinking, and increasing wildness associated with drinking. At one point Boswell returned home after drinking and smashed up all the dining room chairs, throwing them at his wife. Stone recorded that at this time, '. . . a new vice of all-night gambling at cards was growing steadily upon him' (p.366) also. A few months later, he was, '. . . plunged into an endless round of alcoholic excess, all-night card-playing and promiscuous whoring' (p.366). A few years later he was confessing, 'I am really in a state of constant, or at least daily, excess just now' (p.371).

After his wife's death, and the death of Dr Johnson which also deeply affected him, he became, according to Stone, '. . . a habitual drunken lecher, a familiar figure staggering through the less reputable streets of London . . . A man plagued by inherited manic depression, an evident failure as a husband, a father and a lawyer, driven by a lust for female flesh that he was unable to control, constantly more inebriated than was seemly . . .' (p.373).

Stone was impressed by the way Boswell was racked by guilt on the subject, particularly over his infidelity to his wife, the way that he tried unsuccessfully to think the problem through rationally, the way in which he was solemn in discussion on the topic, and the way in which he constantly sought advice: 'No one seems to have been particularly shocked by his indiscretions and infidelities, or by the grossness of his appetite. Dr Johnson advised chastity; General Paoli and Temple marriage, and Rousseau a mystical view of sexual passion which would exclude his brutish couplings' (p.378).

There is, then, sufficient evidence to conclude that excessive heterosexuality exists as a social fact. There is testimony to the fact that some people have sought specialist help because they wished to restrain their sexual behaviour (heterosexual behaviour with adult partners) but were unable to do so. Others have confessed to such dissonance to a professional confidant even though they did not seek help directly for that complaint. And Pepys, Boswell, and Walter are at least three who have written at length of their own excess and at least occasional feelings of dissonance about it. Although there is a great deal of evidence of this kind, it is admittedly in the form of extended clinical and autobiographical anecdote rather than hard scientific evidence. There are two reasons, however, why this evidence should be taken seriously in any debate about the nature of excessive behaviour.

First, the phenomenon of the excessive heterosexual should be expected from what we know of drinking, drug-taking, gambling, and eating. The majority engage in each of these rewarding or potentially rewarding activities in moderation or not at all, whilst a minority show very heavy, frequent, or immoderate indulgence and run the risk of incurring various 'costs' (loss of time, loss of money, social rule-breaking, bodily damage, impairment of performance, etc.). As heterosexual behaviour must be rated one of the most rewarding of activities widely available, it would be most surprising if there were no excessive or 'compulsive' heterosexuals. In China, according to Singer (1974), 'womanizing' was long considered one of the four major 'vices' or 'disasters', along with gambling, drinking, and smoking opium, and immoderate sexual behaviour is often mentioned alongside excessive drinking—for example in the Alcoholics Anonymous 'Big Book' (1955) where 'other women' figure several times as an item that reformed 'alcoholics' should include in their inventory of wrong-doings.

Society has interfered formally in the control of heterosexual behaviour much as it has with drinking, gambling, and drug-taking, and there are examples of the law's involvement in relatively recent British social history. For example, in eighteenth-century Scotland, Trevelyan (1967) tells us, where the law and social conduct was ruled by the Kirk Session and the Presbytery:

> The adulterer or fornicator of either sex was exposed on the stool of repentance in church, to the merriment of the junior half of the congregation, to the grave reprobation of the more respectable, and to the unblushing denunciations of the minister, renewed sometimes for six, ten or 20 Sabbaths on end (p.455).

A century earlier in England, under church law, the 'libertine' had been required to stand publicly in a white sheet for adultery or fornication, and under Puritan lay law an act was passed in 1650 punishing adultery with death (p.246). Controls continue in various guises, including the laws governing marriage and its dissolution.

The second reason for wanting to take what anecdotal evidence exists seriously, is that the phenomenology described in Walter's autobiography and in other accounts is remarkably parallel to accounts of the experience of some excessive drinkers, drug addicts, gamblers, and over-eaters. Each contains reference to the experience of having an 'uncontrollable' desire, or to being 'driven' to activity. Preoccupation with the object of these desires and with the means of consuming or partaking of it is another recurrent theme. The behaviour itself is felt inappropriate and in excess of what the individual or other people or both would consider normal. The activity is often engaged in in response to the experience of unpleasant affect. Of most significance, the experience of conflict and the attendant ambivalence and guilt are described. Attempts at self-control, through a variety of tactics, are usually described as well. These and others are features common to the experience of excessive appetitive behaviour whether the object be the consuming of alcoholic drinks, the placing of bets, or heterosexual activity with an adult partner.

It came as no surprise to learn recently that an organization calling itself Sexaholics Anonymous had been set up in California to help people with 'sexual compulsion' (*Daily Mirror*, 1981). The newspaper article appeared complete with a 20-item self-diagnosis questionnaire ('Do you ever suspect that sex controls you?', 'Does sexual obsession make you careless about your family?', etc.) and a quote from a doctor: 'For sexaholics sex is their undoing whether it takes the form of non-stop affairs or a slavish longing for porn shops.' In fact, this development is probably nothing but a return to one of the preoccupations of the Oxford Group Movement, the forerunner of Alcoholics Anonymous and of modern 'concept houses' such as Synanon and Phoenix Houses for the reform of 'drug addicts' (Russell, 1932).

It is clear also from the various criticisms of the concept of 'hypersexuality', 'nymphomania', etc. which have appeared in the literature, that the phenomenon of dissonant heterosexuality poses conceptual problems and problems of definition remarkably similar to those faced by students of excessive drinking, drug-taking, gambling, and eating. The debate between Marcus and the Kronhausens over Walter's case exemplifies this. Criticisms of reifying the condition as a 'mania' or an 'ism', and of underpinning such concepts by invoking such indefinite 'symptoms' as loss of control and craving, exactly parallel criticisms which have been made of disease concepts of 'alcoholism' and 'compulsive gambling'. Control is a central psychological concept for the understanding of excessive behaviour, but the field of 'alcoholism' studies, for one, has been bedevilled by an all-or-nothing concept of control and uncontrol in precisely the same way as have discussions of excessive sexuality.

Debate over definitions in this area is intriguingly reminiscent of debates on the same subject when drug-taking, drinking, or gambling are under discussion. In none of these areas is there agreement about the precise points on the continuum at which normal behaviour, heavy use, problem behaviour, excessive behaviour, 'mania' or 'ism' are to be distinguished one from another. When reading of the supposed characteristics of the 'real nymphomaniac', one is haunted by memories of attempts to define the 'real alcoholic' or the 'real compulsive gambler'. Was Walter pathological, a 'real hypersexual', or was he merely extremely sexually active and emancipated for his time?

PART II

A Psychological View

CHAPTER SEVEN

Taking Up Appetitive Behaviour

> . . . the principal . . . effects [on drinking and drug-taking in adolescence] come from interaction in or under the influence of those groups which control individuals' major sources of reinforcement and punishment and expose them to behavioral models and normative definitions. The most important of these groups with which one is in differential association are the peer-friendship groups and the family . . . (Akers *et al.*, 1979, p.638).

> How much our findings are bounded by the period in which they were obtained and are specific to that point in history is interesting to contemplate. The interpretation we have made of particular behaviors, and the very notion of problem behavior, depend upon the social and personal meanings that are attached to them. Important changes have taken place in recent history, and their effects on those meanings may well be far reaching (Jessor and Jessor, 1977, p.247).

Part I attempted to show that there are a number of apparently dissimilar human activities which have in common the capacity to create what, in familiar parlance, we call an 'addiction'. What I hope has been made apparent is that this poorly understood state can and very often does involve real suffering, both for the individual and for others. This is not just wilful indulgence or personal preference, and numerous clients of helping agencies and writers of autobiographical accounts have testified to the personal conflict and struggle that they have experienced. What I hope has also been persuasive, and this is more controversial, is that the same phenomenon occurs for drug and non-drug activities. The evidence for excessive heterosexual behaviour is perhaps more anecdotal, but in the case of gambling there is certainly enough evidence to pose a serious challenge to any theory of 'addiction' that can account only for the excessive use of drugs. I hope further, following on from this, that it is abundantly clear already that no simple formulation based on morality, medicine, or societal reaction will suffice. We can put out of our minds at this stage any notion that immorality, illness, or deviance is sufficient to capture what is happening to someone with an excessive appetite. Equally, however, we should rid ourselves of any preconception that any one of these ways-of-looking-at excessive appetites is totally inappropriate. Indeed, I have used the expression 'excessive appetite' throughout this book because it seems to me of all possible expressions to be the least presumptive, as well as serving best the purpose of drawing attention to the social dimension.

The task of the rest of this book is to attempt to develop a unified psychological view of the nature, origins, and treatment of the range of excessive appetitive behaviours introduced separately in the chapters in Part I. This chapter is concerned with causes. To review exhaustively theories and empirical research on the causes of excessive alcohol use, other forms of drug use, gambling, eating, and sexual behaviour would be a task way beyond the scope of this chapter or the abilities of this writer. Rather, the purpose has been to examine selectively some of the major contending theories and some of the research which seems to be the most outstanding, and to use this work to build a unified view of the origins of the types of excessive behaviour with which this book is concerned.

THE JESSORS' STUDIES OF PERSONALITY AND SOCIAL INFLUENCE

There are many possible starting points for this exercise and I have chosen to commence with the work of R. and S. Jessor and their colleagues, from the University of Colorado, for a number of reasons. Their work is typical of a certain kind of research which has been very popular in the study of alcohol and tobacco and increasingly also in the study of the use of other drugs. These are studies of drug-using behaviour amongst young people, usually school or university students, usually resident in the United States, and less often in Canada, Britain, Scandinavia, or elsewhere. Many of these studies, the Jessors' amongst them, are motivated by the special concern, mentioned in earlier chapters, which many feel for deviance occurring in the young. Many such studies are limited to counting rates of problem behaviour in certain localities at certain times and most of these are of little relevance to present interests. Others, however, are concerned with teasing out the antecedents of individual differences in behaviour: Why do some young people use or abuse a drug whilst others do not? Although the authors of most of these pieces of research have few pretensions that their studies have direct relevance for an understanding of excessive behaviour later in life, it is a not unreasonable assumption that the origins of excess lie in adolescence at a time when most people adopt the relevant behaviours for the first time. This is an assumption to which this chapter will return below to examine more critically.

The Jessors' main study, summarized in their book *Problem Behaviour and Psycho-Social Development* (1977), and in several papers (e.g. Jessor *et al.*,

1973), was unusually comprehensive in at least three major respects. First, they recruited subjects at three different ages at school (13, 14, and 15 years) and at college at age 19. Secondly, and of the utmost importance, they followed subjects longitudinally for three years asking questions about the development of behaviour and attitudes yearly, collecting data from subjects on a total of four occasions. Thirdly, and of particular relevance to our present purpose, they did not confine their enquiry, as many researchers have done, to a single form of potentially excessive behaviour, but rather asked about a number. Some of those, namely alcohol use, marijuana use, and sexual behaviour, are forms of behaviour with which this book is particularly concerned, whilst others, such as 'general deviant behaviour' (behaviours including lying, cheating, stealing, aggression, and vandalism), and 'activist protest' or political activism, are of less concern to us. As an aside here, the inclusion of political activism as an object of study in research on adolescent problem or deviant behaviour gives pause for thought. If it is clear that this betrays the prejudices of American research fund-givers in the early 1970s, we should perhaps ask whether the same applies to the other behaviours in their list. The importance of reactions to behaviour, and the way in which these may change radically from place to place and epoch to epoch, is a theme already introduced in the previous chapters.

The limitations of the Jessors' study were those common to almost all studies of this kind, namely reliance upon a self-report questionnaire, less than 100 per cent response rate, and the difficulty of finding methods of statistical analysis which can handle these large volumes of survey data. These limitations aside, there can be no doubt that this study represents one of the most serious attempts to come to terms with the complexity of the determinants of early individual differences in the uptake of a number of potentially troublesome behaviours. Unlike many theorists of social behaviour, the Jessors were persuaded that these behaviours had multiple determinants and in particular that individual differences could be explained in terms of a number of facets of individual *personality* plus a number of different aspects of a person's *environment* as perceived by the individual. Their model, then, was a combinational one, based on the view that neither individual temperament nor a person's social context alone can be held accountable for excessive or 'deviant' behaviour, but that some combination of the two can. The list of main variables which they included as likely correlates of 'deviant behaviour', along with an indication of the frequency with which each of these variables produced significant findings, is given in Table 7.

The Jessors employed multiple regression analysis to explore the best combination of variables for the 'prediction' of a particular criterion. (Note that the word 'prediction' used in a statistical sense here can be misleading, as criterion and 'predictor' variables were, in some analyses, based on data gathered at the same time). The general results of this analysis of their complex data tended to support the Jessors' multivariate view, certainly for high school students. They stated, '. . . the final multiple regression equations for the . . . different problem-behaviour criterion measures . . . *always included at least*

Table 7 Variables included in the Jessors' studies of high school and college behaviour (from Jessor and Jessor, 1977, Tables 5.1, 5.2, 6.1 and 6.2)

Personality system measures	No. of significant findings (out of 16 possible[a]) $p \leq 0.05$	$p \leq 0.001$
Motivational-Instigation Structure		
Value on academic achievement	9	5
Value on independence	4	0
Value on affection	4	0
Independence-achievement value discrepancy	8	5
Expectation for academic achievement	7	4
Expectation for independence	3	1
Expectation for affection	1	0
Personal Belief Structure		
Social criticism	11	5
Alienation	3	0
Self-esteem	0	0
Internal–external control	3	1
Personal Control Structure		
Tolerance of deviance	13	8
Religiosity	9	6
Drinking disjunctions[b]	14	5
Drug disjunctions[b]	15	10
Sex disjunctions[b]	14	8
Perceived environment system measures		
Distal Structure[c]		
Parental support	7	3
Parental controls	3	0
Friends support	3	0
Friends controls	11	5
Parent–friends compatibility	10	6
Parent–friends influence	9	3
Proximal Structure[d]		
Parent approval problem behavior	12	5
Friends approval problem behavior	15	12
Friends models problem behavior	16	14

[a]Correlations with times drunk last year, marijuana involvement, deviant behaviour last year, and multiple problem-behaviour index, for high school and college samples, for males and females separately.

[b]The balance of positive versus negative endorsed reasons for the behaviour.

[c]These scales refer to *general* support and control, and compatibility between and relative influence of parents and friends.

[d]These scales refer to approval–disapproval of, and modelling of, the kinds of problem behaviours considered in these studies.

one personality and one perceived environment variable' (Jessor and Jessor, 1977, p.140, their emphasis).

In the personality domain, results lent particular support to the hypothesis that general 'intolerance of deviance' would operate as an important personality control against indulgence in early drug use, sexual, and other non-conforming behaviours. The measure of intolerance of deviance consisted of questions about 26 forms of behaviour (e.g. 'to take something of value from a store without paying for it', 'to cheat on an important exam') to be responded to on a ten-point scale running from 'not wrong' to 'very wrong'. Students who more often endorsed the view that such actions were wrong consistently tended to be those who reported relatively little involvement in 'deviant' behaviour. It was as if the holding of such views exerted a restraining influence upon certain kinds of behaviour, or at least upon reporting them.

In the course of such exercises in building as comprehensive a picture as possible of the determinants of individual differences in social behaviour, it is possible to play relatively safe by employing variables whose relationship to the criterion social behaviour is 'obvious'. The link between general intolerance of deviant behaviour on the one hand, and 'general deviant behaviour' on the other hand (one of the Jessors' criterion behaviours), is an example of a relatively 'obvious' connection: although such a link cannot be taken for granted it would be somewhat surprising if it did not exist. The connection with alcohol use or sexual behaviour is less obvious. Where the link is obvious, the Jessors termed the 'predictor' variable 'proximal'. The conceptual link between the variable and the criterion was a relatively 'close' one. Other variables were relatively 'distal'. An example of a relatively distal personality variable in their scheme was 'value on academic achievement' (ten questions of the sort, 'How strongly do I like . . . to be considered a bright student by the teachers', with responses to be marked on a scale from 0, 'neither like nor dislike', to 100, 'like very much'). Although the link here is far less obvious, this variable was consistently negatively correlated with criterion behaviours as reported by high school students, although correlations did not reach a significant level for college students.

The distinction between proximal and distal causes of behaviour, which is a useful one for ordering the multitude of variables used by these and other research workers, was employed again in the perceived environment domain. Of all the variables examined by the Jessors, the one which was the most strongly and consistently correlated with criterion behaviour variables was a variable they called, 'friends models problem behaviour' (elsewhere termed 'social support for problem behaviour') a relatively proximal variable concerned with the prevalence of models amongst friends for engaging in drinking, drug use, or sexual behaviour (e.g. 'Do you have any close friends who drink fairly regularly?' 'About how many of your friends have tried marijuana?'). This variable was strongly correlated with the criterion when questioning was limited to friends as models for the particular behaviour in question only (e.g. Jessor *et al.*, 1973). About the only failure of the friends models variable was its failure to correlate with sexual behaviour amongst college students.

Clearly this type of multi-variable picture of the possible causes of behaviour carries more weight if it can be shown that the chosen variables *predict* in the normally understood sense of that word. The Jessors were in fact able to show that within the high school sample many of the same variables which correlated significantly with behaviour at one point in time were also predictive of the occurrence of these behaviours occurring for the *first* time within the subsequent one to three years. For example, those who became users of marijuana for the first time between the third and fourth years had a significantly higher level of 'friends models' for this behaviour at year three than did those who remained non-users at year four. This was true for boys and for girls, whilst value on academic achievement, for example, was significant for girls only (those valuing academic achievement most being more likely to remain non-users). Similarly, girls who valued academic achievement more highly were more likely to remain virgins at year four (again this did not hold for boys), girls with higher 'intolerance of deviance' were more likely to remain virgins (again no difference for boys), whilst a higher level of 'friends models' for this behaviour predicted transmission to non-virginity for both sexes. The Jessors were even able to report some success in predicting the timing of onset of new behaviour. For instance, there was a perfect rank order of five groups (males and females combined) on the 'value on academic achievement' variable, with those who remained non-drinkers throughout the study having the highest average score, those who became drinkers only in the last year of the study the second highest, and so on down to those who reported being drinkers at the first point of enquiry who had the lowest mean score on this variable. Similarly, those who initially reported having used marijuana already had the lowest scores on a scale of 'negative functions of drugs' (the number of reasons against engaging in drug use which were checked by the respondent, e.g. 'it's easy to get too dependent on it, or to go on to trying stronger drugs'), those who initiated marijuana use early in the study came next, those who initiated drug use late in the study next, and finally those who reported remaining non-users throughout the study had the highest scores.

Despite this evidence, the Jessors were well aware of the dangers of attributing causal importance to certain variables where none might exist. They preferred to talk about:

> . . . a transition in social-psychological *status* rather than mere adoption of a particular new behaviour. A *constellation* of developmental changes appears to characterise the process of becoming a drinker, or a marijuana user, or a non-virgin, and the taking on of this pattern of characteristics seems to be involved in making a transition (Jessor and Jessor, 1977, p.205, their emphasis).

In a series of published papers they showed that it was not just a simple matter of personality and perceived environment variables being correlated with the behaviours in question, or of their being able to predict the uptake of new behaviours in the subsequent one to three years. In addition, there was evidence that those who adopted the new behaviours reported *changes* in personality and perception of the environment which were consistent with becoming a drinker or a drug user. For example, Jessor *et al.* (1973) showed that those who became marijuana users between one year and the next also showed significant changes, in comparison with those who remained non-users, in the direction of valuing independence more than achievement, reporting less compatibility between attitudes of parents and peer group, greater use of marijuana by friends, less endorsement of negative functions of marijuana, a greater involvement in general deviant behaviour, more sexual experience, and a higher frequency of drunkenness. These held for both boys and girls in the high school sample, and similar findings emerged when change in drinking status was the criterion (Jessor *et al.*, 1972).

Another way to illustrate their thesis about transition during adolescence is to depict graphically the way in which levels of certain variables changed over a period of years for those who already indulged in a particular behaviour at the beginning of the study, those who showed a transition during the course of the study, and those who did not indulge throughout the course of the study. Two examples are shown in Figures 2 and 3 which concern the onset of drinking in the high school study. A number of things are apparent from these graphs. First, it is clear that changes in drinking status took place against a general

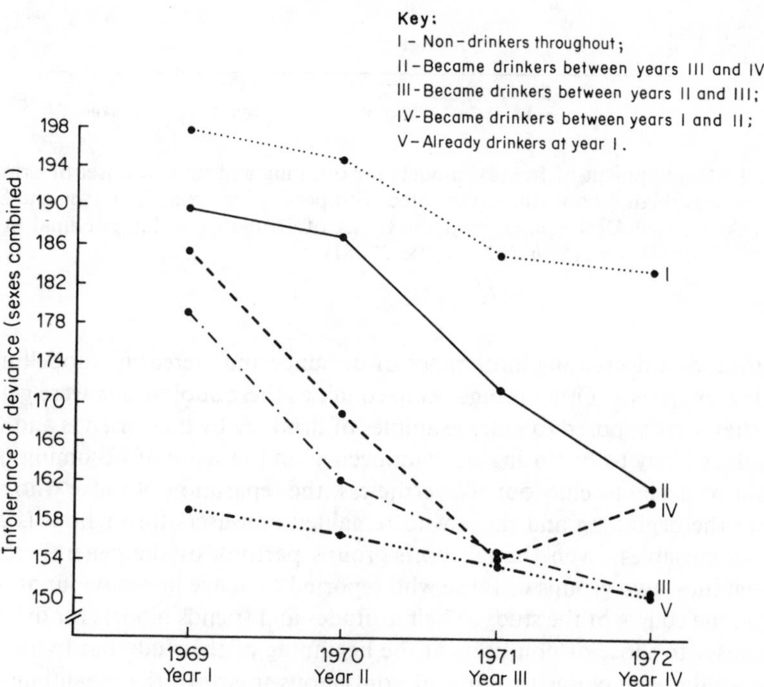

Figure 2 Development of attitude towards deviance and time of onset of drinking in the Jessors' high school study (reprinted with permission from R. Jessor and S. L. Jessor, Adolescent Development and the Onset of Drinking: A Longitudinal Study, *Journal of Studies on Alcohol*, **36**, 1975, 27–51)

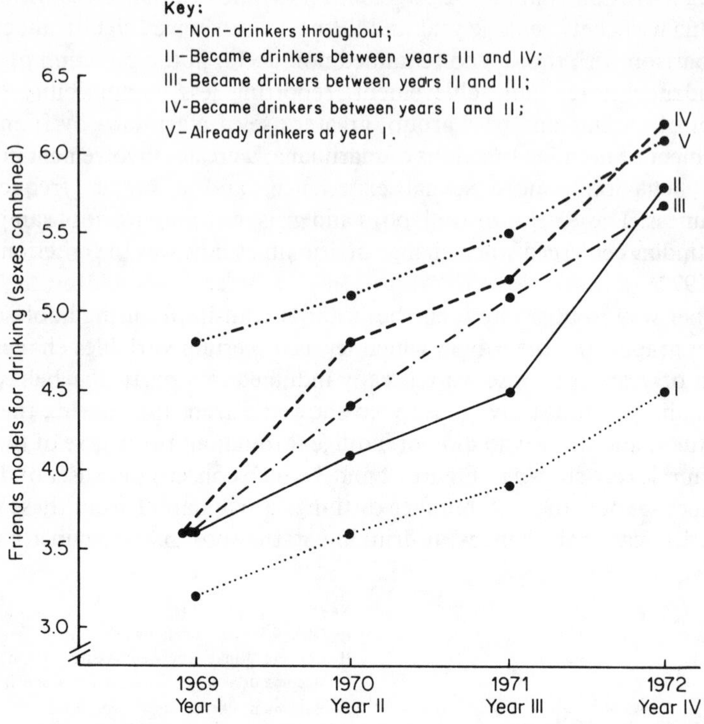

Figure 3 Development of friends' models for drinking and time of onset of drinking in the Jessors' high school study (reprinted with permission from R. Jessor and S. L. Jessor, Adolescent Development and the Onset of Drinking: A Longitudinal Study, *Journal of Studies on Alcohol*, **36**, 1975, 27–51)

background of decreasing intolerance of deviance and increasing modelling of drinking by friends. Other things being equal, as these adolescents were getting older they were exposed to more examples of drinking by their friends and were themselves likely to be 'losing their innocence' in the sense of becoming more tolerant of deviant behaviour. Nevertheless, the separation of those who were users at the beginning and those who remained non-users throughout is clear on both variables, even though both groups partook of the general trends. Between these two groups lie those who reported a change in behaviour at some point in the course of the study. Their attitudes and friends models for drinking were closer to those of non-users at the beginning of the study but by the end of the study were closer to those of continuous users. In the meantime they had shown changes in these variables which were greater than average, and these changes sometimes took place in the year in which they reported becoming a drinker, sometimes they ante-dated this change and sometimes they occurred in the year following.

OTHER STUDIES OF EARLY APPETITIVE BEHAVIOUR

These studies, which have been illustrated in some detail here, are informative on a number of points and set the scene for an acceptable model of the development and the recession of excessive appetitive behaviour. They inform us that the factors influencing development are multiple—no single factor theory is likely to be adequate; that the origins of excess are likely to lie as much in social norms and group pressure as in character and attitudes; that the uptake of new behaviour does not occur in a psychological vacuum but as part of a constellation of changing beliefs, preferences and habits of thought, feeling and action; and that appetitive behaviour cannot be divorced from the demands, both biological and social, of the stage of the life-cycle at which a person finds him or herself.

There are few studies of this kind as comprehensive as the Jessors', but those there are, mainly on alcohol or other drug use, confirm parts of this general picture and some add important points to guide theory. Kandel (1978) has provided a particularly useful review of those studies of youthful drug use, including the Jessors', which involved some element of follow-up and re-interview of subjects. She confirmed that the factors predictive of later illicit drug use—mainly marijuana in these studies—included certain personality variables (rebelliousness, stress on independence, low sense of psychological well-being, low self-esteem, and lower academic aspirations and motivation) but that drug-taking and pro-drug-taking attitudes of friends were, '. . . amongst the most potent predictors of drug involvement' (p.24). One of the studies which looked at this factor in some detail concluded that *choice of* friends with similar interests and *influence by* friends were equally important processes in producing this similarity amongst friendship groups. In any case she noted that, 'Extensive discussions of drugs with peers preceded initiation to all types of illicit drugs' (p.25).

Another review of the factors influencing initial drug use, again largely amongst young people in the United States (Gorsuch and Butler, 1976), found some evidence for the importance of family background (not examined by the Jessors, perhaps because it seemed too 'distal'), and in particular the disruption of normal parent–child relationships for *some* drug users. They also stressed the importance of friends' behaviour and found a number of studies which, '. . . emphasise the central role of social groups in the initiation, development, and maintenance of non-medical drug-use patterns' (p.125). The distinctive contribution of this review, however, and it is one of which we should take special note, was to stress the different 'pathways' which it is possible to take which lead to illicit drug use. Drug-taking may have its origins in an unhappy home background, in peer-group influence, or in medical use, and the personal characteristics which aid or impede progress along these paths will be different from route to route. Leventhal and Cleary (1980) made the same, important point that initial motivation for appetitive behaviour—they were discussing smoking—will probably depend very much upon the age and stage of initiation. Teenage smokers may start to smoke because of the image of toughness and rebellion associated with smoking at that age, whereas someone starting to smoke at exam time at college or university may be more strongly motivated by the need to control work anxiety. The addition of historical and cross-cultural perspectives introduced in Chapter 4 underlines the point that motivation depends upon the social context in which appetitive behaviour occurs.

One of the studies which adds an important theoretical ingredient is Sadava and Forsythe's (1977) study of drug use amongst undergraduate students at a university in Ontario, Canada. They employed the same scheme of 'personal' and 'environmental' variables, both distal and proximal, as the Jessors, and were concerned amongst other things with correlations of these variables with 'range of polydrug use' (a 19-item checklist assessing the sheer number of different drugs tried by the individual). Social support for drug use (including models, reinforcement, and perceived pressures towards illicit drug use), part of the proximal environment system, provided by far the strongest single correlate, and emerged first in their multiple step-wise regression analysis. From the personal system, attitudinal tolerance of drug use emerged as the second strongest correlate.

Where these workers went further in attempting to explore the complexity of the matter was in pointing out that drug-using or other similar social behaviour is likely to be a matter not simply of the *additive* effects of personal factors and environmental influences. Just as in the main stream of research on personality it has been shown that behaviour is correlated with personal and situational factors and with aspects of the *interaction* between the two (e.g. Endler, 1975), so it is also to be expected that the interaction of person and environment will influence drug use. Although, as Sadava and Forsythe so rightly put it, 'The problem of person–environment (P–E) interaction is one of immense complexity' (p.215), they were at least able to suggest the importance of some interaction effects in their own work. For example, social support for drug use interacted with perceived 'fear functions of drug use' (based on a sub-scale assessing the degree to which the person felt that abstinence represented a means of avoiding adverse physical, psychological, legal, and interpersonal consequences—a feature of this study was the use of a number of separate sub-scales to assess different perceived functions of drug use such as instrumental, coping, and ideological functions). In particular, the combination of high fear functions and high social support correlated with a lesser pattern of drug use than would be suggested by a simple additive model: it appeared that beyond some level 'fear' outweighed the positive effects of social support.

Gorsuch and Butler cited another example from a study by Bowers (1968) in which reported alcohol use varied both with individual students' attitudes, but also with the college in which they were studying and the norms regarding alcohol use in the college. Personal opposition to the use of alcohol was a primary, overriding factor which was associated with low use irrespective of college. Positive attitudes, on the other hand, were associated with a relatively greater use of alcohol only when the college atmosphere was relatively permissive.

A simple additive combination of these two variables would not have sufficed.

Studies which strengthen the conclusion regarding the importance of peer-group influence include those by Akers *et al.* (1979), Huba *et al.* (1979), Orford *et al.* (1974), Kosviner *et al.* (1973), and many others. Akers *et al.* studied a sample of 2,000–3,000 12–17-year-old school pupils in seven different communities in three mid-Western States in the United States. The strongest single correlate of both alcohol and marijuana use in this sample was the score on a scale of 'differential peer association': 'A scale of three items measuring how many of respondents' best friends, friends with whom they associate most often, and friends whom they have known for the longest time, use the substance' (p.655). Huba *et al.* found sizeable correlations between 12–14-year-olds' reported own use of one of 13 drugs, including alcohol and tobacco, and the number of known adults who used the drug or used it regularly, the number of the subject's friends who used it, and the number of the subject's friends who had given the subject the particular substance concerned. In our study of the drinking behaviour and attitudes of first year English university students, too, the estimated recent consumption of the respondent's two closest friends provided the strongest correlation with the respondent's own reported drinking.

In Kosviner *et al.*'s (1973) study of cannabis use at three universities in Southern England it was found that those who had ever tried cannabis were much more likely to report having played truant several times at school, having been considered a trouble-maker at school, ever having gambled for money, having no religion now, ever having smoked tobacco (a large difference: 77 per cent of users compared to 33 percent of non-users of cannabis having smoked tobacco), and having been drunk on alcohol more than ten times (one of the most impressive differences: 36 per cent of users versus 13 per cent of non-users). Once again, tolerance of or involvement in generally 'deviant' behaviour appears to have been important. In the area of social influence, friends' use again emerged as the strongest single influence of all: 41 per cent of users estimated that more than two-fifths of their friends smoked cannabis, compared to 3 per cent of non-users. In an attempt to integrate these findings, Kosviner *et al.* suggested that a pattern emerged in which users might be seen as displaying, '. . . looser association with traditional transmitters of "societal morality" ' (p.57).

One of the major limitations of this and other studies reviewed so far is their geographical and cultural circumscription. The Jessors' study was confined to a single mid-Western community, our own study to one English university, and all to the English-speaking industrialized Western world of the 1960s or 1970s. Although in one sense these restrictions serve an important research purpose, namely that of limiting undue heterogeneity of samples so that close attention may be paid to the personality and micro-level social influence variables already discussed, there is no doubt that these studies miss the wider perspective. A recent British study which provided an interesting partial corrective is that of O'Connor (1978), which I shall discuss in some detail because it raises a number of points.

O'Connor's study involved interviews with over 700 18–21-year-olds plus separate interviews with most of their mothers and fathers. The sample was divided into those born of Irish parents, brought up and still living in Ireland; those born of English parents, born, brought up, and still living in England; and a third sample of 18–21-year-olds born and brought up in England by Irish parents who had themselves been born and reared in the Republic of Ireland (the Anglo-Irish group). This study adds considerable further complexity to the picture of the early determinants of appetitive behaviour drawn by studies reviewed so far. In particular, it introduces the idea of *ambivalence*, a concept which has an important part to play in the psychological model of excessive behaviour to be developed in this book, but which is used by O'Connor as a culture-level rather than person-level variable.

O'Connor certainly produced evidence that an Irish upbringing exposed young people to abstinence norms, and that those young people born and brought up in England by Irish parents shared this early experience to some degree. The majority of Irish and Anglo-Irish young men and women in her sample had taken a pledge early in their teens not to drink until the age of 21. No member of the English sample had done so. More Anglo-Irish than English young people had parents who themselves had taken a pledge and who were now abstinent, although in both respects the Anglo-Irish group fell short of the Irish group. On the other hand, more Anglo-Irish fathers drank heavily than was the case in either the Irish or the English groups (rates of heavy drinking were uniformly low for all three groups of mothers).

Despite their pledge-taking, Anglo-Irish youngsters reported starting to drink as often during their teens as did the English (over half the males before their fifteenth birthday, for example) in comparison with a much lower figure for Irish youngsters (17 per cent of males drinking by age 15). Early drinking was hidden from parents most often for the Irish and least often for the English, and Irish youngsters reported hiding their current drinking from parents and feeling guilty and worried about their drinking more often than either of the other groups. Drinking at home occasionally with a meal was much more common an experience for the English. Some large differences emerged in attributed motives for drinking. For example, 15 per cent of Irish young males compared with 8 per cent of Anglo-Irish, and less than 1 per cent of English claimed anxiety reduction as one of the reasons why 'lads drink'. Differences of a similar order occurred when respondents were asked why girls drank, and also when asked about anticipation of adulthood as a motive. Not surprisingly, permissiveness regarding drinking was greatest in English young people and their parents, intermediate for the Anglo-Irish, and lowest for the Irish, young Irishmen in particular having a double standard for boys and girls. This double standard was less apparent for Anglo-Irish young men, and apparently lacking for English young men and women.

When it came to attempting to account for individual differences in the young people's drinking within cultural groups, fathers' drinking as well as both fathers' and mothers' permissiveness or non-permissiveness with regard to their children's drinking (parental attitudes as perceived by the children were rather more significant than attitudes expressed directly at interview by the parents themselves) turned out to be important. Combining all groups and both sexes together, children whose fathers were light drinkers and whose parents both had relatively disapproving attitudes towards them drinking had a 2.5 to 1 chance of being light drinkers themselves, whereas those with heavy drinking fathers and parents who approved of their drinking had more than a 3 to 1 chance of being relatively heavy drinkers themselves. Like all other investigators, however, O'Connor found that the influence of peer support for drinking generally exceeded that of parental drinking and parental attitudes. What is clear from O'Connor's analysis is that by the age of 18–21 drinking was largely a peer-centred activity, that the influence of peers was predominant, and that the Anglo-Irish group of young people born and brought up in England were exposed to roughly the same level of peer-group support for drinking as were the English. Many of the Irish, on the other hand, were exposed to lower levels of peer support for drinking than was usual for all but a very few English and Anglo-Irish.

Thus, Anglo-Irish youngsters in particular were exposed to the conflicting influences of intolerance of drinking by their Irish parents on the one hand and permissiveness towards drinking on the part of their English friends. There was support for those who argue for the importance of cultural ambivalence in the generation of drinking problems in O'Connor's findings that young Anglo-Irish males were more frequently found to be very heavy drinkers (drinking 75 pints of beer or more or its equivalent per month) than were members of the other groups, and that young Anglo-Irish women were much more frequently found to be heavy drinkers (25 or more pints of beer or the equivalent per month—very heavy drinking was rare amongst young women) than the others.

The existence of simultaneously held positive and negative emotional attitudes towards the same object, at both an individual and cultural level, has often been remarked upon by others (e.g. Lemert, 1951; Minkowich *et al.*, 1966). Other examples offered by Lemert in his general discussion of deviance included sons of U.S. immigrants from rural Italy caught, like O'Connor's Anglo-Irish youngsters, between their parents' values and those acquired from their American friends. Another of Lemert's examples, not involving a clash of values between cultures, but rather ambibalence built into the attitudes of a single society, was the intensely ambivalent attitude to sex of young men in societies where full sexual behaviour was postponed long beyond physical maturity, despite much erotic stimulation.

In his book, *The Folklore of Sex*, Albert Ellis (1951) came to the conclusion, on the basis of his analysis of attitudes expressed publicly in the media, in fiction, and elsewhere, that ambivalence and dissonance regarding sex were endemic in the United States at that time. Human sexual needs and desires, social changes in sexual codes and ideas, as well as individualism and secularism discouraging people from uniformly following traditional tenets, all encouraged doubt and ambivalence and, '. . . motivate millions of Americans to act differently than they think and unconsciously to think differently than they consciously permit themselves to think they think' (p.270). As a result, in Ellis's view, the average American was extremely muddled about sex, holding simultaneously contradictory views. Officially, sex views were negative and disapproving; but unofficially, attitudes were much more positive and approving.

It was certainly Ellis's view that this very ambivalence could contribute to promiscuity. The official emphasis upon monogamous sexual behaviour, and public disapproval of sex without affection, could itself make deviance appear more novel, exciting, and adventurous. Anti-sexual attitudes could create, '. . . inattentions and rigidities which encourage compulsive, neurotic outbursts . . .' (p.51). In other words, repression might create compulsion. Don Juanism, he suggested, was most likely due, not to latent homosexuality as orthodox psychoanalysts had suggested, but due to compulsive over-reaction partly as a result of the over-repressive attitudes towards sexual variety in the American culture.

To return to our main theme, the general picture that emerges from the study of drinking and drug-taking so far is confirmed by the results of two major studies of tobacco-smoking amongst young people in Britain. Bynner's survey (1969) of over 5,000 10–15-year-old boys revealed four main influences of which the single most important was the familiar variable of friends' behaviour. The difference between those who said that none of their friends smoked and those who said that all their friends smoked was impressive (none of the former smoked themselves versus 62% of the latter). Of the others, parents' permissiveness towards smoking made a lesser contribution. The others would be termed personality variables by some, one relatively proximal—'whether put off smoking by the danger of lung cancer' (equivalent to the Jessors' and Sadava and Forsythe's negative functions)—the other relatively distal—'anticipation of adulthood' (participation in the activities of older boys such as going out drinking, driving a car, going to coffee bars, dances, and staying out late). In addition, boys who smoked perceived themselves and were perceived by others as lacking educational success relative to non-smokers, and Bynner argued that they were led to compensate by adopting a behaviour, i.e. smoking, which was perceived as symbolic of 'toughness' and 'precocity'.

McKennell and Thomas's (1967) survey of a representative British sample of 800–900 16–20-year-olds and a slightly larger number of adults confirmed some of these findings in these two different age groups. People were more likely to be smokers if most of their friends smoked, if they themselves drank one or twice a week or more, and if they did not go to church regularly. With these three factors operating in the stated direction, 70 per cent of adolescents and 90 per cent of adults reported being regular smokers, and with all three pointing in the opposite direction, 12 per cent of adolescents and 29 per cent of adults were regular smokers. Degree of commitment to religious belief has regularly been found to correlate inversely with drinking and drug-taking (Jolly and Orford, 1983; Gorsuch and Butler, 1976), and correlations between use of different drugs, including alcohol and tobacco, are invariably positive (e.g. Kosviner *et al.*, 1973).

That many of the same influences operate on sexual behaviour as operate on drug-using behaviour is shown by Schofield's (1968) study of the sexual behaviour of 15–19-year-olds in seven different areas of Britain in the early 1960s. There was considerable evidence from Schofield's work that sexually experienced young people conformed relatively strongly to the teenage culture and were relatively less influenced by parents. Experienced youngsters were more likely to be against adult standards and restrictions, were more influenced by other teenagers, drank more often, and, particularly in the case of girls, smoked more cigarettes and went to more unsupervised late-night parties. Parents of inexperienced boys were more likely to know where they spent their leisure time and were more likely to insist that they return home in the evenings at a definite time. There is support here then for the variable the Jessors called 'parents versus friends' influence', a variable they found to be important in some analyses but not in others (the latter, strangely, including the comparison of virgins and non-virgins at high school). The general run of Schofield's findings are also in line with Kosviner *et al.*'s hypothesis on the loosening of influence of those agents of socialization, such as parents and teachers, who generally aim to lead young people in the direction of conventional morality. Other findings which conform to those of other investigators are that experienced boys tended not to go to church, had less satisfactory academic careers, more frequently disliked school, had more school problems, and were more likely to leave school early.

There were some interesting gender differences in Schofield's findings. Perhaps because for teenage girls to be sexually experienced represented a greater degree of social deviance than for boys, it was necessary for girls to overcome greater attempts at family control, and experienced girls showed poorer relations with both parents than did the inexperienced and showed a greater degree of antipathy to family loyalty. Schofield concluded that the personality characteristic of permissiveness was associated in boys with what he called 'outgoing hedonism', whilst in girls it was strongly combined with a 'rejection of family influence'. These differences illustrate an important general point: namely that the characteristics associated with adopting a particular kind of social behaviour will vary depending upon the social meaning of that behaviour to the person concerned and to members of their family, their peer group, and their culture. Associated with different meanings or interpretations of behaviour—e.g. dangerous behaviour, manly behaviour, immoral behaviour, exciting behaviour—are different sanctions, both legal and informal, which further define the social context in which the behaviour will be adopted or not as the case may be. Different kinds of people will be inclined towards behaviour depending upon these varied circumstances. We should certainly not expect to discover unvarying correlates of appetitive behaviour. Other things being equal, sexual experience as a teenager probably had different connotations for boys and girls and for the families of boys and girls even within this one culture at one point in history. We should not expect the causes of early sexual experience to be the same for boys and girls. Even less should we expect precisely the same kinds of people to have been sexually experienced relatively early in life in Puritan or Victorian England as in the eighteenth century, or the same kinds of people to have been drinkers in eighteenth-century England as in the United States under prohibition, or drug-takers in the Fens in the nineteenth century as amongst doctors or their patients in the 1920s or 1930s or in an American university in the 1970s.

That relationships between appetitive behaviour and demographic variables can be very different in different social and cultural contexts is illustrated, for smoking, by Eckholm's (1977) report of the massive difference in male and female smoking in Japan (70 per cent of males versus 9 per cent of females) in contrast to the present picture in Britain and the United States, as well as social status differences in smoking in countries such as India and Uganda where he reports that smoking tobacco is a sign of privilege.

A glimpse of the considerable differences in attitudes towards sexual behaviour which we know have existed in the past and exist cross-culturally now (see Chapter 6) is provided by Iwawaki and Eysenck's (1978) study comparing the sexual attitudes of British and Japanese students. Several hundred Japanese students replied to the same questionnaire used by Eysenck in his study of British students (Eysenck, 1970). Both groups were aged between 18 and 22 years with an average age of 21. The comparison generally confirmed the view that Japan is still relatively Victorian in its outlook to sexual behaviour. Japanese students did not have many friends of the opposite sex, felt more comfortable in the company of friends of the same sex, and had relatively few dates. In addition, there were a large number of differences suggesting that Japanese students found certain aspects of sexual behaviour less acceptable. One of the most extreme differences involved the acceptability of 'petting' (92 per cent of male, 78 per cent of British female students finding such behaviour acceptable, compared with only 16 per cent of male and 5 per cent of female Japanese students). More Japanese students than British were, 'embarrassed to talk about sex' (25 per cent males and 38 per cent females in Japan versus 9 per cent males and 8 per cent females in Britain). There were large differences in response to the statement, 'I think about sex almost every day.' Consistent with these differences were certain differences in attitude. For example, more British students than Japanese thought that, 'the Pill should be universally available', and more British students felt that, 'young people should be allowed out at night without being too closely checked'.

There was a hint too of the importance of ambivalence. A number of Iwawaki and Eysenck's items intercorrelated to form a 'guilt' cluster (e.g. 'have felt guilty about sex experiences'). Women students gave positive replies to such items much more frequently than did male students in Britain, whilst the reverse held true in Japan, where men expressed the greater degree of guilt. Iwawaki and Eysenck could offer no explanation for this finding, but work on cultural attitudes and alcohol use provides a possible answer. Other evidence which they presented suggested that Japanese women students were on the whole quite inexperienced in sexual matters. They were, it seems, rather like O'Connor's Irish girls where drink was concerned, conforming to the relatively non-permissive social rules of their culture—rules that are particularly strict for women. At the other extreme also, so it may be argued, English male students were exposed to a relatively non-ambivalent permissive set of expectations regarding sexual behaviour, and on the whole they conformed to these. Japanese men and British women, on the other hand, might be said to have been exposed, in different ways, to an ambivalent upbringing, rather like the Anglo-Irish in relation to drinking norms in O'Connor's study. Each of these two groups, rather more than would be the case for English young men and Japanese young women, might suffer from being caught between the legacy of Victorian non-permissive attitudes and present-day pressures and encouragement towards sexual experimentation. They would therefore be expected to experience more worry, concern, and guilt regarding their sexual behaviour. There are obvious parallels here with eating. It was noted in Chapter 5 that young women are much more likely than young men to experience concern about the extent of their eating and to attempt self-control over their eating by dieting, even though 'objectively' neither their eating nor their size would warrant it.

TRANSITIONS IN APPETITIVE BEHAVIOUR

For our purpose, one of the possible limitations of most of these studies of individual differences in alcohol use, smoking, other drug use, and sexual behaviour amongst adolescents and young adults is that they largely concern the development of normal or non-problematic behaviours, and that they have little or nothing to say about the development of excessive or problem behaviour, the origins of which may be quite different. This is the criterion problem. It is a problem to which Jessor and Jessor (e.g. 1977) gave relatively little attention in comparison with the meticulous care they gave to their 'predictor' variables. In an effort to learn as much as they could about individual differences, they understandably chose criterion variables which sorted young people into 'active' and 'non-active' groups which were as nearly equal in size as was possible. As a result there was inconsistency in their approach to different social behaviours. Whereas virginity versus non-virginity, and marijuana use versus no use were the criteria in the sex and drug areas, because by a certain age most young people have consumed alcohol, the criterion in the latter area was most often *problem* drinking.

Other researchers have attempted to deal with this problem by examining 'use' and 'misuse' separately. For example, Sadava and Forsythe (1977) examined separately the correlates of frequency of cannabis use, time as a user (in an attempt to measure continued involvement and commitment to using the drug), range of polydrug use, and adverse consequences of use guaged by an 18-item scale assessing the relative frequency of experienced physical, emotional, interpersonal, and behavioural problems attributed to cannabis use. The separate study of these four criterion measures is supported by their finding that the average intercorrelation amongst these measures was a mere +0.23. Not surprisingly under these circumstances, correlations with personality and social influence variables showed considerable variation from criterion to criterion. Sadava and Forsythe used an analytic technique known as canonical correlation analysis in which independent 'canonical variates' are successively extracted starting with the variate which explains the highest proportion of total variance. Each variate is a composite of 'predictor' scores and criterion measures. In their analyses the first variate extracted appeared to reflect moderate use. Amongst the drug-use criteria, time as user and range of polydrug use loaded moderately and adverse consequences of use loaded *negatively*. The only 'predictor' variable with a substantial loading on this variate was social support for drug use, high tolerance for drug use loading moderately in addition. The second variate extracted, on the other hand, was interpreted as indicating 'abuse'. Adverse consequences of use loaded substantially and positively, with time as user loading moderately. A range of 'predictors' was related to this pattern. Social support for drug use loaded again but less highly than for moderate use, tolerance of general deviance now had a stronger loading, and there was a major contribution from initial and increasing expression of fear of the consequences of use. The latter, Sadava and Forsythe suggested, indicated, '. . . conflict within the individual in that the pattern of use represents both a means toward the satisfaction of goals and coping needs, and a source of fear of consequences' (p.236). Conflict has a major part to play in the model of excessive behaviour being developed here and is something to which we shall return in much more detail below.

In our study of English university students we similarly examined correlates of drinking frequency and 'drinking problems' separately. Our measure of drinking problems was obtained by adding scores on five separate scales which assessed, 'concern over drinking', 'experience of intoxication', 'complications of drinking', 'morning after effects', and 'relief of feelings motivation'. Unlike Sadava and Forsythe, however, we were unable to separate 'use' and 'misuse' clearly. Drinking frequency and drinking problems were correlated +0.59 and the first component produced by a principal components analysis combined both use and problem use variables. Correlates of frequency and problems were similar, friends' drinking in particular having substantial positive loadings with each.

Analysis of Eysenck's sexual attitude inventory produced 15 interpretable factors. These were not independent of one another, however, and when analysed further produced two third-order or 'super factors', one relating to 'sexual pathology' (nervousness, repression, guilt, etc.), the other to 'sexual libido' (combining elements indicative of active sexuality and permissiveness regarding sexual behaviour) (Eysenck, 1970).

Although there has been little detailed work of this nature to deal with gambling behaviour, Cornish's (1978) detailed and thoughtful review of the field based on literature that does exist to date, has touched on these issues. He was critical of the frequent assumption that explanations for the initial decision to become involved in gambling serve also as explanations for persistent gambling. He proceeded to treat these two aspects separately on the assumption, equally unwarranted in view of the lack of evidence on this point, that the determinants are separate.

It is clear, then, that the criterion problem is a highly complex one. Being a cannabis user is not the same as being an excessive opiate or polydrug user, even though there is a large body of public opinion in countries such as the United States and Britain that would have it so. Being sexually very active is not the same as being compulsive about sex or running into problems as a result of sexual behaviour. Nor is drinking at a greater than average frequency for one's age group necessarily the same as being a problem drinker. The difficulty does not of course stop there. Having more problems connected with drinking than most other adolescents or young adults is not the same as having a problem sufficiently great to cause one to seek professional help. The types of 'problem drinking' which qualify a person for a relatively high score on scales of problem drinking in studies such as those by O'Connor (1978) and Orford *et al.* (1974) may be thought of as relatively trivial (e.g. being late for a lecture or meeting; being admonished by a friend) in comparison with the complaints of many older help-seekers. Nor can it be assumed that the former is a stage in a predictable process which will lead to the latter, and that those identified as having greater problems than their peers at an early age will be very likely to turn up in the ranks of the excessive alcohol users at a later age. In fact, the logic of the numbers involved is against this possibility. Population surveys of drinking practices (e.g. Cahalan, 1970; Edwards *et al.*, 1972b) show young males in their late teens and early twenties to be the group who reports the highest frequency of drinking problems. The tentative conclusion to be drawn is that many young adults, in the natural course of events, become more restrained in their drinking as they get older rather than moving on to greater levels of excess. There is indeed some evidence, which will be examined more closely in a later chapter, that this conclusion is correct.

The question, then, is whether those predictors of individual differences in early appetitive behaviour are good for predicting later more excessive and problematic forms of the same behaviour? Robins *et al.*'s study (1977) of heroin use and addiction amongst American soldiers returning from the Vietnam war is an important and instructive one in this regard. Robins found that it was very difficult to predict, other than extremely weakly, 'addiction' to heroin after return to the United States on the basis of factors known prior to service in Vietnam such as demographic factors, parental behaviour (including broken homes, parents' arrests, drug use, and drinking problems), own deviance, and even own pre-service drug use. On the other hand, by 'decomposing' the process into three stages—using heroin in Vietnam, continuing to use after Vietnam, and becoming 'addicted' after Vietnam—it was possible to show that transition from one stage to the next could be predicted much more strongly, if still very imperfectly. At the first stage, pre-service drug use (especially use of amphetamines, barbiturates, or narcotics) was the factor most predictive of being a user of heroin in Vietnam. Twenty-eight per cent of those using in Vietnam continued to use heroin on return to the United States—stage two. This was the most difficult stage to predict, although pre-service drug use was positively related as were demographic factors, in particular being black, coming from an inner-city area, and being relatively young. Of those who continued to use after Vietnam, the proportion who became 'addicted' (at least three of the following four criteria had to be met: using at least once a week; feeling dependent on narcotics; having at least two of the classic symptoms of withdrawal when narcotics were discontinued; these symptoms lasting for more than two days) was again 28 per cent. Factors which predicted this last transition, from using upon return to America to becoming a heroin addict, were quite different from those that predicted transitions one and two. First, the factor most strongly predictive of this third transition was one with virtually no predictive power at the earlier two stages, namely 'parental behaviour'. Even more striking was the finding that the direction of prediction was reversed for the scale of demographic factors. Whereas it was the black, inner-city, young soldiers who were most likely to become users in Vietnam and to continue with use afterwards, it was the older, white post-Vietnam heroin user from outside central city areas who was at the greatest risk of becoming addicted.

As Kandel (1978) put it in her review of youth drug studies:

> Whereas most studies compare youths within a total population on the basis of their use or non-use of a particular substance, [these] results . . . suggest a different strategy, namely the decomposition of the panel sample into appropriate subsamples of individuals at a particular stage who are at risk for initiation into the next stage. Because each stage represents a cumulative pattern of use and contains fewer adolescents than the preceding stage in the sequence, comparisons of users and non-users must be made among members of the restricted group that has already used the drugs at the preceding stage. Unless this is done, the attributes identified as apparent characteristics of a particular class of drug users may actually reflect characteristics important for involvement in drugs at the preceding level (p.15).

If Robins had not 'decomposed' her sample of Vietnam veterans in this way, several of her findings might not have emerged because no simple variable was strongly predictive at each and all of the three stages.

The kinds of transitions described by Robins are of course very different from some of those that the Jessors and others have studied. For one thing, Robins' subjects were unusual by virtue of having experienced, within a fairly short space of time, two quite different sets of circumstances, which apart from anything else involved living in two areas of the world geographically quite distant and poles apart with regard to availability of and attitudes towards the use of certain drugs. For another, whilst Vietnam veterans returning to the United States were moving from a culture of high to one of low drug availability, the Jessors' high school students were in a sense moving in the opposite direction. The Jessors', and other studies like theirs, were at least in part studies of the adoption of new behaviours in line with prevailing developmental trends. This is particularly true for such transitions as those from sexual inexperience to sexual experience, and non-drinker to drinker, in which cases they were observing the rate of uptake of new behaviours which in the course of time were to be taken up by the large majority. In one sense at least, Robins was observing the downward arm of a developmental process, whilst the Jessors and others like them were examining the upward arm. This is illustrated by the fact that virtually none of Robins' subjects took up heroin use in the United States who had not also been heroin users in Vietnam. In fact, the natural course of events was in the opposite direction, with over 70 per cent of users in Vietnam reporting giving up on return home. The question of why some people take up drug use can, under those circumstances, be turned around to ask why it is that some people did not follow the normal course of events, which was to give up heroin use on returning from overseas service.

Nevertheless, the idea of a stepwise transition from one status to another, with differing factors predicting different stages, has wide relevance for understanding excessive appetitive behaviour and Robins' sample was not as anomalous as it may appear. After all, when we move from examining transitions that are developmentally normal (from sexual inexperience to sexual experience, for example) to those that represent increased involvement in activities that are non-normal or defined by many as deviant or excessive (using illicit drugs or becoming a regular, heavy gambler, for example), then we are dealing, like Robins, with a diminishing sample at risk. The question is: Why do some people go on to greater levels of deviance or excess whilst many do not?

Similarly, although the geographic change makes Robins sample unusual, there is nothing unusual about major changes in life circumstances, particularly in late adolescence and early adulthood. After all, moving from the single to married state, from adolescence to adulthood, from being a pupil in full-time education to being a worker, each involves large changes in roles, self-concept, and experience of pressures and constraints towards or against indulgence in behaviours of one sort or another, and it is probably at these points of change that the most dramatic transitions in behaviour occur. Vietnam veterans may constitute extreme examples of a very general phenomenon, namely change of behaviour in response to changes in life circumstances.

Kandel and her colleagues also used the technique of decomposing the overall sample in their study of New York State high school students. They found that minor delinquency and use of cigarettes, beer and wine were predictive of use of 'hard liquor'; pro-marijuana beliefs and values and association with using peers were predictive of marijuana use; and that poor relations with parents, feelings of depression, and exposure to drug-using peers predicted initiation into use of illicit drugs other than marijuana. Again partitioning of the sample into those at risk because of having reached the preceding stage, and those not at such risk, enabled these different predictors of entry to the next stage to be revealed. These were 'stages' in the sense that engaging in one of these activities (e.g. drinking 'hard liquor') increased substantially the 'risk' of engaging in the next (e.g. marijuana use) even though only a minority might proceed to the next stage (Kandel, 1978).

One immediate consequence of using this strategy based upon the idea of 'stages' is that variables indicative of personal 'needs' or disabilities start to emerge as important at later stages which did not appear earlier and which, indeed, were totally neglected in studies like the Jessors' which concentrated on normal youthful development. Thus, Robins *et al.* (1977) found unusual home background to be predictive only at the stage of progression from use to 'addiction' on return to the United States; Kandel (1978) reported poor relations with parents and feelings of depression correlated with progression to illicit drugs other than marijuana; and in our study, although we did not use the decomposition strategy, we found that the personality variable *N* (Eysenck's 'neuroticism' or general anxiety—Eysenck and Eysenck, 1969) correlated significantly with drinking problems but not at all with drinking frequency.

In fact, Robins offered an explanation for the striking change in direction of prediction from her stages 1 and 2 to stage 3 in terms of the balance between social or 'extrinsic' support for drug use and 'intrinsic' motives. She argued that inner-city black youths were more likely to use narcotics because of peer encouragement and pressure towards use for social purposes. This is the factor, whether in the guise of 'peer support for drug use', 'friends' use', or 'peer pressure', which emerges from most of the surveys of drinking, drugs, and other appetitive behaviours as the single most important determinant of individual differences at least at early stages. On the other hand:

> Individuals who live in environments in which none of their peers use narcotics are not being urged by friends to use them for social purposes. Indeed, if they use narcotics at all, they are both violating local norms and expending great effort to maintain their supply . . . Presumably, older whites who live outside of the central city and still use narcotics must be driven to this use by an unusual compulsion to achieve euphoria or by serious subjective problems. We infer that use against demographic odds implies a greater need, a need so great that it overrides considerations of discipline and moderation that might prevent addiction (p.35).

Hence, the finding that older, non-urban whites who continue to be users of heroin in the United States are then more likely to become addicted. This is very similar to the type of explanation suggested by Jellinek (1960) to explain the observations made by some clinicians at the time (and unlikely to be true now) that women problem drinkers were more difficult to help than men: if women had had to overcome the odds against them becoming heavy drinkers, odds created by society's double standard for men and women, then they must have had strong intrinsic or personality reasons for becoming problem drinkers.

Robins drew a parallel also with the finding from certain 'dry' states within the Union, that the transition from teetotaller to drinker was comparatively low, but the transition from drinker to 'alcoholic' was relatively high in frequency: those whose drinking was so great as to override local customs presumably had stronger 'needs' to behave in this way.

This brings our discussion of the causes of excessive appetitive behaviour on to the possible nature of the 'intrinsic' personal 'needs' that might be served by such behaviour. Here we move into quite different research territory: one dominated by observation, discussion, and experimentation with people who have sought help, rather than by surveys of 'normal' youths or adults. Each of these two major research traditions is important, providing insights which the other is unable to give.

CHAPTER EIGHT

Personal Inclinations

The mischief is not really in the drug but in people (Dr John Jones, an early eighteenth century physician, in his *The Mysteries of Opium Revealed* (cited by Kurland, 1978, pp.1–2).)

. . . when behaviour is being discussed at the level of the individual a strong inclination exists to regard it as being determined by factors unique to that person and to be found by studying his personality and attitudes. The more intense a person's gambling involvement, the more likely it is to be ascribed to such 'internal' causes—on the assumption that 'external' or situational determinants are relatively constant for all gamblers. Similarly, since heavy participation is a minority behaviour, it is likely to be ascribed to pathological motives (Cornish, 1978, p.152).

APPETITIVE BEHAVIOURS AS MOOD MODIFIERS

A major legacy of the clinical tradition in the study of appetitive behaviour is the tension reduction hypothesis. The reduction of tension is a motive to which people frequently attribute appetitive behaviour, particularly if it is excessive. In the case of sedative-hypnotic and tranquillizing drugs, at least, there exists a pharmacological basis for the expectation that use of these drugs may be functional because they relieve the experience of tension or anxiety. This constitutes the major part of the justification for the very widespread medical use of these drugs. In the case of most of the other appetitive behaviours with which we are concerned, tension reduction is controversial.

For example, the idea that an abnormal appetite for food may be the result of eating serving the function of anxiety reduction was termed by Kaplan and Kaplan (1957) the 'psychosomatic concept of obesity' (note that they accepted, as did most authorities until very recently, that obesity and excessive eating were very closely linked). They assumed that emotional tensions, whether described as a 'fear', 'loneliness', or 'feelings of unworthiness', for example, could be conditioned by association, in childhood, with feelings of hunger for food. Hence, a person might 'feel hungry' when tense. In addition, or alternatively, feeding might be associated with relaxation or tension relief, and hence food might acquire, to use the language of learning theory, extra reinforcing properties in addition to its value as a hunger-reducing reinforcer. In its supposed anxiety-reducing properties, Kaplan and Kaplan likened eating to, '. . . the excessive ingestion of alcohol, masturbation, compulsive behaviour, and interpersonal contact . . .' (p.190). They went on to argue, however, that there was a mechanism additional to those involving conditioning processes, which could partially explain how eating reduced anxiety. They speculated that there might be, '. . . some degree of physiological incompatibility between the act of eating and intense fear or anxiety; it has been demonstrated that while eating, intense anxiety states are temporarily diminished' (p.190). In view of the need for some degree of attention, not to mention social behaviour which may accompany eating, as well as the psychomotor acts of eating and the partly autonomically governed digestive processes, it seems highly probable that this notion is correct.

There may be an important parallel between this 'physiological incompatibility' which the Kaplans believed to exist between eating and anxiety and an incompatibility between anxiety and other appetitive behaviours such as gambling and sexual behaviour, including masturbation. Both involve the focusing of attention in a direction which may be removed from the source of anxiety, and in addition can involve intense cognitive activity in the form of calculation or fantasy, which may serve as effective distractors from anxiety-arousing thoughts or circumstances. In so far as different forms of behaviour have these important psychological elements in common, it may not be so fanciful to think of them as partially equivalent and to speak, for example, of gambling or excessive eating as 'masturbation equivalents'. Is it possible, then, that one of the most significant functions of appetitive behaviour is to provide activity, the exact form of which is unimportant compared with its ability temporarily to distract attention from unpleasant emotion, in the same way that activity can temporarily reduce physical pain (e.g. Ray, 1981)?

In fact, later psychological theories of obesity, for example the external cue sensitivity theory of Schachter *et al.* (1968), have tended to discount the psychosomatic hypothesis. Certainly the experimental evidence, reviewed by Leon and Roth (1977), gives no support to the hypothesis that eating reduces anxiety for the obese. Leon and Roth, however, doubted the conclusiveness of these findings based as they were upon necessarily contrived laboratory situations. Under these circumstances it is difficult to be certain that anxiety has been aroused which is at all comparable to the real world tensions which some people describe as being relieved by eating, and also whether the eating behaviour observed (eating is usually under the guise of a 'taste test') is comparable to everyday eating. There is also the problem, discussed in Chapter 5, of deciding who are appropriate subjects for such research. Clinically obese people, or even the mildly overweight college students frequently used in such experiments (mostly male according to Leon and Roth—a strange choice in view of the overwhelming predominance of women amongst those complaining of overweight or excessive eating), may not be the most appropriate subjects if, as has been suggested by some writers (e.g. Rodin, 1978; Ley, 1980), and discussed in Chapter 5, the tendency to eat excessively is to be found as frequently amongst restrained eaters of normal weight as amongst the obese. In view of the burden of clinical accounts linking food intake and anxiety or other states of emotional arousal, Leon and Roth believed it premature to wholly dismiss the view that excessive eating and the search for anxiety reduction were linked. The question whether eating in fact *successfully* relieves tension at all is a further question which can be complicated still more by asking what kinds of tension are relieved if any, to what degree, and for how long? In fact, Ley's (1980) more recent review concluded that the experimental and survey evidence is mixed in its support for the suggestion that the obese or 'latent obese' (restrained eaters) eat more when anxious or under stress. Amongst the mainly negative experimental findings he finds one study at least (Slochower, 1976) showing significant reduction in emotion following eating by obese people.

The status of tension reduction as a major motive for appetitive behaviour is no clearer when the behaviour in question is the consumption of the major Western recreational drug substances, tobacco and alcohol. In the case of tobacco-smoking, Nesbitt (1969) drew attention to the paradox created by the reports of many smokers that they feel more relaxed when smoking, despite the evidence that smoking *increases* arousal, as indicated by increases in blood pressure, heart rate, acetylcholine release, signs of arousal in electroencephalogram (EEG) recordings, and improved vigilance and reaction time performance.

Schachter (1973) attempted to explain Nesbitt's paradox in two ways. First, a person might feel more 'relaxed' because any increase in arousal which occurred for any other reasons (due to tension within the social group of which the smoker was a part, for example) would be experienced as relatively less arousing if arousal started from a relatively high level as a consequence of smoking (the law of initial values). Secondly, if arousal was attributed to smoking rather than to circumstances, a person might 'feel' less aroused than if an increase in tension could be attributed only to the circumstances in which the person found him or herself. On the face of it neither of these mechanisms would appear to account very satisfactorily for the experience of feeling more *relaxed*.

The findings themselves are in fact more complex than at first appears to be the case. Reviewing the evidence, Paxton (1980) found some evidence for 'dearousal' effects of smoking. For example, some smokers have shown EEG changes that indicate a decrease in arousal, and one study has found clear evidence of skeletal muscle relaxation in the form of depression of the patella reflex which could account for feelings of relaxation. Some experimental work with rats has suggested that both EEG and behavioural arousal is dependent upon dose, with an initial increase in arousal followed by a decrease with larger doses of nicotine. Dose dependent effects are not at all uncommon with psychoactive drugs. The possibility of opposing effects of different dosages provides scope for a drug to be used in different ways and indeed Paxton concluded his review by proposing that smokers may use tobacco to vary arousal levels in either direction.

Much the same thing has been proposed by others, for example by Matarazzo (1973), namely that smoking may be a response to the need to maintain a 'steady state' of arousal, whether this requires an increase or a decrease in stimulation or stress. Incidentally in this context he noted how frequently aggression had appeared in studies on smoking, both as a mood that often triggers smoking and as a trait that has often been found to be more present amongst smokers than non-smokers. The general point for present purposes is that the mood-modifying properties of a variety of appetitive activities should be taken seriously and that attention should not be limited to 'tension reduction', unless we define tension broadly to include anger and possibly a whole range of felt emotions.

These observations on smoking are very significant because they lead directly to a crucial point that can be made about appetitive behaviour in general, namely that behaviour can serve many *different* functions for different people and in addition that it can serve different functions for a single individual. If tobacco-smoking can be shown to produce opposite effects when only arousal of a psychophysiological kind is being examined, how much greater must be the scope for smoking to result in various quite disparate kinds of desired effects when the whole panoply of social, psychological, and physical outcomes is considered. The same can be said of alcohol and other drug use, eating, gambling, and sexual activity. This being the case, we should hardly expect to be able to predict, particularly over any great span of time (from adolescence to middle age for example), who will and who will not gain such reward from appetitive behaviour that they are at risk of initiating, continuing, or escalating the activity.

The recognition that there are important individual differences in accounts that smokers give of their motives for smoking, or the types of occasions on which they smoke, has led a number of researchers to look for different types of smoking. One of the first such typologies was developed by Tomkins (e.g. 1968) who concluded that there were four main types: positive affect (motivated by the arousal of positive feelings), negative affect (motivated by the reduction of negative affects including tension and anxiety), addictive, and habitual smoking. The second of these, negative affect smoking, comes closest to the idea of 'tension reduction'. Ikard and Tomkins (1973) carried out some interesting tests of this typology with some success. For instance, in one study university student smokers who described predominantly negative affect smoking were observed to smoke more than others during the viewing of a documentary film about Second World War concentration camp atrocities. In another study spectators at a public race track were unobtrusively observed during different stages before, during, and after a race. The highest ratio of people smoking to those not smoking was observed during the race itself. However, although the researchers assumed that this would be a time of maximal *negative* affect, there seems intuitively no justification for describing affects customarily experienced during such a time as negative.

A second typology of smoking motives was that developed by McKennell and Thomas (1967) in the course of their survey into the smoking habits and attitudes of adolescents and adults. Their subjects were asked to indicate how likely or unlikely they were to smoke under a variety of different circumstances. Factor analysis of the data indicated seven factors, five representing what McKennell and Thomas called 'inner needs' and two social factors. Amongst the five inner need factors the one coming closest to 'tension reduction' was one which they labelled 'nervous irritation': high scorers on this factor said they were likely to smoke, 'when irritable', 'when anxious or worried', 'when angry', and 'when nervous' (p.63).

Russell *et al.* (1974) attempted to improve on these previous classifications by including the best items from the previous two lists, and by giving greater weight to the possibility of smoking because of 'nicotine dependence', a factor which they believed previous research had underplayed. Their analysis produced six factors, none corresponding to Tomkins' negative affect smoking or to McKennell and Thomas' nervous irritation factor. However, as is well known to those who use multivariate statistics, the results are highly susceptible to the exact nature of the items put into the analysis. When Russell *et al.* repeated their analysis based upon a smaller selection of items a 'sedation' factor emerged to which two items in particular contributed: 'I smoke more when I am worried about something', and, 'I light up a cigarette when I feel angry about something'. Although Russell *et al.* accorded this factor a peripheral status on account of the results of the multivariate analyses they carried out, an inspection of the data on the frequencies with which their subjects applied these items to themselves reveals the importance of this 'motive'. These two items were amongst the most frequently endorsed both by subjects in their main sample (a cross-section of staff of a London teaching hospital) and in their smoking clinic sample. In fact, the first of these two items was the most frequently endorsed of all 34 items in their analysis in the case of the smoking clinic sample, and was ranked second for the main sample (the most frequently endorsed item for the main sample being, 'after meals is the time I most enjoy smoking').

Although it may be argued that self-accounts of reasons for and occasions of smoking, or indeed of any other appetitive behaviour, are misleading, it does appear that the reduction of tension or of other unpleasant affects is part of the reason given by many people for their smoking. The same appears from surveys of drinking habits (e.g. Edwards *et al.*, 1972c; Mulford and Miller, 1960) to be true for alcohol consumption. As with smoking, however, the experimental evidence on the tension-reducing properties of alcohol is inconclusive. Some authors (e.g. Cappell and Herman, 1972) have gone so far as to conclude that the evidence on the whole is against the tension-reduction theory. Their review was based upon an examination of animal studies, and extrapolation to the human case is of course uncertain. In any event, Hodgson *et al.* (1979a) have considered the animal evidence again and have drawn opposite conclusions. They pointed out that a number of distinctions need to be made in order to give the tension-reduction theory a fair test. One of these is that between 'passive' and 'active' avoidance learning. Much of the negative evidence derived from studies in which animals avoided an aversive experience such as electric shock by actively moving when they perceived a discriminating stimulus such as a light or buzzer which had previously preceded the aversive stimulus. Drawing on recent adaptations of learning theory, Hodgson *et al.* argued that animals under these circumstances may not experience tension at all, and hence the demonstration that alcohol has no effect on this behaviour is no test of its tension-reducing properties. A much more adequate test, in their view, is a passive avoidance paradigm in which, for example, an animal is shocked if it *does* respond. Early studies by Conger (1951) and Masserman and Yum (1946) in which rats and cats had to approach a goal box where they received shock in order to feed there (hence setting up an 'approach-avoidance conflict') provided such a test. In these, and experiments carried out since, it has regularly been found that alcohol reduces the tendency to avoid and enables the animal to approach the goal. In such circumstances, Hodgson *et al.* argued, the animal experiences an increasing number of cues that elicit conditioned anxiety as the goal is approached. Hence, tension is aroused and such experiments *do* provide a test of the tension-reduction hypothesis.

There can be little doubt that the matter is equally, and probably more, complex in the human case. Research on the tension-reducing effects of alcohol suggests that effects depend at least on dose, on individual differences, and on such factors as expectation. For example, small doses of alcohol appeared in at least one experiment to reduce anxiety for the college students who served as subjects (Williams, 1966), whilst larger doses produced reports of increased anxiety (i.e. an opposite dose effect to that found for nicotine with rats). Studies by Mayfield and Coleman (e.g. 1968) showed greater tension-reducing effects of alcohol for subjects who were depressed than for others. In general it has proved difficult to demonstrate tension reduction in an experimental setting, but in at least one study (Higgins and Marlatt, 1975) great pains were taken to make sure that social anxiety was aroused (subjects were led to believe that their social performance would be rated by opposite sex peers) and heavy social drinkers were chosen as subjects; this combination did indeed lead to greater drinking.

Hodgson *et al.* (1979a) pointed out that there are learning mechanisms which may explain the development of a drinking habit on the basis of tension reduction, even if it is the case that drinking frequently fails to relieve tension or even increases it. First, each separate drink during a drinking occasion may be followed by a brief period of tension reduction, even though the cumulative effect of drinking heavily may be the opposite. Stockwell *et al.* (1982) have produced evidence that this effect does occur in the case of some people with drinking problems and their study will be discussed in greater detail in the following chapter. Secondly, drinking may be reinforced by tension reduction only intermittently, a case of 'partial' reinforcement known to lead to behaviour which is relatively difficult to extinguish. On the basis of their clinical experience, Hodgson *et al.* preferred a third explanation based on the notion of the relativity of reinforcement. Even if anxiety increases as a result of prolonged drinking, this may still be reinforcing if it is less distressing than the frustration, anxiety, or withdrawal symptoms that the person *expected* to experience if he or she had not continued to drink. In fact, modern adaptations of learning theory place considerable weight upon expectations of the outcomes of different behaviours and we shall consider the role of expectations further in Chapter 9.

Hull (1981), too, points out how very complex is the question of whether alcohol reduces tension. Different studies have suggested that alcohol may increase muscle relaxation even though it does not reduce self-reported anxiety; that in addition to its other effects the realization that one is consuming alcohol may itself increase tension (particularly for people who feel guilty about it); and that it may decrease heart rate, even when self-reported anxiety is unaffected. Hull believes that overall the evidence is not in favour of the tension-reduction hypothesis and in its place proposes a 'self-awareness' model. This proposal grew out of the Hull and Levy (1979) adaptation of Duval and Wicklund's (1972) theory of self-awareness in social psychology. The view is that alcohol reduces the user's level of self-awareness, thereby decreasing sensitivity to information about present and past behaviour. If behaviour is, or has been, inappropriate and liable to self- and other-criticism, then a reduction in self-awareness may provide a source of psychological relief.

Although Hull does not make this point explicitly, it can be seen how valuable this function of alcohol would be to someone experiencing the kind of dissonance and conflict which I have suggested is the hallmark of excessive appetitive behaviours. If Hull is correct, drinking alcohol might be one of the most effective ways of temporarily reducing the discomfort of knowing that one's behaviour is deviant. Hull reviewed an impressive array of research which is consistent with this theory, although it is admittedly difficult to test and many of the results could be interpreted in other ways. Studies included one in which subjects who had consumed alcohol made fewer self-focused statements than those who had consumed only tonic water (interestingly this was one experiment where it was the consumption of alcohol itself which made the difference, and not having been *told* that alcohol had been consumed—see pp.180–181 below); one in which subjects who had been given alcohol gave more shocks to partners in a 'pain-perception' task and gave them less contingently upon the partner's response; and studies showing that those who had consumed alcohol performed less well on various tasks but at the same time were unaware of the inferior quality of their performance. Hull was aware that no single theory could totally account for the use and misuse of alcohol, and that the model proposed was an over-simplification. Nevertheless, it is an important and well thought out attempt to make sense of quite a large body of research and it merits serious consideration.

Before leaving the issue of emotional control and alcohol, mention should be made of the model proposed by Russell and Mehrabian (1978) because it incorporates some features not included by others. Although their views of the way in which drug use affects emotions are undoubtedly over-simple, their model has some undoubted virtues and generates some directly testable predictions. Their general theory of the emotions proposes that most feeling states can be reduced to three dimensions: pleasure–displeasure, high–low arousal, and dominance–submissiveness. In its application to drug use, the theory supposes that felt effects depend upon dose (alcohol perhaps producing pleasure, arousal, and dominance in moderate doses, but less pleasure, reduced arousal, and increased submissiveness in larger doses), and that its effects are additive with features of the setting (the assumption is that settings also can be described as affecting pleasure, arousal, and dominance in one direction or another) and the person's prior mood state. Amongst interesting ideas that can be generated from this model, is the expectation that a drug like alcohol in moderate doses may produce a feeling of 'excitement' (pleasure, high arousal, dominance) in a setting that contributes to pleasure, but that this may easily translate into 'anger' (displeasure, high arousal, dominance) if the circumstances change into ones that promote displeasure. This has a certain appeal, and perhaps begins to help explain how excitement at a sporting event can so rapidly turn into violence under the influence of alcohol, and why some drunks so amenable at the pub or club can be so abusive when they return home.

A complete theory of mood modification and drugs would of course have to include the propensity of different groups of drugs to produce different felt effects. A whole programme of research on this subject has been carried out at the U.S. National Institute of Mental Health Addiction Research Centre using a self-report inventory which includes, for example, one scale referred to as the 'pentobarbital–chlorpromazine–alcohol group'—containing largely sluggish, heavy, drowsy-type items as opposed to the clear-headed, happy-type items of the 'morphine–benzedrine group' scale (e.g. Jasinski *et al.*, 1971).

Where do the other non-drug forms of appetitive behaviour fit into the tension-reduction or mood-control scheme? In the case of gambling it has often been suggested that, far from being a purely instrumental, affectively bland, activity motivated largely by financial reward, it is in fact for many people an emotionally intense and complex experience. Surveys of gamblers reviewed by Cornish (1978) have produced reports of 'excitement', 'thrill', and 'challenge', for example. It has been suggested that gambling is 'stimulus-seeking', or that, as others have suggested for smoking, it serves the need to maintain arousal at some optimum level. Alternatively the uncertain or risky nature of gambling may provide a sought-after 'strain' or 'pleasurable–painful tension' (e.g. Bolen and Boyd, 1968). Gamblers' reports give grounds, then, for supposing that gambling is a potential mood modifier, or psychotropic activity, to borrow the jargon normally reserved for pharmacological agents. It would probably be grossly over-simple to suppose that its major affective function was one of tension reduction, however. Indeed, there would be as strong grounds for supposing the opposite.

Finally, it should be recalled that several of the clinical and autobiographical anecdotes referred to in Chapter 6 suggested that sexual behaviour may serve mood-modifying functions, or at least may be triggered by felt emotion, amongst those whose sexual behaviour is excessive. This raises a further general question which will be considered more fully below, namely whether tension reduction or other mood-modifying functions of appetitive activity are present for some individuals early on in their history of activity or whether they are acquired as a result of a process of generalization that occurs as behaviour becomes more excessive.

Whatever the answer to this question, and from all that has been said so far we should hardly expect a simple answer, it is clear that most and probably all of the appetitive behaviours with which this book is concerned have in common the propensity either to alter mood in various complex ways or at least to offer the expectation that their consumption or use will change mood. These commonalities could partly explain some of the links between different excessive appetitive behaviours noted by Miller, P. (1980). He pointed to findings that dieters, unlike non-dieters, eat more after thinking they have consumed alcohol; that drinking increases smoking rate amongst smokers; that there is a tendency to increase weight on giving up smoking; that smoking often increases for excessive drinkers who give up drinking; and that alcohol use has been noted to increase for heroin 'addicts' who give up heroin. He might have added the tendency of doctors to prescribe drugs with 'dependence potential' to help people overcome drug 'addictions' and other kinds of excessive appetitive behaviour. The explanation put forward by Miller for these commonalities is that they are linked via a common difficulty in maintaining stability of arousal level.

THE PERSONAL FUNCTIONS OF APPETITIVE BEHAVIOUR

Some time has been spent considering the possible mood-modifying functions of appetitive behaviours, but although such theories have an important place in the catalogue of ideas about the causes of excessive appetitive behaviour, they hardly exhaust the possibilities. One of the commonest approaches to appetitive behaviour has been a general functionalist one. According to Sadava (1975) it has been one of the four principal approaches to understanding illicit drug use—the others being the socio-cultural, the psychopathological, and social learning—and is an eclectic position consisting of the enumeration of the reasons or functions underlying drug use. Two main points emerge from his review of work on drugs within the functionalist tradition. First, it is very evident that the list of the functions of drugs reported by users or inferred by observers is a lengthy one and, secondly, the point is strongly made that the functions served by drug use are not universal but to a large extent vary with, and are a reflection of, the age and socio-cultural positions of the user.

To illustrate these points, Sadava culled from the literature the following possible functions of opiate use in urban slums: to achieve detachment; to reduce threats to feelings of adequacy; to reduce drive states; to suppress pain and discomfort; to achieve a state of aloofness and isolation; to protect against depression, psychotic reaction, or sadistic impulses; to forget personal problems; to cope with sexuality; to help control social anxiety; to allow the expression of dependency; to express rebellion or hostility against the dominant culture; to enhance peer status; to relieve a sense of boredom; to provide some sense of purpose in an otherwise purposeless life; to relieve frustration or anxiety; and to expiate guilt by self-punishing behaviour. Thus, even confining attention to one group of drugs within one broad socio-cultural setting, the range of suggested functions is very wide indeed.

The same is true of the list Sadava produced for opiate use by 'physician addicts', although some of the functions in this case are different from those proposed for urban slum use. The list included: to relieve fatigue; to cope with marital problems; to relieve physical distress; to provide an alternative to excess alcohol use and to relieve alcohol hangovers; to relieve role strain inherent in their job; to relieve the conflict between the activity of their job and a basic passivity; and to enhance fantasies of omnipotence. The functions of student psychedelic drug use may be different again, including: to aid the search for meaning; to expand mental experience; to achieve a temporary state of loss of identity; or to help establish personal identity.

To these differences in age and social context should be added the observation that the functions of drugs can be very different for men and women, even though they be of the same generation and social position. This emerged strongly, for example, in Cooperstock and Lennard's (1979) analysis of stated functions of prescribed tranquillizer use. Like U.S. physician opiate users, their Canadian men mainly described drug use to ease the stress and conflict of their work, whilst the more numerous women in their sample emphasized using drugs to help cope with the strains and role conflicts of being wives and mothers. In another study, we have found that women excessive alcohol users are less likely than their male counterparts to refer to the positive social functions of drinking when asked to give their reasons for alcohol use (Orford and Keddie, 1984).

The functions listed above, many and varied though they are, do not include others reported from quite different cultures. Drug use in different parts of Asia, for example, may serve to relieve hunger, to alleviate symptoms of disease, to intensify sexual pleasure, or, as was so common in Victorian Britain, to sedate infants.

Sadava is another who has made the point, agreeing with many others including Robins *et al.* (1977), McKennell and Thomas (1967), and Cornish (1978), that the functions served by later, continuing activity, may not be the same as those served by early, initial use. He further noted, as have others who have studied motives for alcohol use (Edwards *et al.*, 1972c; Mulford and Miller, 1960), that it is a consistent finding that the heavier the pattern of drug use, the larger the number of functions reported for its use. This will be a crucial point in our discussion of the development of *excessive* behaviour in the following chapters.

Kaplan and Kaplan (1957) performed the same task of listing the various functions which it had been suggested might be served, in this case by over-eating. They included the reduction of anxiety, insecurity or indecision, a diversion from monotony, the relief of frustration or discouragement, the expression of hostility, self-indulgence, a way of rewarding oneself for some task accomplished, rebellion against authority and control, submission to authority, self-punishment and self-degradation, guilt-reduction, exhibitionism, to gain attention or care, to test love and affection, to justify failure, to sedate, to avoid competition, to avoid maturity, to substitute for pregnancy, to protect against sexuality, and, amongst the poor, to diminish fear of starvation. These motives might be conscious or unconscious according to the Kaplans and do not include suggested symbolic functions such as 'alimentary orgasm' or 'penis envy'. They suggested that the great range of functions listed, and those mentioned above by no means cover their list, indicates that *any* emotional conflict may be the cause of over-eating and that the psychological factors involved are non-specific.

Bruch (1974), too, was critical of what she called the 'thermodynamic approach' to excessive eating with its prescription of, 'eat less and exercise more' (p.29), because it ignored the many psychological functions to which eating could be put. Her book, *Eating Disorders: Obesity, Anorexia Nervosa, and the Person Within*, was based on her experience with a group of people, admittedly very selective, for whom eating, or not eating in the case of anorexia, served psychological purposes. In such cases of obesity, it was her view that this represented a protection against more severe disorder, an effort to stay well or at least to be less sick. For such people weight loss itself had to be considered a secondary question. In her view, though, food lent itself so readily to such psychological purposes, that these functions of eating were present, in part, for everyone:

> For normal people, too, food is never restricted to the biological aspects alone. There is no human society that deals rationally with food in its environment, that eats according to the availability, edibility, and nutritional value alone. Food is endowed with complex values and elaborate ideologies, religious beliefs, and prestige systems . . . It is these aspects that give to eating habits and food traditions their special cultural and national character, and to the food habits of one's background and family the emotional connotation of warmth and home (Bruch, 1974, p.3).

The many functions which Bruch saw as being potentially served by over-eating are illustrated in another quotation:

> Food may symbolically stand for an insatiable desire for unobtainable love, or as an expression of rage and hatred; it may substitute for sexual gratification or indicate ascetic denial; it may represent the wish to be a man and possess a penis, or the wish to be

> pregnant or fear of it. It may provide a sense of spurious power and thus lead to self-aggrandizement, or it may serve as a defence against adulthood and responsibility. Preoccupation with food may appear as helpless, dependent clinging to parents, or as hostile rejection of them (p.44).

Bruch also stressed the great diversity of eating patterns and personality types to be found amongst the over-weight or obese and regretted the way that many theorists have attempted to generalize. Indeed, she pointed out that the incidence of over-weight was such that not all instances could possibly be due to the same causes or present the same picture. Amongst attempts to make some order of this diversity, she cited Stunkard's (1959) 'night eating syndrome' and 'binge eating syndrome'; Hamburger's (1951) types which included those patients who over-ate in response to non-specific emotional tensions, those who used food as a substitute gratification to solve problems of chronic tension and frustration, those for whom over-eating was a symptom of an underlying emotional illness often depression, and those for whom over-eating became an 'addiction' characterized by compulsive craving for food apparently unrelated to life events or emotions; as well as her own division into three main groups: the developmentally obese, the reactively obese, and those for whom over-weight appeared unrelated to abnormal psychological functioning (p.124).

Bruch's ideas were derived from close knowledge of individuals who had sought help. Such data have advantages and disadvantages as bases for an explanation of excessive appetitive behaviour. On the one hand, they suffer by being selectively based upon clinical cases and by being subject to the biases of the observing clinician. On the other hand, they provide a relatively rich source, often the only such source, of in-depth knowledge of individuals whose appetites have become excessive.

Even relatively superficial surveys, however, suggest the range of motives for appetitive behaviour. Russell *et al.*'s (1974) analysis of self-reported motives for smoking, for example, found that some people reported smoking not for obvious tension-reduction, or sedative, reasons, but rather, 'while busy and working hard', 'to keep going when tired', 'to help think and concentrate', 'to get a definite lift and feel more alert', and 'when rushed and having lots to do'. This they termed 'stimulation smoking'. Others reported smoking most, 'when comfortable and relaxed', 'after meals', 'when having a quiet rest', and 'when I can really sit back and enjoy it' ('indulgent smoking'). That an activity such as smoking may serve other quite simple motives is suggested by the finding that some people reported enjoying handling cigarettes, the pleasure of having something in their mouths, of watching smoke as they blow it out, taking steps to light up, and enjoying the smell ('sensorimotor smoking').

McKennell and Thomas (1967) found two social motive factors which combined in Russell *et al.*'s typology to form factor III (psychosocial smoking). One of these they termed simply 'social smoking', highest scorers being those who said they liked to smoke, 'in company', 'at a party', 'when talking', and who, 'get more pleasure out of smoking when in company than alone'. It is with the second of these two factors that we move further into the realm of more complex personal motivation. Highest scorers on this factor, the 'social confidence' factor, were those who said, for example, that they, 'felt happier with other smokers than with non-smokers', 'smoking helped them to feel more sure of themselves and gave them confidence with other people', that they, 'felt that by smoking they looked more relaxed to others and fitted in better in a group', and in the case of adolescents that, 'smoking helped them to feel more grown up'. McKennell and Thomas in fact found that adolescents scored particularly highly on this factor, but that this motive for smoking became less prominent in smokers' self-reports with increasing age. Bynner's (1969) study of teenage smoking suggested the great importance of a person's self-concept and the image of an activity such as smoking as a means of promoting or enhancing a desired self-image. Although the self-concept and its assessment are complex matters (for example, is it more important what a person thinks of herself or what she thinks *others* think of her?; how many additional 'layers' of the self-concept should we distinguish?), the results of Bynner's study were in general fairly clear. On the whole young people who smoked were seen by themselves and by their peers as more tough and precocious.

Such approaches to the question of personality and appetitive behaviour as the motivational typologies of smokers or Bruch's analysis of different motives for excessive eating are relatively sophisticated approaches in comparison with, for example, the over-simple search for such unlikely entities as 'the alcoholic personality'. The attempt to find a personality type predisposed to excessive appetitive behaviour of a particular form seems at some time or another to have been a preoccupation with each of the forms of behaviour with which we are concerned. Cornish (1978) was rightly critical of, '. . . simple person-centred forms of explanation . . .', which still dominate the relatively new field of gambling research, '. . . at the expense of more sophisticated . . . viewpoints stressing the importance of situational determinants . . .' (pp.88–9). The former, he argued, arise because the unwarranted assumptions have been made, first, that gamblers are similar to one another and different from non-gamblers and, secondly, that gamblers are engaged in a similar basic activity, hence ignoring the evident differences which exist between the various forms of gambling, as others had earlier ignored differences in eating or smoking patterns. Coupled with these assumptions is a third, of which Cornish was particularly critical, namely the assumption that explanations for the *initial* decision to gamble are closely related to those explaining *persistent* gambling. This leads to person-centred concepts stressing motives arising from maladjustments of personality and attitudes. What he said about the tendency to look to 'internal' causes of personality or attitude (quoted at the beginning of this chapter) applies with equal force to any form of appetitive behaviour.

Cornish recognized, nevertheless, that there might be 'expressive' motives for participation in gambling in addition to those that are purely economic or 'instrumental' or mood modifying. Suggestions that have been put forward by those who have studied gamblers or gambling in some form or another vary widely. At one level, for example, it has been suggested that gambling enables people who are lower in status in a competitive society to compensate by 'achieving' in a world where very different skills and abilities operate. A number of observers of gambling, for example Herman (1976) in the case of on-course horse-race betting in the United States and Newman (1972) for East End London betting shops, have similarly proposed that gambling is largely motivated by the opportunities it provides for exercising intelligent choice, the experience of control, the opportunity to discuss with others, and to appear knowledgeable. Against this Cornish pointed out that Dickerson (1974) observed very little discussion and interpersonal contact in betting shops, and Downes *et al.* (1976) pointed out that pools punters on the whole do not discuss their gambling with others.

There seems little doubt though that the appetitive behaviours with which we are concerned can each serve a very considerable variety of functions. Nor can we omit sexual behaviour from this generalization. It too can clearly serve many human personality functions, as Hardy (1964) and Gross (1978) have both reminded us. Gross, for example, has pointed out that sex for men can serve the needs for success (producing a high rate of orgasms in partners being merely the modern fashionable equivalent of achieving a large number of sexual conquests), of control and power (men are still much more likely to be expected to be the initiators of sexual activity, and are expected to be knowledgeable and not to have to seek advice), and for aggression and violence (Gross reviews evidence that some degree of aggression on the part of males in the course of sexual activity is widespread and by no means confined to occasions of acknowledged rape).

It follows, surely, that no theory of the causes of excessive appetitive behaviour could succeed that was based upon the assumption that such behaviour served one particular function, such as tension reduction, for each and every person whose behaviour became excessive. A psychology of excess must take into account the great diversity of purposes to which these behaviours can be put.

THE LIMITATIONS OF SIMPLE PERSONAL EXPLANATIONS

The problem with a great deal of 'personality' research is, as Cornish pointed out, not only that it assumes homogeneity amongst 'gamblers', 'alcoholics', or 'the obese', but also that it has rested upon a crude and now outdated view of what constitutes personality. The search has been for enduring traits without regard either to the large part played by situation and the interaction between situation and person in the determination of behaviour, or to the possibility of a change in a person's standing on a trait dimension during the course of adolescent or adult life. Amongst traits which have been examined in the context of gambling are 'locus of control'—the hypothesis being that people who feel themselves to be 'externally' controlled by fate or circumstance are more prone to gamble than those who feel themselves to be 'internally' in control of themselves—and 'risk-taking'. On the face of it these two characteristics appear to be relatively good candidates to explain at least a proportion of the variance in gambling behaviour: there is at least a clear theoretical justification for them, and they would qualify as relatively 'proximal' personality variables in Jessor and Jessor's (1977) sense. Nevertheless, in view of the many criticisms of traditional personality research, it is not surprising to find that they fall far short of commanding widespread acceptance as factors accounting for why some people gamble and others do not.

Much personality research has been *post hoc*, based upon examination of people whose appetitive behaviour has already come to notice as being excessive. This fact immediately gives rise to the most challenging question: Are we witnessing the causes of excess or its consequences? The individual excessive drinker, for example, may impress people as having a distinctive temperament, and it is always tempting to assume that the causes of his or her excess lie therein, and to extend this reasoning to other excessive drinkers also. Clearly, only longitudinal, predictive research can establish whether certain characteristics existed prior to the development of excessive habitual behaviour. In the case of alcohol use there have in fact been four major studies of this kind (McCord and McCord, 1960; Robins, 1966; Jones, 1968; Kammeier *et al.*, 1973) and there does appear to be a certain consistency between the results. If anything, it was the adolescent boy (with the exception of a smaller sub-study of the Jones study, all were confined to males) whose behaviour was relatively aggressive, impulsive, and difficult for others to control, who was more at risk of later excessive or problem drinking. There are perhaps no great surprises here: the best predictor of future uncontrolled behaviour is present uncontrolled behaviour (a further support for proximal variables). The limitations of these studies should however be borne in mind. Each was North American, and as well as having little or nothing to say about girls and women, the two larger studies concerned special populations of high risk youngsters (McCord and McCord followed up 255 boys thought to be at high risk of future delinquency as part of the Cambridge–Somerville study; Robins examined the Child Guidance Clinic records for 503 childhood attenders of whom a proportion were found to have drinking problems later in life).

A major personality theory of obesity, the externality theory, also illustrates a number of the problems with research on personality and appetitive behaviour. Schachter (1971) proposed that whilst normal people eat largely in response to internal, hunger cues, obese people eat more in response to external or situational stimuli. Schachter and others carried out a series of intriguing experiments which tended to support this view (Ley, 1980). For example, preloading (i.e. feeding a person before an experiment) reduced the probability of eating in the lean but not in the obese; palatability of food had more effect on the eating of the obese than on the lean; in the absence of food-related cues, the obese were less affected by hours of food deprivation than the lean; and eating in the obese was triggered by apparent time while in the lean it was triggered more by real time (the discrepancy being created by deliberately altering clocks or by studying subjects who had travelled across time zones) (Ley, 1980).

To this point the externality theory is one linking the state of being obese with one general aspect of responsiveness to specifically food-related cues or stimuli. It required the next step in order to qualify the theory as a personality theory, and with that step the implication becomes stronger that the tendency towards externality may have predated obesity and perhaps have been partially causative of it. This step was taken by Rodin (1978) who put forward the view that the obese were *generally* 'stimulus-bound' or especially reactive to salient external stimuli, not merely food-related ones. Evidence in support of this view included the findings that the obese were more reactive to electric shock, were more reactive to emotional stimuli, were more affected by distracting stimuli, and were better at incidental learning (Ley, 1980).

As is so often the case in an area short of strong theories, the idea of externality was hailed for some time as offering the key to understanding the often intractable problem of obesity, and the theory stimulated a great deal of research. The consensus of opinion now appears to be that the case for externality was overstated and that the theory certainly requires considerable modification if it is to survive at all (Ley, 1980). The strongest support Leon and Roth (1977) found in their review came from studies of time estimation in which obese people reported longer estimations of elapsed time in the presence of external visual or auditory stimuli or emotionally arousing material. There are also other serious problems with the theory as it stands. Rodin herself (1978) has questioned whether the distinction between internal and external stimuli is as straightforward as had previously been supposed and whether it has not, '. . . outlived its usefulness?'. Her present view is that internal and external factors are interrelated rather than to be thought of as constituting the two opposite ends of a continuum. She reviewed considerable evidence that internal state (level of food deprivation) affects such aspects of the perception of food stimuli as the pleasantness of sweet taste, as well as fantasies about palatable foods and amounts of salivation when palatable food is presented. On the basis of recent evidence, Rodin believes that the opposite direction of influence also holds, namely that external stimuli can directly influence internal physiological state. For example, external and sensory stimuli such as the taste, smell, and sight of attractive food (Rodin has used the presentation of a grilling steak in some of her own experiments) affects not only salivation but also the release of insulin. Another demonstration of the intimate relationship between internal and external factors comes from Rodin's study of patients who had received intestinal by-pass surgery for obesity resulting in a greatly shortened intestinal tract. The preference curve for sweetness intensity of such people changed dramatically after surgery and became indistinguishable from the curve obtained from normal weight subjects.

A second major problem with this work is the one raised in Chapter 5, concerning definitions of excessive eating and the question of the selection of subjects for such experiments. In fact, recent evidence suggests that external responsiveness, far from being peculiar to the obese, is to be found at all weight levels and may be most common amongst those who are slightly over-weight or amongst 'restrained eaters' who may be of normal weight or below but who are deliberately moderating their eating in order to keep their weight down (Rodin, 1978; Ley, 1980).

In view of the general lack of cross-fertilization between research on different appetitive behaviours, it is reassuring to see that the idea of externality, previously confined to studies of obesity, has been thought worthy of testing in the field of excessive drinking. Tucker *et al.* (1979) found, as predicted, that the quantity of beverage consumed in a taste test was less affected by a liquid preload for 'alcoholics' than for 'normal drinkers' (both were prisoners in an American State penetentiary). Furthermore, 'alcoholics' drank relatively more of the 'preferred' as opposed to the 'non-preferred' beverage. It is important to realize, however, that these beverages were non-alcoholic (orange juice and grapefruit juice being the preferred and non-preferred beverages, respectively). What seems to be under study here, therefore, is not external responsiveness to cues directly related to the object of excessive consumption (alcoholic beverages), nor external responsiveness *in general*, but rather external versus internal responsiveness for the consumption of beverages in general. The distinction is important, because of the confusion that has arisen over whether externality is part of a special relationship between some people and the objects of their special interest or excessive behaviour (alcohol for excessive drinkers, gambling for compulsive gamblers, sexual stimuli for the hypersexual, etc.), or whether we are dealing with general external responsiveness as a personality characteristic which might confer some 'addiction proneness'. Tucker *et al.* themselves raise the question of whether their finding has aetiological significance for alcohol 'dependence'. As they wisely point out:

> Though it may be that prior to developing a drinking problem, alcoholics respond differently than normal drinkers to internal and external stimuli related to beverage consumption, it is equally plausible that alcoholics' differential responsivity to these stimuli is a result of their having repeatedly engaged in excessive alcohol consumption. It seems reasonable to speculate after repeated episodes of excessive beverage consumption . . . any control initially exerted by internal bodily cues over that consumption might diminish, whereas the external stimuli . . . associated with that consumption might become more salient (p.150).

Although there is still to be found the occasional argument for an 'addiction-prone' personality (e.g. Owen and Butcher, 1979, who raise again the question of an 'alcoholic personality' on the basis of MMPI studies and the longitudinal investigations referred to above), the general consensus of opinion now is that no single personality type is prone to excessive drinking (e.g. Mendelson and Mello, 1966), excessive eating (Ley, 1980), excessive gambling (Cornish, 1978), smoking (Paxton, 1980), or drug abuse (Kandel, 1978). Two caveats must be borne in mind, however. The first is the distinction to which repeated reference has already been made between distal and proximal personality variables. The search for the 'addictive personality', or species of it, such as the 'alcoholic personality', has largely looked in the direction of distal variables and it should come as little surprise that this search has not been highly fruitful.

The second caveat has to do with the assumptions being made about personality itself. Much of the research has been based upon relatively simple trait models of personality which scarcely do justice to some of the more complex and individual personality notions which have been put forward to explain appetitive behaviour. Amongst such explanations are those in the psychoanalytic tradition. Although psychoanalysts have not on the whole pressed any great claim to understand or to be able to treat excessive appetitive behaviour, there have been sporadic attempts to develop a psychoanalytic view. Bergler's theory of the origins of excessive gambling, for example, have been highly influential. He first put forward his view, in an article in the 1930s, that 'real' or neurotic gamblers had an unconscious wish to lose. There followed several further publications and popularization in several magazines such as *Reader's Digest* in the 1940s, and the theory of the unconscious wish to lose has since been adopted by Gamblers Anonymous.

Bergler was impressed by the excessive gambler's almost fanatical belief in the possibility of success; '. . . his illogical, senseless certainty that he will win' (1958, p.15). He was struck, as others with very different theoretical positions have been when considering this and other forms of excessive appetitive behaviour, by the selective nature of reminiscences, the dwelling on success, and the relative forgetting of numerous failures. Bergler concluded that the motivation for 'real' or excessive gambling must be unconscious. The fanatical, and illogical, belief in success was like the child's feeling of omnipotence or megalomania. Growing up involved replacing these feelings with the 'reality principle' largely instilled by parental figures. Gambling offered the perfect rebellion against this principle, because in gambling chance rules, and the virtues of honesty, logic, reason, and justice—all virtues that parents had taught—conferred no advantage. Hence, gambling revived old childhood fantasies of grandeur and, more important, '. . . it activates the *latent rebellion* against logic, intelligence, moderation, morality, and renunciation' (p.18, his emphasis). It enabled the individual:

> . . . to scoff ironically at all the rules of life he has learned from education and experience . . . Since the child has learned these rules from his parents and their representatives . . . his rebellion activates a profound unconscious feeling of guilt (p.18).

It is this unconscious rebellion against parents that is responsible, in Bergler's view, for the neurotic wish to lose, because, like all acts or feelings of rebellion against parents, whether conscious or unconscious, it produces feelings of guilt and an unconscious tendency to self-punishment.

Although Bergler seems to have been unaware that motivation can change greatly with the development of excess, his is a persuasive argument for one particular kind of expressive motivation for excessive appetitive behaviour. It is of interest that it is the 'wish to lose' part of Bergler's formulation that has been best remembered, although it is by no means the most prominent part of the theory expounded in his book, and it is probably the aspect of his ideas which fits least well with observations made by others about excessive gambling and other forms of excessive appetitive behaviour. On the other hand, his descriptive account of excessive gambling, for example the way in which it precludes other interests, and in particular the way in which it involves distorted thinking, plus his views on the possible function of excessive gambling as rebellion, are well described, and have parallels in others' descriptions of other forms of excessive behaviour.

In 1933, Rado had presented a psychoanalytic view of 'pharmacothymia' (drug addiction) remarkably similar in outline to parts of Bergler's (1958) view of 'compulsive gambling'. Like many others, his view was, '. . . not the toxic agent, but the impulse to use it, makes an addict of a given individual' (p.78 of Shaffer and Burglass, 1981). Drugs which could be classed as 'elatents', either allaying or preventing pain or producing euphoria, could magically restore that feeling of omnipotence associated with infantile narcissistic gratification which is forced to give way to 'the realistic regime of the ego' with increasing age. This 'elation' lasted, however, only a short while, with inevitable return to feelings of depression now exacerbated ('sharpened by contrast') and with the addition of a sense of guilt and increased fear of reality. As Rado put it, '. . . the ego has become more irritable and, because of the increased anxiety and bad conscience, weaker . . .' (p.83). The cyclical state set up what Rado referred to as a 'pharmacothymic regime' standing in contrast to a 'realistic regime', i.e. '. . . this illness is a narcissistic disorder, a destruction through artificial means of the natural ego organization' (p.83). Although couched in the psychoanalytic language of the time, Rado's understanding that the emotional changes associated with drug-taking changed with continued use, producing 'diminishing returns', is not inconsistent with other theories, including the 'opponent process theory' (Solomon and Corbit, 1973), which was developed at a much later date and in a quite different psychological tradition and will be considered further in Chapter 10.

In Freudian terms, obesity has also been explained as a regression, in this case to the early oral level of psychosexual development. Excessive eating therefore represents an infantile, dependent form of pleasure-seeking, in contrast to facing up to adult life frustrations and the need to strike a balance between dependence and independence (Kaplan and Kaplan, 1957).

Psychoanalytic views of 'alcoholism', reviewed by Lisansky (1960), have also revolved around oral narcissism and the 'alcoholic's' inability to cope and a need for easy satisfaction and indulgence. Lisansky acknowledged the point that these characteristics may be more of a consequence of excess than a cause of it.

As a final illustration of psychoanalytic theory, Robbins (1956) described a case of Don Juanism treated by psychoanalysis. The patient had numerous affairs, almost all with married women, and in addition had recurrent episodes of excessive drinking leading finally to an aversion therapy cure for his 'alcoholism'. His treatment exposed deep-seated anxieties, feelings of inferiority, and fears of lack of masculinity and potency. Robbins concluded, as had Rank (1922, cited by Robbins) in his analysis of the legendary Don Juan, that the nucleus of his patient's conflict lay in his desire to possess his own mother and his rivalry with his elder brother and his father.

Some more recent views on the personality functions of appetitive behaviour have been articulated more precisely and in a way that renders them more easily amenable to testing. For instance, McClelland *et al.* (1972) have offered support from a wide range of sources, including observations of drinking parties, responses to projective materials under the influence of alcohol, and content analyses of folk tales from different parts of the world, in support of their theory that a major function of the drinking of alcohol is an increase in feelings of 'personal power'.

Similarly, Barry (1976) has reviewed cross-cultural and other evidence in favour of the view that dependency conflict motivates drunkenness. To the present author's mind, this is one of the most appealing of the personality theories of excessive drinking, but there can be little doubt that the theory is highly complex and that even its strongest exponents can be muddled in its presentation. There is a tendency, for example, to equate such terms as 'assertiveness', 'self-reliance', and 'independence'. At one point in Barry's chapter he implied that 'affectionateness' is the opposite of 'self-reliance' and can be equated with 'dependency'. Nevertheless, the view that as a child develops into adolescence and adulthood he or she is subject to conflict between motives of dependency and of self-reliance, and that alcohol has the capacity to relieve this conflict in a variety of possible ways, is an attractive notion. Barry cited the finding that people with drinking problems are more often the last born in their families than would be expected by chance as evidence for the dependency conflict theory, and also the evidence from the longitudinal studies referred to above suggesting that 'pre-alcoholics', are often '. . . assertive, uninhibited, sometimes hostile, and compulsively anti-social in behaviour . . .' (p.255). From anthropological work, he took the finding that there is a, '. . . low or inconsistent degree of reward for dependency characteristics in infancy and early childhood in societies with a high frequency of drunkenness' (p.255), and that in these same societies self-reliance is rewarded and dependency punished in later childhood and adult life. Quite apart from the difficulties of definition in such work, the evidence is hardly as strongly supportive as Barry made out, but there is enough suggestive evidence to make the theory a strong contender. However, like the power theory, this hypothesis is more directly relevant to men's drinking than women's, based as it is upon the assumption that men as adults have to suppress from consciousness any overt behaviour signs of dependency.

It is of course possible to generate a whole set of differing hypotheses to explain the consumption of alcohol, based upon discrepancies between different aspects of self-concept—between ideal and real, between conscious and unconscious, or between different aspects of the conscious self (Leland, 1982). The Wilsnacks, for example, carried out a series of studies (e.g. Wilsnack, 1973; Wilsnack and Wilsnack, 1978) to test their hypothesis that women are motivated to drink by a discrepancy between conscious feminine identification and unconscious masculinity, a conflict which is reduced by drinking, hence making women feel more feminine. They have indeed produced some support for this view, although Leland (1982) has pointed to a number of qualifications which need to be made. For one thing, the Wilsnacks' own later work suggested that younger women who drink heavily are more likely to consciously reject the traditional female role than to identify with it. There is other evidence, too, that women who develop drinking problems relatively early in life are different from those who develop problems only later on: the former, according to Gomberg (1979), being 'overtly rebellious' and having impulse control problems, a description which is intriguingly reminiscent of the characteristics found to be predictive of later problem drinking amongst men in those few longitudinal studies which exist. Of even greater importance, perhaps, is the qualification which must be introduced once data from individuals are considered separately rather than *en masse*. It appears from the Wilsnacks' and other studies that only a minority of women who drink excessively show the particular pattern of sex-role conflict which they had predicted. This proportion may be higher than that to be found amongst control groups of women, but the majority of excessively drinking women show *other* forms of sex-role conflict (often at no higher a rate than that to be found amongst controls) or no obvious conflict at all.

Once again, then, we have an individual personality-based theory of the origins of excessive behaviour which turns out on close examination to have no more than limited value, and once again this should come as no surprise. The multiple-variable approach used to good effect by Jessor and Jessor (1977) and others (see Chapter 7 above); the longitudinal element which they, Robins *et al.* (1977) and others have introduced and which shows how appetitive behaviour changes as part of a wider personal, developmental process, and how different personal and social factors are predictive at different stages in an 'appetitive career'; the huge number of different personal functions which appetitive behaviours can potentially serve; as well as the historical and cross-cultural perspectives introduced in the early chapters in Part I and which show clearly how the psychological meaning and use of a drug or activity varies from time to time and place to place, all should alert us to the futility of the search for personality variables, other than the most 'proximal' to appetitive behaviour itself, which provide more than a very partial explanation of excessive forms of appetitive behaviour in general. Such theories may, however, be valid as explanations for the transition, or lack of it, from one stage of a developmental process to the next, for certain individuals in a certain socio-cultural position at one historical moment in time. Conflict over sex-role identification may be part of the reason why a woman does not diet when she has become over-weight, and dependency conflict may be a partial explanation of why a man continues with heavy gambling after he and his wife have had their first child (note that most of the personality theories are as applicable to one form of excessive appetitive behaviour as to another), but neither is sufficient as anything like a total explanation of excessive eating or gambling as a whole.

ENVIRONMENT AND BIOLOGY

Much space has been devoted to personality theories despite their shortcomings. This is because they have been, and continue to be, so influential, and hence it is important to place them in perspective. Whilst it would be an error to give too much credence to any one particular theory, it would equally, in this author's view, be mistaken to dismiss personal explanations totally as some have tended to do. Nonetheless, Cornish (1978) was almost certainly right in attempting to correct what he saw as a previous imbalance in their favour. The purpose of the remainder of this chapter is, equally, to restore some semblance of balance by briefly reminding the reader of the importance, in the total picture, of environmental, and more briefly still, of biological factors.

On the basis of the wide-ranging evidence which he collected regarding the possible determinants of gambling, Cornish concluded that this almost total reliance upon person-centred forms of explanation had resulted in neglect of the importance of situational determinants. His own view rested heavily upon the importance of availability and 'ecologic opportunity', as he termed it. He referred to numerous studies showing the concentration of gambling outlets in working-class areas, for example, plus the influence of the visibility and acceptability of opportunities for gambling of different kinds. The free busing of customers to Nevada casinos, the attempt to establish off-course betting facilities at cricket, golf and other sporting events, and the placing of gambling machines in public houses, all are commercial attempts to increase the visibility and accessibility of opportunities for gambling. There are, furthermore, structural characteristics which render different gambling activities differentially attractive and some more prone to elicit excess than others. Cornish did not use the term 'dependence potential', but he came close to it when he stated that:

> . . . forms of gambling which offer participants a variety of odds and/or stake-levels at which to make bets, and hence choose the rate at which their wins or losses multiply are likely to appeal to a greater variety of people . . . When the opportunity to use longer-odds bets or higher stakes in order to multiply winnings or recoup losses rapidly is combined with a high event-frequency and short payout-interval, participants may be tempted to continue gambling longer than they might otherwise do (p.168).

The range of odds and the range of the possible stakes—what Weinstein and Deitch (1974) called 'multiplier potential'—was just one of the structural variables which Cornish considered important. Others, which together make up a structural 'profile' of the forms of gambling, include the interval elapsing between betting and paying out (the payout interval), the degree of active involvement of the bettor and the amount of skill involved, the probability of winning an individual bet, and the 'payment ratio' or average winnings per unit amount staked. An important consideration in Cornish's view was, '. . . the extent to which different forms of gambling create conditions which encourage the suspension of those forms of judgement which participants normally exercise in their daily lives' (p.171). The sumptuousness or artificiality of the surroundings may contribute additionally to this.

Although Cornish leant towards an environmental or 'ecological' position himself, he made a good point when he acknowledged that the presently available forms of outlet may reflect responses to the personal or expressive needs of former 'generations' of gamblers and that the structural and the intrapsychic may thus not be as independent as might be supposed.

In general it seems that we may currently be passing out of a period during which individual, intrapsychic, or psychopathological explanations of excessive behaviour were fashionable (when the 'diseases' of 'alcoholism', other forms of drug 'dependence', and 'compulsive gambling' were 'discovered'), and into a period in which far greater weight is given to the availability of opportunities for appetitive behaviour on a social and national level.

There is no better illustration of the move away from individual-centred explanations than the recent shift in thinking about the origins of excessive drinking. Note has had to be taken of the epidemiological finding that the average rate of consumption of alcohol within a population covaries with the number of heavy drinkers within that population and with the estimates of the amount of harm, at least of some kinds, generated by drinking in that population (Kendell, 1979). For example, correlations in excess of 0.90 have been found between liver cirrhosis death-rates and variations in average consumption both across time (e.g. the years 1954 to 1973 in Britain) and across different countries for the same year (Schmidt, 1977). These findings and others like them have been examined with a view to the probable effects of public control policies, the argument being that the numbers of excessive drinkers or drug-takers in a population can only be reduced, not by the treatment of individuals, but by somehow reducing the average level of consumption in the population as a whole (Smart, 1971; de Lint and Schmidt, 1971; Royal College of Psychiatrists, 1979).

Other relevant examples of analyses at the level of whole neighbourhoods or nations include Chein *et al.*'s (1964) now classic account of heroin 'addiction' in New York and Russell's (1973) investigation of price and tobacco consumption (see Chapter 4). In their book, sub-titled *The Road to H*, Chein *et al.* noted the highly disproportionate concentration of known cases in certain census tracts of the city, largely those with high Negro and Puerto Rican populations, high rates of family breakdown, and, for the most part, high rates of delinquency. Theirs is one of the very few analyses of *excessive* appetitive behaviour, as opposed to those of youthful, largely non-excessive appetitive behaviour, which attempts to combine environmental availability, family factors (non-cohesiveness), and personality (alienation, 'dysphoric' mood, and delinquency orientation).

Russell's (1973) demonstration that small increases in the price of cigarettes made little permanent difference to consumption because of the general trend towards cheaper cigarettes as the value of the pound fell, provided a good illustration of a society making one particular form of appetitive behaviour readily available to its members. It is an obvious point, but one easily overlooked when the focus is upon differences between individuals within one culture, that different activities are very unequally available in different societies. It is an often-expressed, but moot, point however whether it is the case that every society has its own brand of favourite 'addiction'. Barry (1976) certainly maintained that one of the factors, other than a low level of dependency conflict in a culture, which might limit the amount of excessive drinking was the availability of alternative behaviours that might serve some of the same functions. Other drugs such as kavakava, a mild sedative cum exhilarating drug used in parts of Melanesia and Polynesia, and tobacco used by North American Indians, may have been alternatives in the only two areas of the world not using alcohol prior to European contact (Marshall, 1976). Gambling could be another alternative: Adler and Goleman (1969) found the extent of drinking inversely related to the extent of gambling across more than 100 societies. The ancient Aztecs and the modern Jews are two examples of societies that have apparently abhorred excessive drinking but have exercised much greater permissiveness towards gambling, perhaps because each valued the clear-thinking associated with sobriety and the competitiveness necessary for gambling? (Adler and Goleman, 1969; Wasserman, 1982).

The Chinese provide another such example, and in this case there may be genetically determined biological factors at work which might partly explain a relatively low consumption of alcohol. Indeed, this is a good point at which to make brief mention of the possibility of genetic mechanisms in the transmission of excessive appetites. Since it is almost a truism to say that human behaviour is determined both by heredity and environment, and since a polarization of views concerning the predominance of one or other type of influence has proved sterile in other fields (such as the field of mental abilities), it would be odd indeed if heredity had no influence at all upon predisposition to excessive appetitive behaviour. Nevertheless, it is easy to neglect its influence. The case of excessive drinking may be used as an example, since there has been a resurgence of research on the familial transmission of drinking problems in recent years. The earlier assumption that heredity was of negligible importance has been overturned by research, particularly that carried out by Goodwin and his colleagues and reviewed by Goodwin (1979), Murray and Stabenau (1982), and Davies (1982). Amongst other things, children of 'alcoholic' biological parents showed a higher rate of excessive drinking in later life than other people, even when they had been adopted at an early age by substitute parents without drinking problems. Concordance rates for 'alcoholism' have been reported to be significantly higher in monozygotic than in dizygotic twins. A further study of half sibs (Schuckit *et al.*, 1972) found that the factor of having had an 'alcoholic' biological parent was more influential in determining later problem drinking than was the factor of having lived with an excessively drinking parent during childhood. Davies (1982) cautiously concludes that, '. . . *to some degree*, alcoholism can probably be transmitted from one generation to the next by a genetic mechanism. Its effect is to *increase the probability* that offspring will encounter problems with alcohol in later life' (p.77, his emphases).

Whether the process of genetic transmission, however important this may be, involves personality or physiology is unknown. There is evidence that female first degree relatives of individuals with drinking problems are at an unusually high risk for depression (Behar and Winokur, 1979) and there are known to be variant forms of dehydrogenase, the enzyme responsible for breakdown of alcohol in the liver. It has also been shown that there are racial differences in rates of metabolism and in responses to small amounts of alcohol, and this is where the Chinese come in. Studies have regularly found Oriental people to metabolize alcohol faster than individuals of European descent, and it is now well established that 75 per cent or more of Orientals display a hypersensitivity to alcohol which consists of flushing and dysphoria, hot stomach, pounding in the head, tachycardia, muscle weakness, dizziness, sleepiness, exhaustion, nausea, and diahorrea (Schaefer, 1979). This reaction is present in infants prior to social experience with alcohol and half-Orientals and American Indians, distant relatives of the Chinese, have the same but diminished effects. Comparisons of North American Europeans and Orientals have shown that the latter metabolize alcohol significantly faster. There have been speculations that this hypersensitivity and faster metabolism affords protection against excessive drinking, and might go some way towards explaining the reported low levels of alcoholism amongst the Chinese (Goodwin, 1979; Schaefer, 1979). However, Schaefer raised the question: Why should American Indians have the *high* levels of problem drinking which have been widely reported? He took this to be evidence that, '. . . in some cases social, psychological and cultural factors may transcend the "protection" ' (p.230). Davies (1982) also stressed that a genetic predisposition can be neither a necessary nor sufficient condition for excessive alcohol use. Nevertheless, it is important that psychologists and others, fearful of the charge of 'reductionism', should not take a high-handed and neglectful view of biological processes in the excessive appetites. The complex and fast-moving field of research on endorphins—naturally occurring opioid peptides found at sites in the brain which, when stimulated, give a reduction in pain responsiveness comparable to the effects of a large dose of morphine (Watson and Akil, 1979)—provides another obvious example of developments with which students of excessive appetites should be familiar, and research on food metabolism and energy balance is another (Garrow, 1978). The possibility of a genetically determined 'set point' for body weight was mentioned in Chapter 5.

INCLINATION AND RESTRAINT IN RAJASTHAN

To conclude this chapter, and to prepare the way for the next, I have chosen a piece of anthropological writing which I believe offers one of the best descriptions of how different groups may use differing substances for related purposes. It also illustrates what is probably the major theme of this book, namely the balance which has to be struck between appetitive inclination and restraint. This is Carstairs' (1954) account of the use of daru (a potent form of distilled alcohol) and bhang (an infusion of the leaves and stems of Indian hemp—cannabis) which he observed during a year spent in a large village in the state of Rajasthan in Northern India. His portrayal will be summarized at some length because it contains a wealth of points which bear upon the psychology of drug use and excess. These two forms of intoxicant were not the only ones used in the village. Opium had traditionally been used, particularly by warriors before battle, but had become too expensive for widespread use, and in addition villagers frequently spoke of the intoxication produced by drinking cups of sickly-sweet tea infused in milk. In fact, 'Some went so far as to blame the breakdown of traditional piety on this modern indulgence in "English tea" ' (p.220).

It was the contrast between the drug use and associated opinions of the two highest and most privileged caste groups, the ruling or warrior caste (the Rajputs) and the religious leaders (the Brahmins), which struck Carstairs most forcibly. As fighters, the Rajputs had the privilege of being allowed to eat meat and drink alcohol, and from Carstairs' account it appears they took full advantage of both, and their use of alcohol very frequently produced obvious intoxication associated with sexual and aggressive disinhibition. By contrast, the Brahmins unequivocally denounced the use of daru as being quite inimicable to the religious life. Holy men insisted that a darulia (an 'alcoholic') was beyond salvation. Yet Carstairs witnessed time and again respectable Brahmins drunk on bhang, a state of intoxication which they believed not only to be no disgrace, but actually to enhance the spiritual life.

Carstairs made it his business to talk to as many villagers as possible about their views on daru and bhang. What struck him here was that whilst the Brahmins were unanimous in their negative views on daru, the Rajputs displayed towards this alcoholic beverage the same type of ambivalence with which we are familiar in large parts of the West. Many Rajputs were proud of drinking with discrimination. For example, 'My father used to drink a fixed quantity of daru from a small measure, every night. It was his niyam, his rule' (p.226). Restraint, and the use of small measures, were stressed in discussion, particularly when emphasizing religious values and observances. On the other hand, during evening hospitalities, and in association with fighting, these restraints seemed easily forgotten. As one informant said, 'In time of war, when the drum beats, only opium and daru drive out fear' (p.227). Age was probably a significant variable in the village of Carstairs' observations, as elsewhere. For example, 'Sahib, I am not interested in these things. These religious matters, usually one begins to be interested in them after the age of 50' (p.228).

In contrast to their emotive, but markedly ambivalent, attitude towards daru, the Rajputs held a phlegmatic and seemingly more objective view of bhang. For example, '. . . its not a thing I like. It makes you very sleepy and turns your throat dry . . .' (p.228). The Brahmins too were matter of fact rather than lyrical, but much more positive, about bhang, seeing it as an aid to devotional acts, the practice of austerities of one kind or another, and a general asceticism. The Brahmins were the leaders in Hindu beliefs with their stress upon karma (predestined lot), and dharma (right conduct), observance of which led ultimately to moksh (liberation from the cycle of reincarnation). In the attainment of moksh, '. . . asceticism, . . . self-deprivation, . . . trying to eliminate one's sensual appetites, is a basic theme' (p.231). These values impinged upon both Rajputs and Brahmins, although the latter were obliged to observe them all the time.

In discussion of his observations, Carstairs wrote of the Rajputs' and Brahmins' situation in terms of factors promoting and restraining excessive drug use. Promotional factors for Rajput daru use were strong, and restraints, in the form of a knowledge of offence against the Hindu code of asceticism, existed but were weak. These restraints weighed heavily with Brahmins, however, and inclination in the form of possible release of sexual and aggressive feelings was probably less because of their ready sublimation in the form of religious exercises which played such a large part in the Brahmins' lives. Appetitive indulgence, as well as the expression of sexual and aggressive needs, was played down in favour of obedience to a common, impersonal, set of rules of Right Behaviour (p.235). As we shall see in the following chapters, this way of viewing behaviour as the resultant of opposing forces, some promoting, others restraining, has since become popular in the form of social learning theory and is particularly relevant to appetitive behaviour.

The finale to Carstairs' intriguing paper, written in the early 1950s, is startling when viewed from the perspective of the 1980s. He observed that bhang use by the Brahmins was far less socially disruptive than daru use by the Rajputs and yet he admitted that the use of bhang was so alien to his own culture and personality that he much preferred daru. He thought this was likely to be the case for all Westerners, and thought Aldous Huxley (1954) was unrealistic to think that Westerners might take to mescalin:

> If the thesis of this paper is valid, Westerners have refrained from taking mescalin (which has long been available to them) because its effect does not accord with their desires. Unless there is an unforeseen reversal of their basic values, they are as little likely to follow Huxley's advice as are the Brahmins to abandon bhang in favour of the Rajputs' daru, or vice versa (p.236).

Carstairs could not foresee the changes that were to take place in patterns of drug use in the West within a very few years, changes that illustrate a cardinal theme in the psychology of appetitive behaviour. Such behaviours have inordinate capacity to serve a wide variety of human functions, and to adapt to meet the particular needs of a specified time, place, and person. The factors promoting appetitive indulgence are many and powerful and we are continually being caught off guard by some unfamiliar or neglected activity or substance.

Most societies are aware of the dangers of those appetites with which they have been familiar, and have taken steps to prevent excess. Indeed, it is a central tenet of the view to be taken here that the very potency of appetitive objects and activities, their potential for excess, gives rise to restraining and controlling forces which can be seen at work in the form of legal controls, social group sanctions, and personal self-restraint. It is to these naturally occurring controlling mechanisms that we must now begin to turn our attention.

CHAPTER NINE

Overcoming Restraint

> The causes of acquired disease are sometimes small, gradual, and accumulative, and so are those of vice. By continuous use and repetition diseased conditions become inveterate, and so do vicious ones, indeed, by far the more so. . . . In some extreme cases, or even in many or all cases if you choose, the will is helpless. This is not necessarily or probably the effect of disease. For it is in the nature of vice to become inveterate . . . It is important to observe that all vices partake of the nature, and exhibit the phenomena of drunkenness, to a greater or lesser extent; yet it is not pretended in the case of any other of them that there is disease . . . (J. E. Todd, *Drunkenness a Vice not a Disease*, 1882 (cited by E. M. Jellinek, *The Disease Concept of Alcoholism*, 1960, pp.208–9).)

> Never underestimate the strength of a habit (Reinert, 1968, pp.37–8).

CONFORMITY, DETERRENCE AND RESTRAINT

One of the cornerstones of the new public health approach to the prevention of excessive drinking has been the now often repeated observation that alcohol consumption by individuals within a population is distributed along a skewed frequency distribution curve of the kind shown in Figure 4 (de Lint, 1977). Quite apart from what such curves may tell us about the likely effects of increasing or decreasing national consumption upon rates of excessive drinking, which is a hotly debated area (e.g. Grant *et al.*, 1983), a curve of this kind stresses the continuity of the variation from light to heavy drinking and takes the focus right away from a disease view. Even though it may not be intended, disease models, by contrast, suggest qualitative differences between those who suffer the disease and those who do not.

There has in fact been much controversy about the exact form of the alcohol consumption frequency distribution curve. Ledermann (1956) proposed that mathematically the curve corresponded to a lognormal distribution, although others have pointed out since (Duffy, 1977; Skog, 1977) that there exists a whole family of lognormal distribution curves (which differ in degree of dispersion around the mean), for any one value for the average consumption within the population. These contributors to the debate point out that it was necessary for Ledermann to make unwarranted assumptions in order to fix the shape of this curve in one particular lognormal form in a way that enabled a prediction to be made of the number of excessive drinkers to be found in a population (for example, the number consuming more than 8 ozs of spirits a day) from the average consumption of the whole population. For example, he assumed that the proportion of people consuming more than 1 litre of alcohol a day must be small and he proceeded on the basis that 1 per cent of the population consume in excess of this quantity. Not only is the evidence against

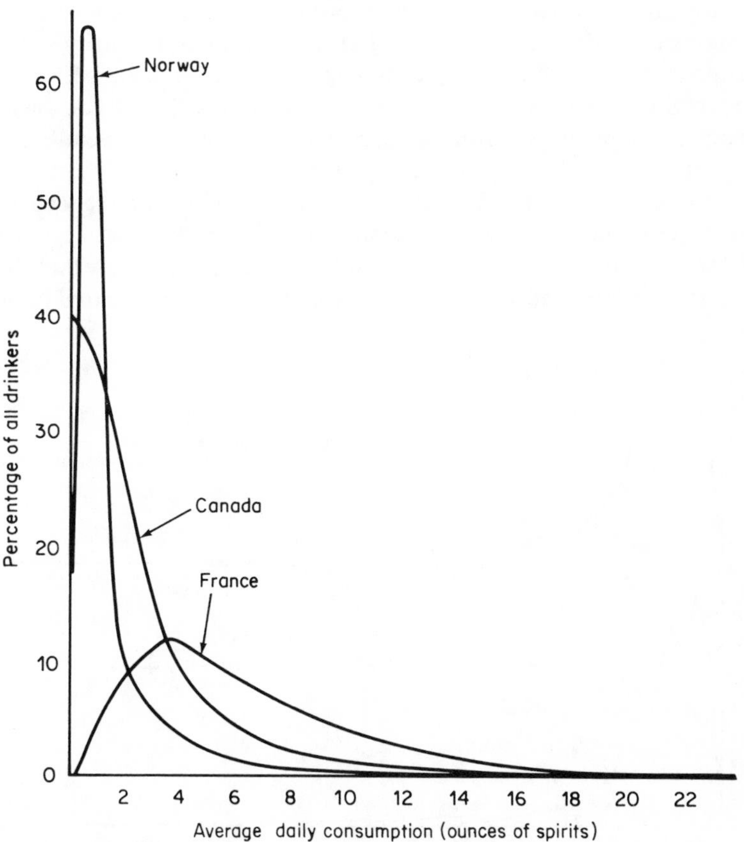

Figure 4 Typical skewed population frequency distribution curves for alcohol consumption in Norway, Canada, and France in 1968 (reprinted with permission from Miller and Agnew, 1974)

Ledermann's exact mathematical formulation, but there is doubt even that the curves obtained take a lognormal form at all (Hyman, 1979). All that can safely be concluded is that alcohol consumption frequency distribution curves are regularly found to be smooth, unimodal, and markedly skewed towards the higher consumption end of the distribution: the majority of people are found to conform more or less to a relatively moderate norm (or in certain sub-populations to an abstinence norm) with smaller and smaller proportions of people displaying consumption in excess of this norm to a greater and greater degree.

There is some evidence that such a distribution may be a feature of a number of the forms of appetitive behaviour with which this book is dealing. Although personal alcohol consumption provides the best documented example, frequency of sexual outlet is another variable following a similar distribution curve (Kinsey *et al.*, 1948, p.200, for males). (The curves that can be drawn from these data are shown in Figure 5.) The distributions show a peak at the low frequency end of the range (with a mode at one to two outlets per week), with a long and continuous tail to the curves showing ever decreasing proportions of people reporting increasing weekly frequencies up to 10 to 20 times a week. A similar curve for number of partners with whom boys aged 15–19 had had sexual intercourse can be drawn from the survey data provided by Schofield (1968, p.88), but here the data are less complete.

Smart (1971) has produced similar curves for drug use in three separate high school populations in Canadian towns. The distribution for Toronto High School students is shown in Figure 6. It will be noted immediately that the norm in this case is not one of moderation, as was the case for the sexual outlet data

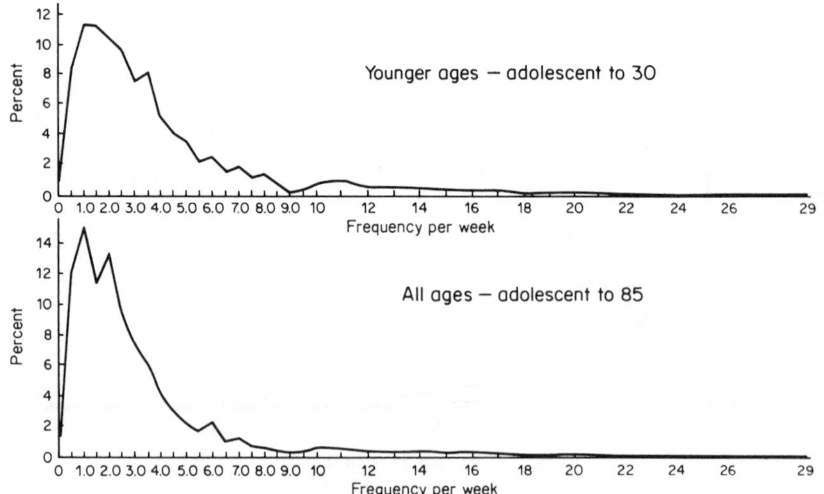

Figure 5 Distribution of frequencies of sexual outlets for U.S. males (Reproduced by permission of the Kinsey Institute for Research in Sex, Gender and Reproduction, Inc.)

produced by Kinsey and the alcohol consumption data produced by Ledermann and others, but is one of abstinence. Furthermore, it may be thought that the distribution obtained is an artefact of the rather complex method Smart used to obtain 'drug use' scores. These scores represented the sum of frequency of usage ratings for ten separate drugs. Respondents were required to categorize their use of each drug on a four-point scale and these responses were assigned 'mid-point' scores as follows: 1–2 times = 1.5; 3–4 times = 3.5; 5–6 times = 5.5; and 7+ times = 7.5. The exact meaning of such scores is therefore not

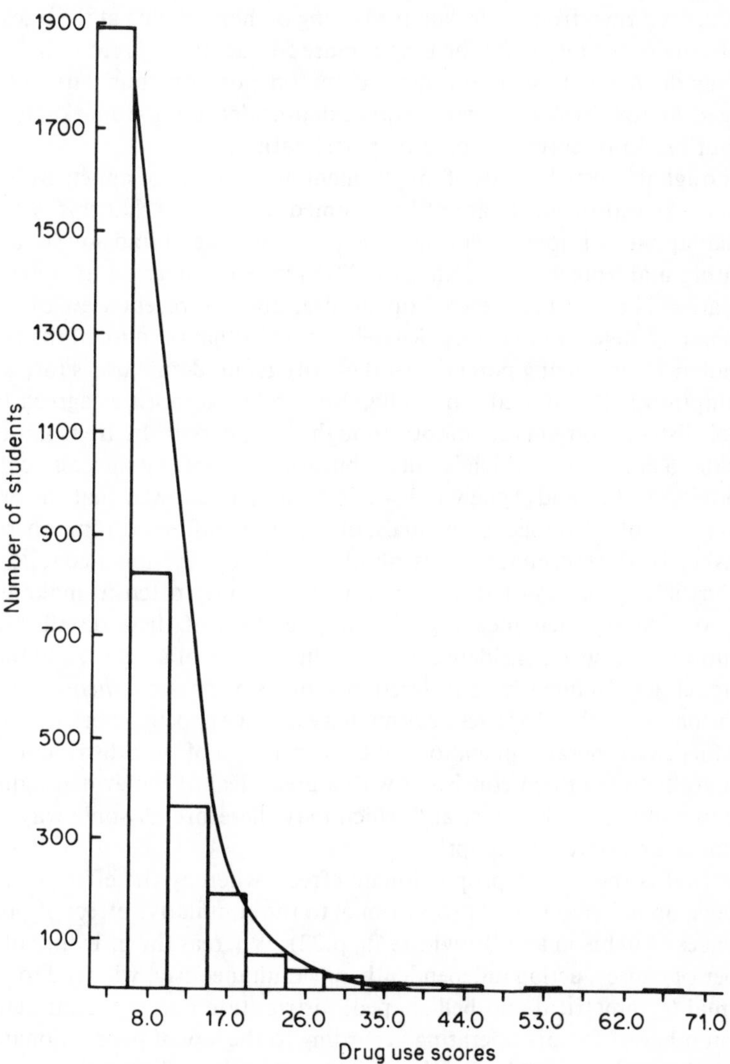

Figure 6 Drug use among high school students in Toronto (Reprinted from Smart (1971), p.401, by courtesy of Marcel Dekker Inc.)

immediately obvious. However, Smart reported drawing curves for individual drug usage on the basis of data from a later study in which subjects were asked to say 'exactly how many times' they had used certain drugs. Frequency distributions for marijuana, LSD, 'speed', other stimulants, solvents, tranquillizers, and barbiturates, corresponded to the skewed, approximately lognormal, form.

In the case of gambling, the only data which lend themselves at all to the drawing of a 'consumption' curve are those produced in the course of the survey carried out by Kallick *et al.* (1979) in the United States. Figures 7 (a) and (b) show curves drawn from their data for betting on horse racing at the track (much more frequent for men) and for Bingo (more frequently engaged in by women). Once again 'abstinence' is the most common position, but participants are arranged as for drinking, drugs, and sexual outlet along a markedly skewed distribution representing volume of participation.

Although the distributions of involvement in a number of appetitive activities take this skewed form, it cannot be assumed, of course, that this is a general rule that applies without exception. I have been unable to find any suitable data for eating and, interestingly, Smart (1971) made no mention of tobacco, nor of opiates. The popular view of opiate use, and the recent view of tobacco-smoking now held by many (e.g. Russell, 1971), is that because of the powerful 'dependence'-producing potential of these drugs, moderate use is rare and that consumption is distributed bimodally. Nor are all authorities agreed that the alcohol distribution curve, smooth though it appears to be in broad outline, illustrates a continuum which is only arbitrarily divisible into excessive drinkers and others. Miller and Agnew (1974), for example, showed that the existence of a minority of 'alcoholic' individuals, qualitatively different from others, could be masked by the consumption distribution of the larger 'non-alcoholic' group.

Nevertheless, curves of this kind recur sufficiently often to make it worth while considering their meaning. The implications of these distributions for prevention have been considered, but only in the case of alcohol, and they have been much less frequently considered as sources of possible *theoretical* insight into the nature of the processes determining excessive appetitive behaviour. There are in fact two general explanations of the generation of such distribution curves which are between them consistent with a great deal of the evidence discussed in the previous two chapters, and which may therefore go some way towards explaining excessive consumption.

The first is the law of proportionate effect, whereby the effect of any one influence upon behaviour is proportional to the cumulative effect of preceding influences (Aitchison and Brown, 1966, p.22). Whereas the influence of a large number of causes, acting independently or simultaneously, will tend to produce a normal (symmetrical and bell-shaped) distribution curve, the influence of a large number of factors operating according to the law of proportionate effect will produce a lognormal, or at least a markedly skewed, distribution. All the evidence is that appetitive behaviour of each of the kinds considered here is determined not by a single causative factor, or even by a few factors, but rather

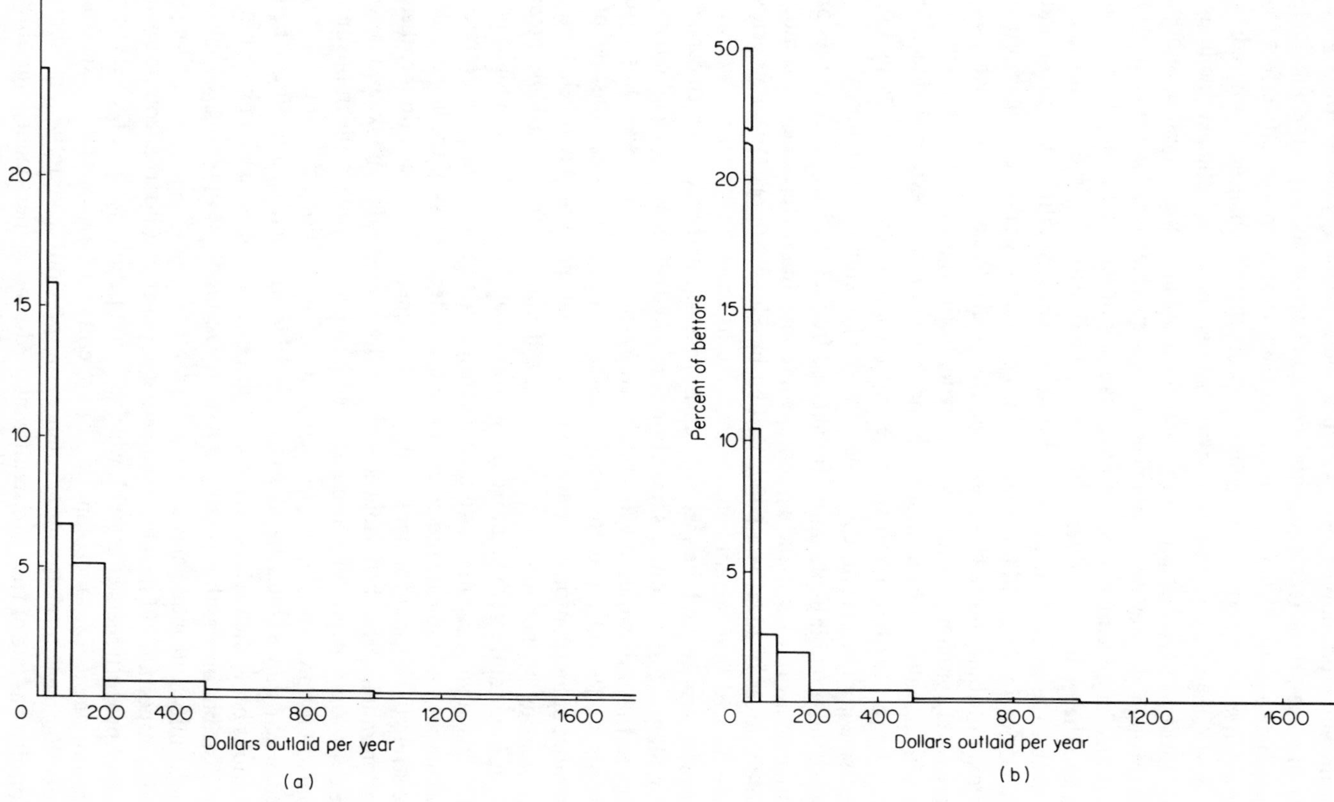

Figure 7 Annual outlay by U.S. bettors on (a) Horses at the track, and (b) Bingo (*Source*: Kallick *et al.*, 1979, p.11)

by a very large number of influences of biological, psychological, and sociological kinds. Furthermore, because we are dealing here with human social behaviour which develops slowly within a social context, perhaps through a number of stages, these factors are not acting independently or at the same time.

To produce a skewed curve according to the law of proportionate effect we require a *developmental* theory, one that supposes that the chances of proceeding to the next 'stage', or of responding to the next positive influence inclining towards further 'consumption', are greater the more previous 'stages' have been passed through or previous influences have been effective. Learning theory explanations for appetitive behaviour are examples of one kind of developmental theory and they will be considered in some detail shortly. Any theory, however, which relies on an accumulation of influence would qualify. Aitchison and Brown (1966) in fact built a machine which sorted grains of sand into a lognormal distribution by a clever arrangement of dividers which gave each grain a progressively greater probability of moving to the right depending upon the distance it had already been moved in that direction by previous dividers. It may not be too far fetched to suppose that those who experience the pull of an excessive appetite are in the grips of a similar kind of mechanism.

The second possible explanation for skewed frequency distribution curves of appetitive behaviour lies in the psychology of conformity. Here one of the most valuable sources of ideas is a paper written by Floyd Allport (1934) 50 years ago. He noticed that certain behaviours, such as times of arrival for work or for a church service, and the speed of vehicles across intersections which carried Halt or Slow signs, followed skewed or reversed J-shaped frequency curves. He argued that this would always be the case when behaviour was subject to social control. Provided this control was effective to some degree, most people would more or less conform to the norm, rule, or law governing that behaviour, and decreasing proportions of people would deviate to an increasingly great extent. A mode at the zero point would indicate an abstinence, or non-indulgence norm, whilst a non-zero mode would indicate a moderation norm. The steepness of the curve would indicate the precision and/or effectiveness of the law or rule, or the strength of the informal social processes operating to restrain members of the community from behavioural excess. Allport referred to the skewed curve as the *conformity curve*, and he considered it to be the result of the imposition of conformity processes upon people's inclinations to do such things as stay in bed when they should be at work, or drive fast across junctions (these inclinations being themselves variable quantities). The position of an individual on the distribution was thus presumed to be the result of the opposing tendencies to conformity and indulgence.

In this important but now little remembered paper of Allport's, coupled with the law of proportionate effect with which it is compatible, we have the necessary basic components for an explanation of appetitive behaviour and its excessive forms. We have already met evidence, in previous chapters, that social conformity was one of the most significant predisposing 'personality' variables, at least within the culture and times in which most of the research reviewed was carried out. This evidence came from research on the inverse relationship between religious views and drug and alcohol use and sexual behaviour, work correlating scores on various scales of social conformity and drug and alcohol use, work such as the Jessors' on attitudes towards deviancy in general and their correlations with appetitive behaviours, and correlations between radical and non-conformist political and social views and drug use. Although it must be presumed that Allport's assumptions that conformity acts always to restrain, and that biological influences act always in opposition to restraint, are too simple, the basic idea of forces in opposition is, I believe, essential to an understanding of excessive appetites. The perspective on excessive drinking, excessive gambling, drug-taking, and other similar forms of excess, to be developed in the remainder of this chapter and the rest of the book, rests heavily upon the idea of opposing tendencies towards restraint versus appetitive inclination, the counter-balancing of incentive and disincentive, and the moral conflict between deviant excess and conforming moderation.

Ledermann conjectured that alcohol consumption obeyed the law of proportionate effect on account of a mechanism which he termed the *boule de neige* effect. Alcohol consumption gathered momentum, like a ball of snow rolling downhill, on account, he argued, of two factors, namely the 'addictive' properties of alcohol, and social contagion. The skewed frequency distribution curve confirmed his belief that alcohol consumption spread in a contagious fashion like certain infectious diseases. Although the boule de neige explanation is now generally reckoned to be over-simple, the emphasis upon processes of social interaction is generally considered more or less correct, and is in keeping with a great deal of evidence, reviewed in Chapter 7, that the behaviour and attitudes of a person's peers and the support which they give a person either towards or against appetitive behaviour, are amongst the strongest correlates of appetitive behaviour.

It should be noted here that contagion theories have had some popularity in explaining the uptake of drug use. In Britain, de Alarcon (1969) charted the spread from individual to individual of heroin use in a new town area in the 1960s, and Hunt *et al.* (1979) have described an 'epidemic' of drug use in one county in California in the early 1970s by examining the changing prevalence and age distribution of use year by year. Crawford *et al.* (1978) have described how the way heroin use may spread in an area where use is endemic is rather different from the way use spreads in an area experiencing a new 'epidemic'. In contrast to epidemic areas, where most 'initiators' of others were friends who had recently begun to use heroin themselves, in two of Chicago's 'old dope' neighbourhoods the large majority of initiators were already addicted. Although most were friends or relatives of the new user, their ages ranged widely and many were middle-aged. This approach, treating heroin or other drug use as if it were a kind of infectious disease, the spread of which can be traced and hopefully eliminated, is much criticized by those such as Brecher (1972), Westemeyer (1978), and Jacobs (1978), who believe that legal and social responses to heroin use have created most of the harm that is usually, wrongly, attributed to the drug itself.

Returning to the appetitive consumption distribution curve, Hyman (1979) has pointed out that contagion alone cannot explain the positively skewed shape of the curve and that some other factor must be involved. He pointed out that similar distributions are obtained for purchases of non-durable goods such as meat, clothing, and fuel, for economic variables such as inheritances, bank deposits, total individual wealth, numbers of employed persons in industries, and industrial profits, as well as for certain geographical variables such as numbers of inhabitants in towns, distances between cities of the same size, and even the numbers and lengths of streams in river systems. Certain social variables such as numbers of surviving children and ages at first marriage are also distributed in a similar fashion. He put forward the hypothesis that the underlying theme of all such distributions (he called them para-lognormal to underline the point that they do not all conform mathematically to the lognormal distribution) is that of, 'major deterrences nipping the evolution of a phenomenon in the bud (though not entirely suppressing it)' (p.345). Just as there are a number of impediments to the further development of a river tributary (competition from other tributaries, insufficient rain, excessive evaporation, hard rockbeds, etc.) or the size of cities (competition from other cities, inability to generate exports, inability to provide a wide range of services, etc.), so the evolution of appetitive behaviour to higher levels of consumption might, he argued, be impeded by a variety of deterrences including (he was considering alcohol use) gastric distress, headaches, and dizziness, a psychological makeup which makes intoxication seem unpleasant, family and friendship norms that proscribe heavy drinking, competition from other activities for time and money, etc. Although, as already stated, Allport's ideas focused solely upon conformity to rules or norms as the factor nipping deviance in the bud, the overall similarity between the two positions is striking. The idea basic to both is that of inclination restrained: in the one case by social conformity, in the other by deterring forces of various kinds, social and otherwise.

The idea of deterrence or control has a long history in criminology and its relevance to an understanding of excessive appetitive behaviour has recently been seen, for example by Akers *et al.* (1979), in the context of adolescent drinking and drug-taking. Deterrence theory, they pointed out, has some relevance, but is limited to the real or perceived likelihood of legal punishment for crime, as well as its swiftness and severity. Hirschi's (1969) control theory has wider application, however, concerned as it is with the constraining influence of informal social bonds to groups and institutions. Cornish (1978) also made use of Hirschi's thinking in developing his own theory of gambling behaviour. Amongst the factors associated with non-gambling, which he cited, were frequent church-attendance, Protestant or sectarian beliefs, conjugal role-sharing, involvement in work-centred leisure activities such as studying at home, and involvement in political or community activities (Downes *et al.*, 1976). These exercised inhibitory control over gambling not only because of the attitudes and social bonds antithetical to gambling which they implied, but also because they restricted 'freedom' to gamble on account of, '. . . activities, interests and social roles making prior calls upon a person's attention, time and income' (Cornish, p.158). One of the components of Hirschi's control theory was 'involvement': some people are just too engrossed in conventional activities to engage in delinquency. To Cornish it was a question of using time and money in ways incompatible with gambling. Certain ages and stages in life, in youth for example, might provide a temporary 'leisure vacuum', with fewer competing uses of resources.

Other constraining or regulatory factors are inherent in the activity rather than the person or his or her life-style. In the case of gambling, Cornish argued, controls are exercised over frequency of participation in certain forms of betting because access is limited (e.g. on-course betting), membership is required (e.g. gaming), play is supervised (e.g. Bingo), or participation is necessarily spaced (e.g. pools betting). These obstacles in the way of greater participation may be placed by national or local statute but they operate at the individual level by entering into the attraction–deterrence equation which determines the behaviour of each individual.

Others who have explicitly applied the notion of deterrence or control to explaining variations in drug use include Staats (1978) who, following Becker (1963), explored the possibility that marijuana users were deterred from greater use by limitations of supply and access, the need to keep use hidden from non-users, and the conventional belief that drug use was wrong. Some support was forthcoming in his own study for the first two of these three 'controls'. Staats was critical of the assumptions contained in alternative theories that drug use can only be explained by positing some strain propelling a person to use drugs, some function served by use, a deviant learning process, or the incorporation of societal reaction to use. Viewed from the control theory perspective:

> . . . deviance is taken for granted; it is conformity which must be explained. The assumption is that without controls many would not remain conformists. Conformity is assured through controls and when they weaken, the probability of deviance increases (Staats, 1978, p.392).

An important implication of this emphasis upon restraining or deterring factors is that much research, of the type that has compared people whose appetitive behaviour is already known to be excessive with others, has been misdirected. Hyman's view was that 'normal' drinkers were merely a, '. . . diverse potpourri of people who have not further "evolved" as heavy drinkers for numerous reasons or combinations of reasons'. Similarly, 'alcoholics', '. . . might be looked at as a residual category, i.e. they are those people for whom one or another potential deterrence did not succeed in deterring' (p.346). From the perspective of deterrence theory, the interesting question is not: Why do some people become excessive in their appetitive behaviour? But rather: Why are most people not excessive?

Although Ledermann and others used the word 'contagion' in relation to alcohol consumption to draw an analogy with a contagious disease, some social psychologists have used the word in a different sense but one which makes the use of the word quite apposite if the notion of restraint or deterrence is correct. Wheeler (1966) suggested that the term 'contagion' be distinguished from other terms referring to forms of interpersonal influence upon behaviour, such as 'imitation' and 'conformity', by confining its use to circumstances in which influence operated by removing controls or restraints upon behaviour. He conceived of contagion as the process whereby a person who is instigated towards a particular behaviour but does not perform this behaviour because of certain restraints, is released from this conflict by interpersonal influence, typically by observing another person perform the behaviour in question. In theoretical terms: '. . . behavioural contagion . . . is mediated by the lowering of the observer's avoidance gradient in an approach–avoidance conflict' (p.185). This is a key theoretical statement for the development of the psychological explanation put forward in this book, and the theme of approach–avoidance conflict is one to which we shall return in the following chapter.

The opposition of instigating and restraining forces is an idea inherent also in general social learning theory approaches to human behaviour. Such approaches (e.g. Phares, 1972; Bandura, 1977) differ from most animal models of learning in their emphasis upon the cognitive expectation of future failure or punishment, or of future success or reward, as opposed to the strengthening of behaviour by reinforcement, and by their emphasis upon individual needs and values and attitudes toward the self which determine which events an individual defines as rewarding and which as punishing. Thus, they combine an emphasis upon adaptive learning of social behaviour through experience, with due attention to phenomenological and individualistic factors (personality), in a way that renders them fitting contenders for the task of explaining the types of complex human behaviour described in Part I of this book.

The particular aspect of social learning theories which needs to be focused on in the present context is the opposing nature of inclination and restraint. Put at its very simplest, the prediction of social learning theory (at least that variation of Rotter's, 1954, social learning theory outlined by Phares, 1972) is that the outcome of a behavioural choice (to pass the betting shop or to go in and place a bet; to eat or not to eat a second cream doughnut; to buy a packet of cigarettes or not) is the result of the balance of expectations of positive outcomes over negative outcomes (rewards over punishments) for engaging in rather than desisting from appetitive behaviour. The equation may be a complex one, with entries varying from those that represent intrinsic rewards and punishments (the pleasure of genital stimulation or a drug-induced altered state of consciousness; the punishment of a flushing response to alcohol ingestion or the loss of money on a failed bet), to those that represent expectations of extrinsic, social reward or punishment. Other entries will correspond to a process of moral self-regulation, derived from notions of right conduct or socially approved behaviour, rather than regulation by others or by biologically and intrinsically rewarding or punishing events (Bandura, 1977).

A particular variety of social learning theory has been put forward by Akers *et al.* (1979) to explain drug use and abuse. The particular flavour of Akers *et al.*'s view derives from its origins in the *differential association* theory of delinquency (Sutherland and Cressey, 1970) with its emphasis upon the norms and behaviours to be found in the social groups with which an individual associates. Akers *et al.* stated their theory as follows:

> The reinforcers can be non-social (as in the direct physiological effects of drugs) as well as social, but the theory posits that the principal behavioural effects come from interaction in or under the influence of those *groups which control individuals' major sources of reinforcement and punishment and expose them to behavioural models and normative definitions.* The most important of these groups with which one is in *differential association* are the *peer-friendship* groups and the *family* but they also include schools, churches, and other groups. Behaviour (whether deviant or conforming) results from greater reinforcement, on balance, over punishing contingencies for the same behaviour and the reinforcing–punishing contingencies on alternative behaviour. Definitions are conducive to deviant behaviour when, on balance, the positive and neutralizing definitions of the behaviour offset negative definitions of it (p.638, their emphasis).

Here Akers *et al.* were concerned with the initial taking up of drug use, but the following passage, concerned with *increasing* drug use, also makes clear the importance given to the balance between incentive and disincentive:

> Progression into more frequent or sustained use and into abuse is also determined by the extent to which a given pattern is sustained by the combination of the reinforcing effects of the substance with social reinforcement, exposure to models, definitions through associations with using peers, *and by the degree to which it is not deterred* through bad effects of the substance and/or the negative sanctions from peers, parents and the law (p.639, emphasis added).

This balance or conflict, which will be a central and continuing theme in the following chapters, can be expressed as a matter of moral philosophy as much as of social psychology. In an address at a research meeting in 1939, Myerson (1940) linked sexual behaviour and the use of alcohol in terms of the deep ambivalence which there is about each of them in Western thought, and in particular in terms of the conflict, which each gives rise to, between the opposing principles of hedonism and asceticism. Appetite, argued Myerson, was easy to understand, producing a, '. . . native pleasure which once experienced becomes consciously sought for' (p.13), and in the case of the ingestion of food or the sexual act it is biologically functional. Asceticism, on the other hand, '. . . is a trend which, at least on the surface, runs counter to desire and satisfaction which is a denial of pleasure and its validity . . . Pleasure in and of itself is stigmatized as unworthy except for the pleasure of renunciation and self-denial' (p.13). Alongside the myriad images of pleasurable indulgence, have been various ascetic cults including the Hindus, the Essenes of the Jews, groups of early Christians, primitive Buddhists, and Puritan leaders, conducting a, '. . . revolt against all desire . . . so that the ultimate goal becomes the extinction of appetite and the disappearance of the individual in a non-desiring and non-desirous infinity' (p.14).

The result was that each person brought up in a Western culture was, in the case of alcohol use and sex, bombarded by these two opposing sets of forces. Myerson used the idea of conflict between inclination and the pursuit of pleasure on the one hand, and anti-hedonistic restraint on the other, to suggest an explanation why Jewish people, and women in general as opposed to men, had many fewer alcohol problems. Both, he suggested, were exposed to stronger inhibitory influences, the one because of their traditions which were sternly against excessive use of alcohol, the other because of sex roles which exposed women to much more severe pressure against excessive indulgence:

> . . . sobriety is not expected so much of the Gentile as of the Jew; sobriety is not expected so much of the man as of the woman; and punishment for inebriety is not meted out in equal measure to the Gentile as to the Jew, to the man as to the woman (p.19).

This argument, that excessive appetitive behaviour is merely behaviour that has not responded to the pressures for conformity, is a compelling one. It is consistent with the shape of the consumption distribution curve, and with a great deal of survey evidence that suggests that those who indulge certain appetites more than others tend to be non-conformists in other ways. However, in this writer's view it is only part of the explanation. It explains certain excesses, such as over-eating and difficult-to-give-up tranquillizer use, less well than others, and takes no account of the development of excess in a way that would satisfy the law of proportionate effect.

Not that all students of excessive appetites believe that a developmental, progression, or 'exposure' element is necessary for an adequate account. Alexander and Hadaway (1982) have in fact done us a useful service in clarifying this issue. They have discerned, within the, '. . . chaotic and bewildering' literature on opiate 'addiction' which, '. . . teems with theories in the vocabularies of all the major branches of psychology as well as psychiatry, sociology, and physiology' (p.367), two broad and apparently contradictory approaches. As we have found with most that has been written about drug 'addiction' or 'dependence', their statement serves equally as well whether the 'addiction' concerned is to opiates, alcohol, tobacco, other drugs, sex, eating, or gambling. One of the, '. . . fundamentally different orientations', which they described, and it is the one which they favoured and believed had been relatively neglected, they termed the *adaptive* approach. This covered any explanation of drug use which saw it as a response to *pre-existing* distress or deficiency of some kind. The distress or deficiency might be personality related, it might involve pain or fear which could be situational, it might be more a matter of inadequacies of family or community or opportunity, or it might even be a physiological deficiency. Whatever the source, the assumption was that drugs were being used to *cope* with something else, and that the 'something else' constituted the more central 'problem'. Although it might fail, drug use was at least an attempt at adaptation.

The orientation which they believed has dominated the field to its detriment, they termed the *exposure* orientation. What I have called 'developmental' theories would fall within this orientation. 'Addiction' is held to be a consequence of exposure to the drug, pre-existing causes of individual or environment are relegated to a position of secondary importance, and the drug's availability is reckoned of prime importance in providing the means of 'addiction'. Amongst evidence which they cited against this perspective was their own recent animal work suggesting that the apparent 'addiction' susceptibility of rats and monkeys in earlier experiments might have been at least partly a function of the isolated and restricted conditions under which they were housed (e.g. Alexander *et al.*, 1981), and recently accruing evidence that there are casual heroin users who are not 'addicted' despite their exposure (e.g. Zinberg and Jacobson, 1976).

Although Alexander and Hadaway were right in stating that the literature on opiates had been dominated by an over-simple exposure view which saw anyone exposed to heroin as almost inevitably enslaved thereafter, once we consider other drugs, and certainly once we consider a broader range of potentially excessive appetitive activities, a simple one-sided exposure orientation ceases to have much credibility at all in any case. At the same time, even Alexander and Hadaway who leant heavily towards an 'adaptive' view themselves, did admit that this orientation needed some modification to deal with the often progressive nature of opiate 'addiction', and it is a main plank of the argument of this book, developed further in the following chapter, that the idea of 'addiction' does have some substance. There are, in the present author's view, powerful processes at work which can, under the right circumstances, reduce an individual's freedom to choose whether to indulge in an activity or not. These processes which can come into play as a result of exposure, may be fuelled by, and are probably rarely fully independent of, any pre-existing distress or deficiency which contributed to initial exposure, but they are additional and vitally important in their own right.

Of course any attempt to separate out factors existing prior to and consequent upon 'exposure' breaks down when we move from heroin use to activities which are acceptable to society in moderation and where acceptable and unacceptable use are difficult to distinguish. We have also seen in previous chapters the limitations of a simple cause-and-effect model of appetitive behaviour. Not only are the antecedents and consequences of a development in appetitive behaviour so inextricably intertwined that they are almost impossible to separate, as the Jessors' (1977) longitudinal investigations showed, but the successful 'decomposition' models (e.g. Robins, *et al.*, 1977; Kandel, 1978) also showed that different predisposing factors become important at different 'stages' in a developmental process, with the kinds of distress and deficiency factors that Alexander and Hadaway have written about probably being important only at later stages. For various reasons, then, neither a simple 'adaptation' nor a simple 'exposure' model can be adequate alone.

LEARNING THEORY

An obvious candidate for 'developmental' or 'exposure' theory is some variety of learning theory, in particular operant learning theory. The basic tenet of operant theory is well known: behaviour is controlled by its consequences. Consequences which increase the frequency of the behaviour are termed reinforcers, and the behaviour which was instrumental in producing those consequences is said to be reinforced thereby. It hardly needs to be demonstrated that food acts as a reinforcer for a food-deprived animal, or that the opportunity for sexual behaviour acts as a reinforcement for one deprived of sex. Food and sex have 'reinforcement potential'.

In recent years it has been demonstrated that various classes of drug can have reinforcement potential also, at least under laboratory conditions. In a typical experiment, an animal with a catheter chronically implanted in a vein would increase the frequency with which it pressed a bar if bar-pressing was followed by infusion of a dose of certain drugs (Kumar and Stolerman, 1977). For example, rats' and monkeys' bar-pressing is reinforced by infusions of many central nervous system stimulants, including amphetamine, methamphetamine phenmetrazine, cocaine, and caffeine (Kumar and Stolerman, 1977; Pickens and Thompson, 1971). The same is true of the opioids. Demonstrations of the reinforcement potential of opioids have included morphine, heroin, etonitazene, pentazocine, codeine, and methadine, and studies have involved oral, intraperitoneal, and intravenous routes of administration in both rats and monkeys (Schuster and Thompson, 1969). Although opioid self-administration appeared not to be characterized by the same degree of precise regulation of dosage as was the case for stimulant drugs, extinction of behaviour following withdrawal of the drug has been shown in some experiments to be particularly slow.

An advantage of this type of artificial laboratory study of drug-taking behaviour in animals is that conditions can be altered relatively precisely to test various hypotheses about the factors controlling drug-seeking behaviour. For example, although it has been shown that alcohol (ethanol) and sedative-hypnotic drugs such as the barbiturates have reinforcement potential for animals, Kumar and Stolerman were able to conclude that these drugs were less powerful reinforcers of behaviour than were stimulants or opioids. They based this conclusion on such findings as the relative difficulty of establishing self-administration of these drugs in the laboratory, the great difficulty of getting animals to self-administer ethanol orally, and the greater sensitivity of sedative-hypnotic and alcohol self-administration to increases in the effort required to obtain the drug. When animals were required to work under a schedule of reinforcement which produced a reinforcing administration only every ten or twenty responses, then the animals failed to learn the behaviour. It also proved particularly difficult to establish self-administration of hallucinogenic substances and non-hypnotic tranquillizers, although there has been some suggestive work with phencyclidine, chlordiazepoxide, and inhalation of hashish smoke (Kumar and Stolerman, 1977). In this connection Kumar and Stolerman write:

> It might be supposed that only man could appreciate the complex perceptual and emotional experiences induced by hallucinogenic substances, but one has to remember how relatively recent have been the demonstrations in animals of dependence on stimulants, opioids, alcohol and sedative-hypnotics. Previously a variety of exclusively human motivational, emotional and personality factors had often been considered essential for dependence upon even these drugs (p.24).

Although operant analyses of behaviour draw heavily upon studies with animals for their empirical and theoretical foundation, they are of course by no means confined to the animal world in their applications. Indeed, such work serves as an important reminder that biologically the human animal is not totally unlike all lower animals in every respect, and hence it forces us to ask what animal studies have to teach us about human excessive appetitive behaviour. Cornish (1978), for example, in his review of the literature on gambling rested heavily on learning theory in his discussion of the determinants of continued participation once the initial decision to gamble had been taken. He reviewed evidence from experimental studies of simulated gambling showing that a favourable ratio of wins over losses leads to an increased frequency, or at least to the maintenance of the current rate, of gambling, the suggestion being that financial reward constitutes at least part of the reinforcement for gambling behaviour.

Although it may appear difficult for learning theory to account for continuing participation once gambling has started on the basis of financial reinforcement alone when it is so apparent that commercial gambling is organized to make a profit for the promotors and the gambler is likely to show an excess of losses over gains in the long term, learning theory is in fact ideally suited to explain this paradox, as well as the apparent paradox of all excessive appetitive behaviour—that the behaviour persists despite apparently producing for the person concerned more harm than good.

There are three basic features of the process of operant learning which are known to all first year psychology students, which probably go a long way towards explaining the insidious development of strongly habitual appetitive behaviour. One is the *partial* nature of much reinforcement: inconsistent reinforcement results in behaviour even more resistant to extinction than that produced by consistent reward. Second, it is *probabilities* that are affected in learning. It is not a matter of one response taking the place completely of another, but rather of certain acts gradually becoming more probable. Third, there is the *gradient of reinforcement*, a phenomenon which serves to help explain such paradoxical behaviour as the consumption of substances which appear to produce harm or punishment in the long run. Behaviour may have both rewarding and punishing consequences, but it is the immediate consequences that are the most important in shaping habitual behaviour.

Thus occasional, immediate financial reward would be expected to promote future gambling more than the later realization of insufficient money for other purposes would restrain it. Indeed, the process of staking money or token chips or counters, and sometimes receiving concrete reward, seems to resemble operant experimental procedures used with animals to such an extent as to positively invite a learning analysis of gambling. This is particularly so since staking behaviour is not reinforced by a win on every occasion, and the particular schedules of reinforcement in operation are similar to VR schedules (variable ratio schedules: the probability of winning being dependent on the number of times a person stakes, the ratio of wins to number of times staked being made *variable* at least over the short run) which have proved capable of maintaining a high level of responding in animal experiments and rendering the behaviour in question relatively highly resistant to extinction. Cornish cited one example, the American 21-bell 3-wheel fruit machine, set to give a 94.45 per cent return on money inserted, which allowed players to make a win of some denomination on only 13.4 per cent of plays—'a very intermittent VR reinforcement schedule' (pp.181–2). Lewis and Duncan's research (1958, cited by Cornish) certainly demonstrated that resistance to extinction of behaviour by subjects who were trained to pull a lever on a modified 'fruit machine' was *inversely* proportional to the percentage of attempts resulting in reinforcement being given during the training period.

As further support for the idea that intermittent reinforcement schedules are at least partly responsible for inducing new behaviour early on which is then very hard to break off later, Cornish drew upon clinical reports such as those of Bolen and Boyd (1968) and Moran (1970) that 'compulsive' gamblers are likely to have experienced a particularly large early win or a streak of luck at the beginning of their gambling careers. He also cited Dickerson's (1974) report that 72 per cent of those most involved in gambling in his survey sample had had early luck as against 15 per cent of those least involved. The argument is that such experiences 'enrich' otherwise very intermittent early schedules of reinforcement.

From his observations in 'betting shops', Dickerson (1974) concluded that there was a powerful training process in operation there which in operant theory terms could best be described as an FI schedule of reinforcement (reinforcement at fixed intervals) imposed upon a VI schedule of the kind discussed by Cornish.

Regular gamblers were much more likely to stay on the premises for a number of races and to take advantage of the information (and probably, judging by their accounts of their feelings, affected by the excitement) provided by the commentary (the 'blower') relayed from the race track, so as to place their bets near to the start of a race. Dickerson proposed that the race commentary provided reinforcement of betting at fixed intervals and that the gambler's behaviour was gradually shaped, just like that of an animal in a Skinner box, so that he remained in the close environs of the 'shop' whilst the reinforcement contingencies were in operation, betting repetitively at the fixed intervals determined by the pattern of the race meetings. Adaptation to the thrill provided by the race and the uncertainty of winning or losing, plus the incentive to 'chase' previous losses, encouraged the betting of larger stakes as time goes on.

Explanations of appetitive behaviour of this kind are of course open to the criticism that, as a consequence of emphasizing the biological similarity of man and other animals, they relegate humanistic aspects to an inappropriately negligible role. As Cornish pointed out:

> Descriptions of learning through reinforcement contingencies (such as VR schedules) have tended to ignore or explicitly to deny, the relevance of people's subjective expectations or other 'mentalistic' variables to explanations of behaviour. This essentially passive view of the individual as merely a respondent has recently been strongly criticised by more sophisticated cognitive social learning theorists . . . (p.191).

Not only, Cornish argued, are cognitive factors important in gambling because features of gambling settings can lead the punter to make errors in computing probabilities (for example the well-known 'gambler's fallacy' whereby the gambler believes the probability of winning on a purely chance event, such as 'heads', increases the less it comes up, i.e. after a series of 'tails'), but in addition cognitive factors probably play a more active role. In particular, if a gambler adopts a skill-orientation or problem-solving 'set', constructing hypotheses about the determinants of winning, particularly where the gambler can obtain relevant information (as in horse racing for example), the achievement of a win may be more highly valued, strategies may be reinforced in a 'superstitious' fashion by the fortuitous juxtaposition of response and reinforcement, and the anticipation of future winning may be enhanced as a result of experiencing 'near misses'. Interestingly, the designers of commercial gambling machines have been aware of the value of such 'intermediate' reinforcers. Cornish cited Strickland and Grote (1967) who noticed the following design feature:

> . . . in the fruit-machine three-wheel spin when a coin is inserted and the lever pulled. These wheels stop in a 1-2-3 order, from left to right, displaying in a machine's window one symbol from each of the wheels. The player reads off the combination and refers to

> the chart of winning combinations. The researcher noted that, on the machine they studied, the symbols did not appear equally frequently on all the wheels, wheel one having a fairly large proportion of potential winners, the second wheel fewer of these, and the third, fewer still. Since as they point out, the wheel stops in a 1-2-3 order, the player is most likely to see a winning symbol early in a sequential presentation of results (Cornish, pp.194–5).

Carrying out an experiment with a modified slot machine, Strickland and Grote were able to show that this design did indeed result in players playing the machine significantly longer than if winning symbols occurred relatively later in the display.

Discussions of operant learning approaches to drug use (e.g. Kumar and Stolerman, 1977; Teasdale, 1973; Dews, 1973) have pointed out that there are other operant processes which could be responsible for the acquisition and maintenance of drug-seeking behaviour. A major contender is the action of a drug, whether instead of or in addition to its action as a primary positive reinforcer, as a 'negative reinforcer' owing to its ability to enable an animal to *escape* from or *avoid* altogether the distress of tension or other unpleasant affect. Avoidance conditioning has been shown to render animal behaviour particularly resistant to extinction, and is therefore a particularly strong contender for explaining the persistence of drug-seeking behaviour. Whether appetitive activities are used for purposes of tension reduction, and if so whether they are effective in this role, was discussed at length in Chapter 8. The distress caused by the withdrawal of a drug to which the nervous system has adapted is a special case, and the possibility that a powerful source of additional motivation is provided by the use of a drug to escape from or avoid withdrawal distress is discussed below.

A further addition to relevant operant theory is introduced by the idea of control by antecedents. Although the importance of the *consequences* of behaviour is central, to most operant psychologists the basic paradigm has three terms: antecedents, behaviour, and consequences. Antecedents are those stimuli which provide the organism with information about the reinforcing consequences of behaviour to be expected under those circumstances. Behaviour may be as much under the control of antecedent or 'discriminative' stimuli which signal the likelihood of reinforcement following behaviour. For example, in his operant analysis of smoking behaviour, Paxton (1980) referred to the 'well known' fact that many smokers can identify setting conditions which make their smoking likely. The arrival of coffee or tea after a meal, or the consumption of alcoholic drinks, would be examples.

Discriminative stimuli which elicit behaviour, as well as other stimuli which accompany reinforcement, may acquire conditioned or secondary reinforcing properties as a result of their association with reinforcement. For example, it was demonstrated by Schuster and Woods (1968, cited by Kumar and Stolerman, 1977) that monkeys would respond more rapidly for saline plus the presentation of a red light than for saline alone, after being trained to bar-press for a morphine infusion accompanied by the red light. The red light was operating as a 'secondary reinforcer'. The opportunities for stimuli to acquire secondary reinforcing properties as a result of association with appetitive reinforcement in humans are clearly legion. The sights, sounds, odours, and flavours associated with the consumption of alcoholic drinks, for example, are many and are frequently highly distinctive and memorable. The graphic account of the characteristic 'stimuli' of the gambling casino provided by Dostoevsky in *The Gambler* (see Chapter 3) is another case in point. The importance of secondary reinforcement again lies in its apparent potential for increasing behavioural persistence. If an activity no longer meets with the original primary reinforcement or with reinforcement of the withdrawal relief type, or if reinforcement is delivered on a very intermittent schedule, the provision of secondary reinforcement might be expected to be an important element in maintaining behaviour.

Hardy (1964) proposed a learned appetite theory of sexual motivation based upon the notion of an accumulation of positive affective sexual experiences. He was aware too of the additional importance of conditioning by association:

> A new set of associations or meanings is formed. The activities which lead up to the initial erotic arousal now have a tendency to serve as cues leading to the arousal of sexual desire. Furthermore, as erotic experiences are repeated (a) the greater the association values of the cues to sexuality, and (b) the wider the range of cues to sexuality (p.11).

The chain of circumstances leading up to or surrounding the consumptive act itself, along with the experience of its affective consequences, may be repeated in similar form many times. For instance, a cigarette smoker may repeat the smoking sequence 10,000 times or more a year. Hence the habit is greatly 'over-learned' (Hunt and Matarazzo, 1970).

A much-quoted theory proposed by Wikler (1973) in order to account for relapse back to drug-taking on the part of users who had given up for a period of time, is based upon the premise that stimuli associated with drug-taking can acquire conditioned properties as a result of repeated association with drug-taking settings. Wikler's view was that relief of the distress occasioned by withdrawal constituted the main reinforcement for the consumption of narcotic drugs, and that withdrawal symptoms might become conditioned to aspects of situations specifically associated with the availability of these drugs. Hence, withdrawal distress, or something resembling it, might be experienced long after giving up and would act as a 'trigger' for further drug-taking reinforced by relief of these 'symptoms'. His work with rats, made physically dependent and then withdrawn from morphine, suggested that 'symptoms' such as 'wet dog shakes' (shaking like a wet dog, a symptom observed to be associated with morphine withdrawal in rats) were experienced more frequently, after withdrawal, in locations previously associated with morphine consumption.

Teasdale (1973) has argued that Wikler's theory of relapse was unnecessarily complicated. Because anxiety is frequently a component of drug withdrawal distress (studies of alcohol withdrawal in humans also show how difficult it is to discriminate between the symptoms of alcohol withdrawal and general anxiety—e.g. Hershon, 1977) it is only necessary to hypothesize that *anxiety* becomes conditioned to drug-taking settings. This is important because it would follow that any situation giving rise to anxiety or tension could provide the motivation for relapse.

Whatever the precise mechanisms involved, it is clear that operant theory provides a very plausible explanation of how appetitive behaviours may become strengthened through repeated use. There are those, indeed, who believe, that schedules of operant reinforcement offer a complete explanation. Dews (1973), who is one of these, pointed to the infinite variety of scheduling, by time or responses, which animal experiments have shown are possible, many of which produced results at once dramatic and unexpected, and many of which provided considerable control over behaviour for long periods of time. So convinced was Dews of the adequacy of an operant explanation of excessive appetitive behaviour, that he totally eschewed rational or purposive explanations. He concluded his contribution to a symposium on 'psychic dependence' as follows:

> Psychic dependence is nothing more or less than schedule control of drug-taking behaviour . . . The addict is compelled to take the drug . . . not by direct physical constraints, but because evolution has produced subjects who are controlled by schedules . . . Although the mechanisms are normal, they operate in a mechanistic way, so the consequences may be detrimental to the subject, according with the well recognised 'irrationality' of drug-taking. One can make no progress in the understanding of drug-addiction while one insists in finding some 'good' or 'pleasure' connected with the drug which more than balances the manifest bad consequences; there is no such rational balancing of consequences. It has been the search for the rationality of the drug-takers' conduct that has inhibited suggestions of behavioural mechanisms, leading to the paucity of constructive suggestions . . . The addict's account of how he came to his condition should not be taken any more seriously than a cancer victim's account of how he came to be so afflicted; in both cases, processes are involved into which the subject has no particular insight (p.45).

COGNITIVE PROCESSES

This is an extreme position, very contrary for example to the social learning theory of Akers *et al.* (1979) towards which the evidence of the previous two chapters led, and it is not one to which this writer holds. In fact modern adaptations of learning theory (e.g. Gray, 1975) place a far greater emphasis on cognitive factors such as expectations, than was the case with earlier, more mechanistic, and more purely behavioural learning theories. In the case of alcohol effects, there has been increasing experimental evidence in recent years that a whole range of effects depends as much upon placebo as upon pharmacological action, at least where relatively small doses of alcohol are concerned. The typical experiment takes a 2 × 2 'balanced placebo' group design in which half the subjects are given a small dose of alcohol and the other half a placebo drink designed to mimic alcohol (e.g. tonic compared with vodka and tonic). Half of each group is told they have been given an alcoholic drink (thus a quarter of subjects are *correctly* told they are receiving alcohol and a quarter are incorrectly told the same) whilst the other half of each group is told they are receiving a non-alcoholic drink (correctly for a quarter of the subjects, incorrectly for the remaining quarter). Thus, it is possible to test whether receiving alcohol is more or less important than being *told* that one is receiving alcohol. Results fairly uniformly show that being told one is drinking alcohol is the more powerful factor. For example, Vuchinich *et al.* (1979) found 'expectancy' (as being told one is consuming alcohol is normally called by these experimenters) to be more important than receiving alcohol in producing laughter and mirth; Briddell *et al.* (1978) found the same for arousal to sexual stimuli; and Marlatt *et al.* (1973) found that being told one had received alcohol produced more continued drinking ('loss of control' as they, possibly misleadingly, called it) than actually receiving alcohol.

These experimental findings are consistent with the thesis of MacAndrew and Edgerton (1970) who collected together anthropological material on drinking and behaviour associated with drinking in different cultural groups around the world. They argued that the social behaviour associated with drinking is so varied from culture to culture that the effects of alcohol must be mediated more strongly by social expectations than by pharmacological effects. If the meaning of alcohol to a particular group is such that aggressive behaviour is *expected* to follow its consumption, then consumption is more likely on occasions when aggressive behaviour is otherwise promoted, and aggression is the likely result. For other groups alcohol may have quite different meanings, be consumed in different settings and on different occasions, and produce different effects. Demonstrations that people drinking in groups become more friendly and euphoric and less unhappy and bored, whilst those drinking alone are affected differently, feeling less clear-headed and dizzier (Pliner and Cappell, 1974); and that business school students invited to drink while discussing their work created stories in response to a projective test which involved the meaning of life or other major experiences, while members of fraternities invited to drink whilst studying the effects of a party atmosphere on fantasy wrote stories with strong themes of sex and aggression (Kalin *et al.*, 1965); are amongst experimental findings that support these anthropological insights.

Although there is now ample evidence from both experimental psychopharmacology and from anthropology that emotional and behavioural changes following at least moderate consumption of a drug such as alcohol are influenced as much by the user's expectations of the effects plus the social context surrounding use as by the pharmacological action of the drug itself, there is still much room for debate about the psychological mechanisms involved, as Vuchinich and Tucker's (1980) review indicates. They wished to distinguish between 'expectancy' on the one hand and 'cognitive labelling' on the other. The first is adequately tested using the balanced placebo design already described. Although cognitive labelling, whereby a person attributes or misattributes non-specific arousal produced by a drug in terms of the circumstances surrounding drug use (Schachter and Singer, 1962), is often assumed to operate, the balanced placebo design does not test it, according to Vuchinich and Tucker. This requires the kind of manipulation used in Schachter and Singer's classic experiment in which some subjects injected with epinephrine were given an adequate explanation of the effects of the drug whilst others were not.

In their own study of mirth, Vuchinich *et al.* (1979) used a combination of the balanced placebo design with the Schachter and Singer-type addition. Being told that alcohol had been ingested was most influential, influencing both laughter and self-reports of positive feelings. In addition, the actual ingestion of alcohol increased reports of feelings, although it did not influence laughter. Although expectancy theory was supported, cognitive labelling was not, as the giving or withholding of information about the effects of alcohol to be expected had no influence, and being told that alcohol had been ingested did not influence physical sensations reported. Although it seems conceivable that the cognitive labelling manipulation may be relatively ineffective for alcohol, to which most subjects would be well used, and perhaps more effective for other drugs and activities, the results as they stand certainly support expectancy rather than cognitive labelling.

Whatever the precise mechanisms involved and their relative importance from one activity to another, the crucial importance of cognitive events and processes is now fully acknowledged, even by those whose model of man is largely behavioural or physiological. This welcome trend in psychology was strongly influenced by those such as Schachter and Singer who demonstrated the importance, for an understanding of how emotional states are produced, of the events and states to which a person *attributes* physiological arousal, and Meichenbaum (1977) who adduced much evidence for the importance in therapeutic processes of such cognitions as self-instructions, self-deprecatory or self-referential thoughts, and appraisal processes. No psychological theory of the development of appetitive behaviour would be complete without reference to factors of this kind. It was Bruch's (1974) contention, for example, that eating could come to serve the many possible symbolic functions which she listed (see p.142, above) as a result of mislearning, usually starting in the family in the early years of life, leading to an inability to discriminate real 'hunger' from other signals of discomfort and from states of emotional tension. Eating for these, 'wrong', reasons resulted in short-lived and unsatisfying eating 'cycles' in which eating afforded temporary relief from anxious or depressive feelings mistakenly experienced as the 'need to eat'. In this way, '. . . the nutritional function can be misused in the service of complex emotional and interpersonal problems' (p.50).

Similarly, Rook and Hammen (1977) have criticized previous research on sexual behaviour for concentrating on sexual acts alone or upon the more biological components of sexual response. They attempted to provide a corrective by offering a cognitive perspective which in particular emphasized the way in which people appraise physiological responses and attribute them, or not, to sexual arousal. Extrapolating from Schachter's (1964) theory of emotion, they argued that both physiological arousal and 'erotic labelling' were necessary for the subjective experience of sexual arousal. Because, particularly in the early phases of the sexual response cycle, physiological responses are non-specific and in many ways resemble the types of response elicited at other times, wide latitude is possible in explaining arousal by attributing it to sexual feelings or by explaining it in some other way. Not only would this lead us to expect wide differences between social and cultural groups, but this might also help to explain traditional gender differences in frequencies of sexual behaviour and ranges of sexually arousing situations reported by males and females (Kinsey *et al.*, 1948, 1953; Eysenck, 1971b). The greater size and ease of accessibility of genital organs in the male, the less ambiguous signs of sexual arousal afforded by erection and emission, the greater degree of initiative in sexual behaviour expected of males, and the more common male norm for talking about and emphasizing sexual arousal and sexual acts, all may contribute to a sexual socialization process which affords young males far more opportunity than young females for learning to label physiological arousal as sexual.

Rook and Hammen also cited experiments suggesting that 'misattribution' occurs, as would be expected theoretically. For example, men have been shown to give evidence of becoming more sexually aroused than control subjects as a result of physical exercise followed by the viewing of an erotic film and, in one experiment, when being approached by an attractive woman on a fear-arousing suspension bridge! The argument is that both experiments provided a context (the film in one case, the attractive woman in the other) in which physiological response aroused by other means (exercise in one case, fear in the other) could be attributed to sexual arousal. Along similar lines they suggested that drugs of many sorts might acquire their pharmacologically unjustified reputations as aphrodisiacs because they act like placebos which are not totally inert but which produce a range of non-specific physiological arousal cues which, under the right circumstances, people may readily attribute to sexual arousal.

Rook and Hammen's paper contained a number of additional, and highly persuasive, speculations which if correct would have important implications for the development of individual differences in appetitive behaviour. People who have a relatively low threshold for sexual arousal, or who are sexually aroused by a wide range of stimuli, may find sexual arousal easily augmented once they perceive evidence that what they believe is sexual arousal has begun. By contrast, people who apply sexual cognitions more sparingly may run the risk of experiencing arousal-reducing cognitions (guilt, disgust, failure, etc.) at times when sexual arousal is attempted or a sexual partner is aroused, for example. An important ingredient of modern sex therapy techniques (e.g. Masters and Johnson, 1970; Kaplan, 1974) may be the opportunities they afford for learning to reattribute sexual feelings to non-genital stimulation (e.g. the popular 'sensate focus' technique). The important point for present discussion, however, is the suggestion that there may be processes at work which over time augment initial individual differences. Rook and Hammen's ideas are thus useful additions to the general theme of this and the following chapter, that excessive appetitive behaviour has a developmental aspect to it; that whatever its origins in personality, social environment, or biological differences, it can become something more sinister as a result of learning and other processes.

Rook and Hammen pointed out that their perspective need in no way be specific to sexual behaviour, indeed they had to draw upon research most of which lay outside that particular field of study. To underline the point it is only necessary to cite a highly influential sociological account of marijuana use, that by Becker (1963), who wrote of the importance of the *meaning* attributed by users to sensations experienced when using the drug. Becker concluded that the social group in which the drug was used was crucial in supplying the ideas out of which the novice user constructed his or her meaning of the marijuana experience and the pleasure it gave. Some would argue (e.g. Laurie, 1967) that these events may be particularly important with marijuana because its pharmacological effects are weak—early experiences with the drug may be described as pleasant, unpleasant, or disappointing—and that the experience is therefore an ambiguous one requiring interpretation which, if the drug is taken in a social setting, as is often the case, the social group will most likely provide.

The cognitive processes under discussion may operate outside or on the borders of consciousness. Writers such as Meichenbaum (1977), however, have been as much concerned with self-talk, self-statements, and the use of self-instruction, which, like instructions from other people, occur overtly and are perceived consciously. Indeed, he has been particularly at pains to develop a technology for therapeutic purposes which very explicitly uses such cognitions. Just as it can be shown that children can acquire the ability to perform certain complex tasks more quickly by talking to themselves (self-instructions) at appropriate points, so it may be the case that man's capacity for language contributes to the acquisition of excessive appetitive behaviour, quite apart from the role of language in social communication. The human being has the ability, lacking in other animals, to tell herself that she is becoming sexually aroused, that he is looking forward to a forthcoming drink, that a particular horse in the next race is a good bet, or that she is feeling hungry. In the language of learning theory, this might be expressed by saying that man has opportunities for 'rehearsal' of anticipated positive outcomes from behaviour, or for reinforcing him or herself in between times by covert thought processes involving imagination and fantasy (Feldman and MacCulloch, 1971). Reference was made in an earlier chapter to Bergler's (1958) observations about 'compulsive gamblers': that they often showed an almost fanatical belief in the possibility of winning and that their recollections of past gambling were highly selective in favour of recalling successes and forgetting losses. Cornish (1978) too included amongst a number of possible reasons why a gambler might not respond to the inevitability of financial loss from gambling in the longer term, various false beliefs (e.g. the illusion of control or the importance of skill), cognitive biases (e.g. the 'gambler's fallacy'), and information-processing problems which may distort perception of probabilities and pay-offs. The same kinds of process operate as other forms of appetite develop. For example, McGuire *et al.* (1966) showed that excessive drinkers anticipated that drinking would be associated with relaxation and sociability to a far greater extent than was in practice the case, and linked drinking in their thoughts with, for example, sexual prowess and freedom from family surveillance, to an unrealistic degree. The role of fantasy in the anticipation of the pleasures of sexual behaviour is obvious. Masturbatory fantasies have been held partly responsible for the development of some forms of sexual deviance and 'reconditioning' by redirecting such fantasies has been prescribed.

Appetitive activities may become 'over-valued' in these ways, offering more in anticipation than in fact. Such processes are arguably an important part of the development of excess. Not only must it be supposed that cognitions, in the form of a range of general and specific beliefs and self-instructions, are part of the motivational system encouraging appetitive behaviour (Ellis, 1975), but a general tendency towards affective–behavioural–cognitive consistency doubtless operates as well (Ostrom, 1969). Thus, increases in appetitive behaviour and positive affective experience associated with increasing habit strength, are likely to be accompanied by increasingly frequent thoughts serving to bolster habitual behaviour at a new increased level. Such bolstering thoughts may take a variety of forms, including self-statements such as, 'Doing X is the only way I get to feel . . .', 'All men like me do X', 'If he's going to be like that then I'm entitled to X', 'If I didn't do X, then I'd probably do Y', 'X is one of the best things in life'. Such thoughts may be publicly stated, kept private, or may scarcely be within awareness much of the time.

Thus, man's capacity for formulating plans, for thinking ahead, for having wishes and expectations, for evolving strategies and tactics may enhance the human potential for excessive behaviour. By the same token, though, these same abilities might be expected to offer man unusual opportunities for setting up a resistance against excesses to which he is biologically prone.

Human cognitive and linguistic abilities undoubtedly expand the scope for learning on the basis of vicarious experience. Cornish (1978) pointed out how children may receive 'instruction' from parents and others long before they have the opportunity to take part in gambling themselves. At a more general level:

> . . . the televising of races, together with details of market prices, information on, and discussion of 'form', tipsters' selections, exciting

> commentaries, and information on results and potential payoffs, provides opportunities for practically the whole population to be introduced to the mechanics and potential reinforcements of some forms of gambling (pp.186–7).

Each of the forms of behaviour considered in this book has its own 'literature', sex (in the form of educative books and pornography) and eating (in the form of cookery books) perhaps the largest. No one grows up without some knowledge of most of these behaviours and, with the exception of eating, early knowledge long predates the first experience of consumption. Teasdale (1973) has pointed out that few come to their first drug experience completely naive, and Hardy (1964) pointed out in his paper, 'An Appetitional Theory of Sexual Motivation', how early sexual motivation might be based on imagination and fantasy helped on by indirect social influences such as reading a romantic novel. Although few societies allow the privilege afforded Pilaga Indian children (Henry and Henry, 1953, cited by Hardy) of openly watching parental sexual intercourse, the multi-faceted process of acquiring the 'facts of life' is a lengthy one which starts early in life. Similarly, it has been demonstrated that children have already acquired definite concepts of alcohol use and its connotations by the age of eight (Jahoda and Cramond, 1972). Leventhal and Cleary (1980) argued similarly that the stage of preparation for smoking, and this might be a lengthy stage, should be taken into account in considering the whole process of taking up smoking. As they say, it is likely that 'smoking' begins well before the person tries the first cigarette, and that quite young children develop attitudes about smoking and have images of what smoking is like long before they try it for themselves.

In summary, then, we can point to the existence of a compelling process which, with moderate encouragement and not too many impediments, can be capable of fashioning an excessive appetite out of modest beginnings. To this process, various schedules of positive or negative operant reinforcement, and an abundance of discriminative stimuli acting as secondary reinforcers, along with a nexus of expectations, attributions and misattributions, fears, and fantasies, all contribute. Thus, the inclination towards appetitive consumption need not be static, but under the right circumstances can grow into an attachment less easily resistable than formerly. At the same time we must constantly remind ourselves of the cost–benefit type of social learning model which suggests that any leaning towards appetitive indulgence must contend with opposition from biological, social, moral, and other constraints acting to nip any such proclivity in the bud.

CHAPTER TEN

The Development of Strong Attachment

The habit has extended its roots deeply into many aspects and facets of . . . daily life. [There occurs a] complicated interwoven pattern of habits, of needs gratified, of pleasures derived and tensions released (Hochbaum, 1965, cited by Reinert, 1968, pp.41–2, to show the similarities between the smoking habit and excessive drinking.)

When she was depressed, the embrace of a new man gave her a lift. When she was happy, such an embrace constituted the perfect way of accenting and highlighting her happiness. When she was turned down for one job, sex soothed the injury. When she got another job, sex added to the celebration (Morse, 1963, p.43).

. . . the morbid growth upon the opium-eater of his peculiar habit, . . . once rooted in the system, and throwing out *tentacula* like a cancer . . . (Thomas de Quincey, *Confessions of an Opium Eater*, 1897, (orig. 1822), p.417).

DISCRIMINATION AND ITS EROSION

Although the learning and other mechanisms which could account for the development of excess are fairly well understood, the precise ways in which their influence is manifest in the early stages are not. This is the large grey area between acceptable, moderate indulgence and highly troublesome and noticeable excess. I would propose that for help in understanding here we need look no further than the long-familiar psychological ideas of discrimination and generalization. The constraints that are influential in curbing natural tendencies towards increased or excessive behaviour have their impact, let us suppose, through *discrimination*. For most people, training in appetitive conduct is a matter of discrimination. The rules to which socializing agents expect others to adhere are rules about settings and conditions under which consumption is appropriate. The variables in terms of which drinking, gambling, eating, and heterosexuality may be defined as appropriate or inappropriate include time of day, company, day of the week, the meaning of the occasion (celebration, etc.), quantity consumed, and so forth. Appropriateness may be defined in terms of quite complex combinations of such variables. For example, what is considered appropriate drinking at a Saturday night party with certain people present (or not present) may be quite inappropriate with other combinations of day of the week, company, and occasion. The overall rule guiding appetitive behaviour may be that it is acceptable 'in moderation', but this rule is likely to be made operational by a whole set of specific restraints inculcated by detailed discrimination training. The impelling sense of the wrongness of excessive behaviour is particularized by an impelling sense of the wrongness of behaving in a whole variety of very specific ways in a host of specific settings.

The majority of people at the moderate end of the consumption curve are discriminating; they know that there is a time and a place for everything. When the circumstances are right for the development of a strong habit—when incentives are strong and disincentives relatively weak—then there will be a tendency for discrimination to be eroded and for behaviour to generalize to a range of additional stimuli or settings. The stronger the inclination to consume or approach under appropriate circumstances, the greater the tendency to do so under other circumstances also. Indeed, it is arguably the generalized inappropriateness of appetitive behaviour, or the failure to keep it within the confines of normal expectancy that lead to it being branded as 'excessive' or as an 'ism'. It is, for example, the lack of discrimination in the sexual behaviour of Boswell (Stone, 1979) and other 'hypersexuals' (Levitt, 1973) that draws comment. 'Moderate' or 'controlled' use on the other hand is characterized by rules of discrimination, usually promoted by the social groups or wider community of which a person is a member.

These rules are probably fairly general in kind and not dissimilar from one appetitive behaviour to another, even though some forms of behaviour are more widely acceptable than others. It seems, for example, that the ways in which some opiate and other 'drug' users control their use, even in present-day prohibitionist America, are not dissimilar to the ways most drinkers control their alcohol use. This conclusion is based on the work of Zinberg *et al.* (1977, 1981) who studied controlled illicit drug use. They reported on interviews with 99 controlled users (96 being present or past controlled users of marijuana, 52 of psychedelics, and 47 of opiates). They found controlled use to be characterized by rituals and social sanctions:

> All subjects tend to maintain regular ties to social institutions, such as work-place, school, and family . . . Controlled users maintain ordinary social relationships with non-drug users (1981, pp.284–5).

> Virtually all . . . required the assistance of other controlled users to construct appropriate rituals and social sanctions out of the folklore of practices of the diverse subculture of drug-takers (p.293).

With this maintenance of normal ties with non-drug users and with controlled users went the ability to discriminate between approved and disapproved ways of using the drug of choice, and rituals and procedures for drug use which kept its use within limits:

> . . . our subjects demonstrate an ability to keep drugs on hand for some time without using them, and to continue their leisure activities (p.285).

> Rituals . . . may include methods of procuring and administering the drug, selection of a particular social and physical setting for use, and special activities undertaken after the drug has been administered . . . (p.290).

In general the many rules that informants adopted were reminiscent of the rules and regulations surrounding normal alcohol use. In general they served to define moderate use and to condemn compulsive use, to limit use to settings conducive to positive experience, to reinforce the notion that 'dependence' should be avoided, to assist in interpreting the 'high', and to support non-drug-related obligations and relationships.

Zinberg *et al.* were critical of the previously held assumption that controlled use, if it occurred at all, was only a stage on the route to excessive use (witness the terms 'chipper', 'experimenter', 'neophyte user', 'casual user', 'honeymoon stage'). Many of their controlled users had been using for periods of up to ten years or more, the average length of controlled use was four years, and for heroin alone 3.6 years, and none of the groups selected for interview had shown a shift to less controlled use despite a variety of stresses and strains of normal living. In the terms of our cost–benefit type of social learning theory, the social groups and activities within which this controlled use was embedded constituted an important and valued part of life that made control desirable and excess potentially costly.

A principal element in the behavioural treatment of excessive eating, as recommended by Stuart (1967), appears to be the reinstatement of discrimination in eating pattern. Clients are advised, for example, to confine eating to set meal times and, very significantly, not to pair eating with other activities such as watching television, reading, working, or cooking. The same principle lies behind procedures for helping excessive drinkers reinstate control over their drinking (Heather and Robertson, 1983).

The same can be said of those attempts at control exercised on a national level which fall short of total prohibition. Our system of controls on drinking in public according to age and time of day as well as the system of measured amounts of different alcoholic beverages administered by Customs and Excise has the effect of promoting discrimination in drinking. Legislation in the Yemen confining the use of the drug khat to weekends and holidays is another example, and Henry VIII's attempt to confine card-playing to Christmas (France, 1902) and Muhammed's early proscriptions about alcohol (Baasher, 1981) are further historical examples.

Despite informal and formal social rules which invite restraint, not everyone retains control, and some never establish it in the first place. Reinert (1968) described the increasing preoccupation with the 'addicting' substance which occurred in his experience when a person had once had control and had then lost it. He appreciated, in this writer's view correctly, the important role of what learning theorists would call stimulus generalization:

> Among many regular users of alcohol, a great variety of situations, modes, feelings and activities have become linked with alcohol in such a way that a greater or lesser feeling of discomfort is felt if alcohol is absent from the situation. This or that feeling, situation, party, event or hour of the day 'calls' for a drink. In the case of the alcoholic, the situation does not merely 'call for' but 'demands' a drink, and he cannot carry on without one. The analogy to the smoker who cannot write a letter, think, make a decision, drive a car, play a hand of bridge, conduct an interview, converse or drink a cocktail without lighting up a cigarette seems remarkable. Alcoholics drink for the same reasons anyone else does but they gradually come either to use a greater variety of the reasons or establish particularly strong connections between alcohol and a few of the reasons (p.41).

It is, for example, part of the anecdotal wisdom of Alcoholics Anonymous that any event (whether apparently unpleasant or pleasant) is an excuse for drinking for the 'alcoholic', and as previously mentioned survey evidence confirms that heavy drinkers endorse a greater range of drinking motives as applying to themselves than do lighter drinkers (e.g. Edwards *et al.*, 1972c; Mulford and Miller, 1960). Descriptions of other forms of excessive appetitive behaviour frequently stress the cure-all function which behaviour serves for the person whose appetite is excessive. The example of one kind of female 'sexual promiscuity' given by Morse (1963), and quoted at the beginning of this chapter, is one instance.

A most significant part of this generalization process may be the increasing misattribution of meaning to internal psychophysiological states. Thus, internal cues that might otherwise be interpreted as fatigue, tension, or confusion, or else not labelled at all, may be interpreted as indicating a need to go and place a bet, if 'habit strength' for betting is high, for example. It may reasonably be argued that the stronger attachment becomes, the more salient or 'pre-potent' relevant acts (sexual, eating, drug-taking, etc.) become amongst all possible actions, and hence the more likely it becomes that emotional arousal will be interpreted in terms of need, desire, or craving for that substance or activity. In general it may be proposed that excessive appetitive forms of behaviour are always widely cue linked, and that amongst the cues to which such behaviour is linked are psychophysiological arousal cues which are not normally stimuli for non-excessive behaviour of the same kind. This is consistent with Allport's (1961) well-known notion of the 'functional autonomy' of habitual behaviour: that action has become independent of whatever originally motivated it.

Reinert (1968) was struck by the similarity between drinking and smoking in these respects:

> In the description of the smoking habit by Hochbaum (1965), one could easily substitute the word 'alcoholism' for 'smoking'. Smoking, he points out, is not a single, simple habit unrelated to the rest of a person's life and daily activity. In the heavy smoker, 'The habit has extended its roots deeply into many aspects and facets of his daily life'. There occurs a 'complicated interwoven pattern of habits, of needs gratified, of pleasures derived and of tensions released. It is this fact, quite apart from any true pharmacological addiction that may exist, that makes it so very difficult to break the smoking habit' (Reinert, 1968, pp.41–2).

It was the increasingly automatic and generalized nature of behaviour, coupled with decreasing awareness and increasing dependence upon secondary rather than primary rewards, which Hunt and Matarazzo (1970) stressed in their outline of habit mechanisms in smoking. They referred to, 'habitual, affectless behaviour', and to, 'the blandness of habit', and asserted, 'The maintenance of habit in the drug area is largely a matter of learning principles rather than of physical dependence or addiction' (p.73). Interestingly enough it was the lack of conscious thought about behaviour which George Kelly (1955), noted more for his personal construct view of personality than for any interest he may have had in excessive behaviours, stressed when considering what he termed 'impulsivity'. He wrote:

> The field is pre-empted. A choice point is established. A decision is made. Action ensues. The characteristic feature of impulsivity is that the period of circumspection which normally precedes decision is unduly shortened . . . Thus . . . he looks at the situation in a multidimensional manner for a short period of time only. He quickly narrows down the issues and makes a choice which commits him to a course of events. He may then follow this decision by an attempt to retreat to a point where he can look at the decision multidimensionally again and perhaps retract his decision . . . All people behave with a measure of impulsivity . . . [and are] likely to be more impulsive about some matters than others. Some . . . spending

> money. Some . . . like to gamble, some . . . [to become] intoxicated . . . Many . . . are impulsive in their sexual behaviour. When confronted with the possibility of having sexual intercourse they find it difficult to examine the situation multidimensionally over a protacted period of time (pp.526–8).

If it can be accepted that the increasing preoccupation with the activity of choice, so often described in clinical and other theoretical accounts of excessive behaviour, can be equated with an increasing 'commitment' to the activities concerned (one speaks of becoming 'a confirmed smoker' for example, although the positive moral connotations of being 'committed' have probably precluded the use of this word in association with excessive forms of behaviour), then a whole body of experimental social psychological research becomes relevant to our understanding. Much of this work suggests that commitment alters motivation. In one experiment of this kind subjects came having fasted, and in other cases having gone without water, for a number of hours. Those who then voluntarily committed themselves to a further period of hunger or thirst without monetary or other external incentive, described themselves as less hungry or thirsty than those who were not asked to make such a commitment, and the experimenters were able to demonstrate behavioural effects also. When a later opportunity was provided to consume food, or to drink, those who had made a voluntary commitment ate or drank less. Other experiments showed physiological effects of commitment. In one experiment, using plasma-free fatty acids as an index of hunger, it was possible to show that voluntary commitment to a further period of fasting reduced hunger (Zimbardo, 1969).

In yet another experiment of this kind, those who committed themselves to the longest period of further abstention from water (24 hours), with least external justification, not only rated themselves as less thirsty and subsequently consumed less water, but also on testing chose fewer thirst-related words and produced fewer 'drive-related' themes in response to a projective story-telling test (Zimbardo, 1969).

These experiments, convincing though they are, only involved short-term commitment for up to a single day. It can only be supposed that the effects upon both psychological and physiological systems would be much greater if commitment, either to continued appetitive behaviour or to abstention or reduction, was for a far longer period. What we are offered in these experiments, as in Rodin's (1978) demonstrations that subjective hunger, palatability of food, salivation, and insulin release were intimately linked (see p.147, above), is a clear message that alterations in motivation of the kind we have been discussing in this chapter, involve the total system. This is of the utmost importance to the development of a satisfactory psychology of excessive appetites as a whole, because debate in the past has often foundered on the assumption that only drugs with their physiological effects could give rise to 'addiction' proper and that other forms of 'dependence' must be purely 'psychological'. Clearly, no such convenient separation is possible in the light of work such as that on commitment.'

ALTERED BIOLOGICAL RESPONSE

The idea that 'dependence' can be, '. . . psychic and sometimes physical', is enshrined in the World Health Organization definition of drug 'dependence' of 1964, and the view that 'addiction' is only a real driving force when it has a 'biological' basis is widely held. The hallmarks of physical, or biochemical, 'dependence' are generally taken to be, first, tolerance, i.e. a decrease in potency upon continued administration of a drug and secondly, a withdrawal or abstinence syndrome, i.e. a definite, characteristic, and time-limited set of symptoms which appear when the drug disappears or is disappearing from the body.

The existence of 'biochemical dependence' defined in this way is best established in the case of opiate drugs (drug dependence of morphine type), but is also well accepted in the case of certain other drugs, including those of barbiturate type. A good description of the opiate withdrawal syndrome was given by Kurland (1978, pp.23–4) who cited from Light and Torrance's picture, given in 1929, depicting the restlessness, yawning, alternate feelings of hot and cold, 'cold turkey' skin, running nose, drowsiness, stomach cramps, vomiting and diarrhoea, perspiration, and tremor which are classically associated with withdrawal. A review of biochemical theories of these kinds of 'dependence' is beyond the scope of this book. Suffice it to say that most theories suppose that drugs of 'addiction' alter the balance of biochemical neuro-transmitters at synaptic junctions between nerve endings within the nervous system. Whatever the biochemical mechanisms involved, what is important for the present discussion is that there is little dispute that tolerance and withdrawal symptoms occur as a result of the taking of *some* psychoactive drugs.

The undisputed occurrence of these events in the case of some drugs nevertheless raises a host of questions concerning their links with appetitive behaviour. Do they occur in the case of other drugs? When they occur, how important are they in comparison with other factors in accounting for excessive drug use? How can they help, if at all, in accounting for non-drug forms of excessive behaviour? In the case of other drugs, it has not been at all easy to separate out the effects of a possible withdrawal syndrome from such confounding factors as the reasons for discontinuing drug use, the reasons for which drug use was started in the first place, the psychological effects of stopping, and additional complicating factors such as nutritional deficiency brought about by inadequate diet during a period of drug use. Nevertheless, it is now fairly well established that an alcohol withdrawal syndrome exists, commonly characterized by anxiety, restlessness, and tremor, and more rarely by delirium and grand mal seizures. On the other hand, the view is generally held that 'physical dependence' upon cannabis does not occur. A range of other drugs occupy an intermediate and indeterminate position, even though their capacity for being used to excess is not in doubt. Chapter 4 documented the debate that has taken place in the past over whether tobacco, for example, is 'addictive' in this biochemical sense, as well as the present controversy over whether we must include the 'minor' tranquillizers in this category also.

If it can be established that a particular drug can produce such biological changes in the nervous system as a consequence of repeated use over a period of time, it cannot be supposed that we have thereby established the 'real' reason why that drug is sometimes used to excess. The question that does arise is how important this developmental process is in altering a person's motivation in comparison with the learning processes already outlined. A number of medical authorities have placed the development of an altered biological response to alcohol, for example, at the centre of the stage when it comes to explaining excessive drinking. Jellinek (1960), for example, considered that only 'gamma', 'delta', and 'epsilon' forms of 'alcoholism', characterized by tolerance and withdrawal symptoms, constituted *diseases*. Other forms, such as 'alpha alcoholism', characterized by psychological but not physical 'dependence', he considered were less central.

This element of biological change appears to have a central role also in the recently formulated 'alcohol dependence syndrome' (Edwards and Gross, 1976) on which our discussion touched in Chapter 2. The importance of biochemical changes in this formulation is shown by the use of the word 'core' which the authors used to qualify the word 'syndrome', and the listing of 'altered psychobiological state' (experience of withdrawal states, drinking for relief of withdrawal, tolerance) as one of three general signs of the syndrome. On the other hand, the word 'syndrome' is defined as, '. . . a number of phenomena tend[ing] to cluster with sufficient frequency to constitute a recognisable occurrence' (1976, p.1364) and it is stressed that some signs of 'alcohol dependence' may occur without others, and that it can be of variable degree. The deliberate looseness of the syndrome concept is emphasized. Most importantly, nowhere is it made clear whether 'altered psychobiological state' is a necessary condition, or whether the other two hallmarks of the syndrome, namely 'altered behavioural state' (culturally inappropriate drinking, heavy drinking, etc.) and 'altered subjective state' (heightened desire for drinking, preoccupation with drinking, etc.) may alone amount to a high level of 'dependence'.

The implication is that 'dependence' is unlikely to reach its fullest extent without some element of altered biochemical response to alcohol as a drug. Drinking for relief of withdrawal symptoms is a crucial element in this formulation because it provides the necessary link between altered biological response to the drug and increased motivation for consumption. The reasonable supposition is that the experience of unpleasant withdrawal symptoms creates the possibility of learning, through a process of operant conditioning additional to any such process that may have gone before, to perform any act which is followed by relief of this distress. Taking a further dose of the same drug is one such act. If the sequence of withdrawing, experiencing stressful withdrawal symptoms, taking a further dose, and experiencing relief of withdrawal, is followed repeatedly, the motivation to consume the drug regularly will be much increased either because drug-seeking responses are strengthened (according to operant theory) or because expectancies for the relief of distress have been created (according to social learning theory). It has further been suggested that this process is not confined to a late stage in the development of excessive drinking or opiate use but that relief of minimal withdrawal symptoms, not obvious either to the person affected or to others, may be an important source of reinforcement much earlier in the drug-taking history of experimental animal or human 'addicts' than might be supposed (e.g. Teasdale, 1973).

Although few would wish to deny that this process occurs for some people who are regular takers of opiates, alcohol, or barbiturates, relatively little is known about the speed and reliability with which it occurs. How many people experience withdrawal symptoms, perhaps of relatively mild degree, without 'learning' to relieve them by further drinking or drug-taking? Although part of the instigation towards withdrawal-relief drug-taking may be biochemical in such cases, the act is behavioural and a host of factors, some of which will be social, must operate both for and against the use of the drug for withdrawal relief. The balance of these factors must affect the way in which the experience of withdrawal is translated into regular withdrawal-relief drug-taking. Amongst other factors, the attribution of symptoms as experiences deriving from cessation of drug use must play a part, and social and other constraints may also operate in important ways. It must be supposed, for example, that constraints, both internal and external, must be overcome in order to drink alcohol regularly first thing in the morning in order to relieve symptoms that have arisen since stopping drinking the previous night, or to inject opiates or barbiturates intravenously in order to relieve withdrawal symptoms more rapidly. On the other hand, societies that are relatively permissive regarding tobacco-smoking may offer fewer restraints upon a pattern of smoking which is so regular that it ensures virtual continual freedom from nicotine withdrawal during the day.

Some of these complexities were understood by Lindesmith (1947), whose 'sociological theory of drug addiction', with its emphasis on the use of a drug for the relief of withdrawal symptoms, was remarkably similar to the psychobiological part of the much more recent 'alcohol dependence syndrome'. His view was that 'addiction' developed rapidly once a person *interpreted* withdrawal symptoms as being caused by the absence of opiate drugs, and thereafter the drug was used for the consciously understood purpose of alleviating or suppressing these symptoms. To illustrate the need for this element of interpretation, he cited several examples of the therapeutic use of opiates where symptoms, although present, had not been attributed in this way and where 'addiction' had not resulted—an example of what used to be called 'morphinism' at one time in Germany and France in distinction to 'addiction' or 'morphinomania', a use of terms that did not catch on in other countries.

Incidentally, it is of interest that Lindesmith, writing in the 1930s, should have described as 'sociological' a theory which today would be criticized by many as being too limited and overly 'medical'. Interesting also is the way in which he decried any personality view of excessive drug use as 'moral' rather than 'scientific'. He included as moral many of the social psychological factors studied by the Jessors (1977) and others, including the ideas that 'curiosity' or 'bad company' were causative factors.

Understandably, the 'alcohol dependence syndrome' has excited a great deal of comment and criticism. Shaw (1979), for example, has taken exception to it, believing that the WHO's support for it was partly a political decision motivated by a desire to uphold the powerful role of the medical profession. One of Shaw's concerns is of central importance. He pointed out, correctly in this author's view, that no evidence had been presented, '. . . to demonstrate co-variation between psychobiological factors and the other two hypothesized "altered states" ' (p.341). This is of course the nub of the matter. No one is seriously doubting that under the right circumstances a person's biochemical response to heroin, morphine, and a number of other drugs can be altered by their repeated use. The question is: How centrally important is this factor? It is, on available evidence, still possible to take one of two extreme views on this question, or to adopt any intermediate position. One extreme view, towards which the proponents of the alcohol dependence syndrome lean, is that 'biochemical dependence' is of crucial importance: whatever degree of compulsion existed before, the development of withdrawal symptoms and the habit of relieving or avoiding them with further administrations of the drug adds so significantly to the picture that the drive to consume the drug is now vastly increased. The opposite view is that such biochemical change is merely an epiphenomenon—a side-effect, which is likely to occur when drug use has been heavy and prolonged for whatever reason.

Chick (1980) has attempted a direct test of the unidimensionality of the alcohol dependence syndrome by correlating the replies of 109 men receiving treatment in an 'alcoholism' treatment unit to 21 questions designed to cover all aspects of the proposed syndrome including altered behavioural state and altered subjective state. His basic conclusion was that a single underlying dimension could not be demonstrated. Multivariate statistical analysis (principal components analysis with oblique rotation) produced at least three virtually independent factors, each of which captured some aspects of the syndrome. However, the results are sufficiently complex that proponents of all points of view can draw some comfort from them. The first factor was undoubtedly fairly general, comprising aspects of withdrawal (frequency of tremor, retching, sweating, morning tension), subjective need (restless without drink, cannot think of anything else), and the salience of drink (missing meals, organizing the day around drinking). However, two items designed to assess impaired control over drinking (having difficulty keeping to a limit, and difficulty in avoiding getting drunk), considered by Jellinek (1960) and others to be hallmarks of 'alcoholism', contributed to a second factor rather than to the first, and two items designed to assess 'narrowed drinking repertoire' (a change from drinking less on a weekday to 'drinking the same or more nowadays'; a change from drinking according to mood, to 'not drinking according to mood nowadays') contributed to a third factor rather than to the first two.

However, multivariate statistical techniques are notoriously dangerous mathematical tools for testing psychological hypotheses. It looks very much as if Chick's results may partly be attributable to the inclusion within his set of items of two pairs of questions (two intended to assess impaired control, and two narrowing of the drinking repertoire) none of which was particularly valid but each of which correlated highly with the other member of its pair, hence producing in the analysis what looked like a separate factor. On the other hand, champions of the unidimensional syndrome view can have drawn little comfort from the fact that the first unrotated component accounted for less than a quarter of the total variance within the correlation matrix.

The complexity of the matter is illustrated further by work on tobacco-smoking, another example of behaviour involving the ingestion of a drug now agreed to have the potential for inducing altered biological response, but which it is recognized is used for a range of reasons. Earlier reference has already been made to the work of Russell *et al.* (1974) who attempted to classify smokers according to self-reported motives. Elsewhere, Russell has argued for the importance of viewing smoking as a 'dependence disorder' (1971), and he and his colleagues drew support for this view, and for the importance of the pharmacological or biochemical component, from the results of their studies of motives. Two broad clusters of motives emerged, which Russell *et al.* labelled 'pharmacological' and 'non-pharmacological'. Motives indicating smoking for 'stimulation', 'addictive' smoking, and 'automatic' smoking, contributed to the first factor, and 'psychosocial' and 'indulgent' smoking contributed to the second. The three types of smoking motive which contributed most to the pharmacological dimension were those reported more frequently by clients of a smoking clinic than by members of the general population, and the same motives tended to be positively correlated with age, and had the stronger correlations with amount smoked.

Russell *et al.* drew a most important conclusion, and one which is strikingly similar to that which appears to have been advocated in the case of alcohol by Edwards *et al.* (1977), when they wrote:

> We suggest that it may prove more useful to classify smokers according to their position on the single dimension of pharmacological addiction to nicotine rather than in terms of their profile on the six types of smoking (p.332).

Once again, however, it is important to advocate caution in extrapolating in such a way from such complex mathematical techniques. For a start, the amount of variance in the matrix of correlations amongst the six motive dimensions which was accounted for by the two higher-order factors (pharmacological and non-pharmacological) was again just one-quarter. Furthermore, there were some interesting details of the results which are not totally in keeping with the simple unidimensional conclusion reached by Russell *et al.* The items most strongly definitive of the pharmacological factor were not those contributing to the first-order 'addictive' component but were rather the following 'stimulation' and 'automatic' items:

I smoke more when I am rushed and have lots to do (stimulation);
I like smoking while I am busy and working hard (stimulation);
I smoke automatically without even being aware of it (automatic);
I find myself smoking without remembering lighting up (automatic).

The so-called 'addictive' smoking items occupied a less clear position, contributing as a group almost as much to the non-pharmacological factor as to the pharmacological. The two items most definitive of the 'addictive' component were:

When I have run out of cigarettes I find it almost unbearable until I can get some.

I get a real gnawing hunger to smoke when I haven't smoked for a while.

A further most important question which arises in connection with any biological theory of excess asks how it is that individuals can arrive at a point at which their drug use is of sufficient quantity, frequency, or regularity to bring about pharmacological tolerance and an abstinence syndrome. The idea of *progression* from drug use motivated by social and other non-pharmacological rewards and incentives, to later use motivated in the end as much by relief or avoidance of withdrawal as by other reinforcements, is inherent in many models of excessive drug behaviour. Russell *et al.* themselves presented the model shown in Figure 8 on the basis of their work on motives. Note that they proposed three very broad classes of reward from smoking. The first, characterized by psycho-social and sensorimotor smoking in particular, is truly non-pharmacological: the fact that tobacco smoke contains a drug, nicotine, is quite incidental. The second broad class relies upon the positive psychopharmacological effects of nicotine which may underlie part of smokers' reports that smoking has relaxing, sedating, or stimulating effects. Finally, it is proposed, smoking may progress to a stage where it is, in learning theory terms, *negatively* reinforced, i.e. relief or avoidance of unpleasant withdrawal effects is contingent upon smoking. Thus, much simplified, the proposal is that the drug nicotine takes a stronger and stronger hold, as smoking progresses, on individuals who initially smoked for reasons unrelated to the pharmacological properties of the drug.

Although such a model is attractive, and makes intuitive sense, sufficient has been said already to indicate that the research on which it is based hardly supports such a detailed formulation. This is not to deny that there may be a general process of roughly this kind occurring for some individuals. In their survey, McKennell and Thomas (1967) found that craving for cigarettes ('frequently, when I haven't got any cigarettes on me I feel a craving for one'), as well as being correlated with amount smoked, was also correlated with reports of 'nervous irritation' smoking (smoking when irritable, when anxious or worried, when angry or when nervous), but was scarcely correlated at all with social smoking (smoking in company, at a party, when talking, when drinking, etc.) or with smoking for social confidence. It was social confidence smoking

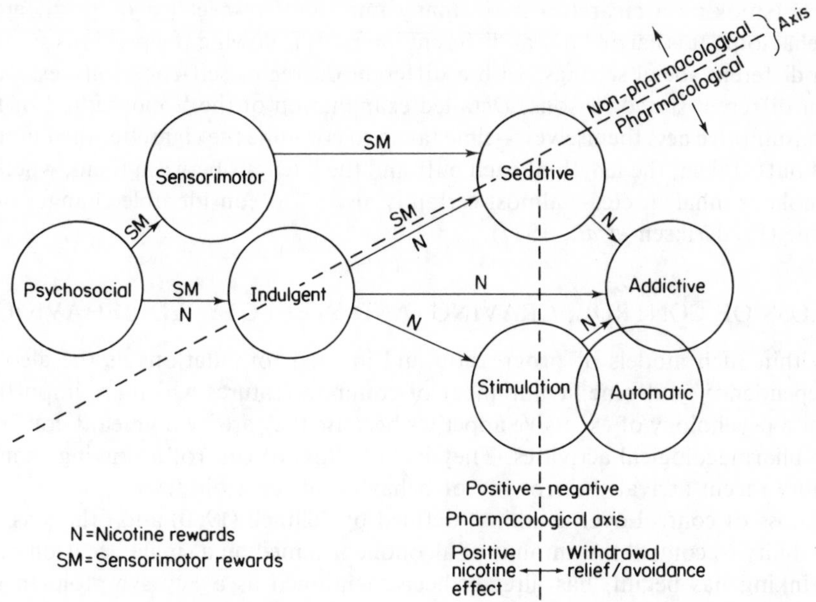

Figure 8 The Russell model of smoking types and progression (reprinted with permission of the author from Russell *et al.*, A Classification of Smoking by Factorial Structure of Motives, *Journal of the Royal Statistical Society*, **137**, 1974, 313–46)

in particular which was found to be high amongst adolescents, and which was reported less and less with age. Nervous irritation smoking, on the other hand, increased rapidly within the first two years of taking up smoking.

There is in fact considerable evidence in McKennell and Thomas's findings to support a general progression theory, with motives for behaviour changing over time—in the case of smoking over a relatively short time. They found that the proportion of young people reporting ever having smoked went up sharply between approximately the thirteenth and sixteenth birthdays. Reports of first becoming a regular smoker (one cigarette a day or one ounce of tobacco a month or more) went up sharply between approximately the fifteenth and eighteenth birthdays. These changes corresponded with a changing pattern of reported motives and also with reported changes in the manner of smoking and its accompaniments. For example, 26 per cent reported inhaling tobacco smoke when first smoking, 60 per cent at the start of regular smoking, and 89 per cent at the time of the survey. Similarly, 26 per cent reported having the occasional solitary smoke at the time of first becoming a smoker, 53 per cent when first becoming a regular smoker, and 69 per cent currently. McKennell and Thomas concluded that it takes on average two to three years from first smoking to become 'addicted'. Certainly there seems to be substantial support here for the view that for many people changes take place over a comparatively short period of time, such that behaviour which appears superficially to be the same as it was (smoking a cigarette) is, in many important respects, a quite different behaviour. It is carried out at different intervals following the previous smoke, in different social settings, with a different degree of self-consciousness, and for different stated reasons. Detailed examination of the 'topography' of the consumptive acts themselves—time taken to consume the cigarette, the number of puffs taken, the length of each puff and the intervals between them, whether smoke is inhaled, etc.—almost certainly also show considerable changes over time (Frederiksen *et al.*, 1977).

LOSS OF CONTROL, CRAVING, AND STEREOTYPED BEHAVIOUR

Within such models of progression and in such formulations as the alcohol dependence syndrome lie a number of common features which are important for a psychology of excessive appetites because they are by no means confined to pharmacological activities. They include 'loss of control', 'craving', and a more recent arrival, 'narrowing of behavioural repertoire'.

Loss of control over drinking, defined by Jellinek (1960) and others as the inability to control the amount of alcohol consumed on a single occasion once drinking has begun, has already been mentioned as a key symptom in the psychobiologically based *disease* concept of 'alcoholism'. Like irresistable craving it represents a poorly defined and highly subjective experience, and until research work began in the 1960s which involved observing what actually happened when people with drinking problems consumed alcohol, their presumed importance rested upon self-accounts given in clinical settings. Laboratory-based experimental studies and priming-dose experiments, reviewed recently by Heather and Robertson (1983), have put matters in a very different light. The results of many of the studies, for example those carried out by Mendelson and Mello (1966) and their colleagues (e.g. by Cohen *et al.*, 1971, and by Bigelow and Liebson, 1972), are summed up by Heather and Robertson as showing that the same kinds of laws operate over the drinking behaviour of excessive drinkers observed in these settings as operate over normal drinking and other behaviour. Although excessive drinkers tend to drink large amounts when given the opportunity to do so, their drinking is controlled, in the sense that it remains to some degree responsive to the balance of incentives and disincentives in operation at the time. For example, in a number of experiments the amount of alcohol consumed was shown to be a function of its 'cost'; this being either the amount of effort required to earn a certain quantity of alcohol, or the difficulty of the task required to earn alcohol. As an example of a study showing the operation of a delicate balance between incentives and 'costs', Cohen *et al.* (1971) showed that drinking 'alcoholics' would remain abstinent for a period of time if paid a certain number of dollars to do so. Either a delay in payment, or the provision of a priming dose of alcohol, disrupted this abstinence, but an increase in payment re-established it.

Hodgson *et al.* (1979b) and Stockwell *et al.* (1982) have more recently carried out careful experimental studies which appear to demonstrate the importance of 'degree of dependence' as estimated by their own Severity of Alcohol Dependence Questionnaire based upon the alcohol dependence syndrome concept. Hodgson *et al.* found that a relatively strong priming dose (about three double spirit drinks) produced relatively faster subsequent drinking (speed of drinking being in their view a good behavioural measure of craving) in 'high dependence' subjects relative to 'moderate dependence' subjects, although the principal effect appears to have been that moderately dependent subjects actually drank more slowly after the high priming dose (Heather and Robertson, 1983). Stockwell *et al.*, in a complex experiment that involved measurements of speed of drinking, subjectively reported craving, and psychophysiological measures such as heart rate, appear to have shown that whilst expectation may be the principal determinant of craving amongst those who are moderately dependent, the actual alcohol content of the priming dose was probably the principal determinant in those with higher levels of 'dependence'. Although Heather and Robertson believe that this evidence, '. . . must be accepted as having revived the possibility of the physiologically-based craving in severely dependent alcoholics . . .' (p.108), they point out that this difference between highly and moderately 'dependent' subjects may nevertheless be due to differing learning histories rather than biological changes in response to alcohol amongst the highly dependent.

With these modern experiments have come more sophisticated concepts of such traditional ideas as craving and loss of control. These newer ideas make the task of integrating different appetitive behaviours, some pharmacological and some not, far easier. Hodgson *et al.* (1979c), for example, have defined craving in such a way that it leaves open the possibility that this experience may arise via a number of different routes. Drawing a useful analogy with similar concepts such as fear, they explained:

> Craving, like fear, can be considered to be a system of inter-related responses involving subjective, physiological, behavioural and biochemical components. For example, as part of his treatment, we recently persuaded an alcoholic who was wanting a drink to sit with an open bottle of whisky and sniff it without indulging. He did this for half an hour and did not drink, but he did express anger, he did stare at the bottle and then deliberately turn his back on it, he did beg for a drink and, moreover, hand tremor was pronounced and his pulse increased from 90 to 125. This state we are labelling 'strong craving' whether it is caused by drink or by any other physiological or psychological event. Only by studying craving as a complex system can we fully understand the phenomenon of compulsive drinking (p.344).

Attempts to integrate an altered biological drug response and learning in the explanation of craving have been made by Wikler (1973) and more recently by Leventhal and Cleary (1980), and in both cases the models proposed can be expanded with little difficulty to encompass non-drug forms of appetite. As already outlined (pp.179–180) Wikler hypothesized that relapse amongst opiate addicts was frequently provoked by withdrawal-like symptoms conditioned to circumstances in which addicts might find themselves which were similar to those which they had previously experienced during withdrawal from opiate drugs. Ludwig and Wikler (1974) extended this hypothesis to the case of alcohol and much enlarged the range of cues that it was thought could produce the conditioned withdrawal syndrome. For example, they stated that any physiological state resembling withdrawal or any situations associated with prior heavy drinking or with the psychological effects of withdrawal might precipitate a 'sub-clinical conditioned withdrawal syndrome' and hence provoke relapse. Indeed, it appears as if Ludwig and Wikler were saying that any state of arousal, whether or not it produced a sub-clinical conditioned withdrawal syndrome, could produce craving. A further complication is introduced when the question is asked, under what circumstances a person labels an internal state (whether one of arousal, conditioned withdrawal, or both) as indicating desire for the appetitive object or substance.

Leventhal and Cleary (1980) reviewed work by Schachter and Russell and their colleagues (e.g. Schachter *et al.*, 1977; Russell *et al.*, 1976) suggesting that heavy smokers, at least, were motivated to regulate or titrate the amount of nicotine in their bodies. They pointed out, however, that this model of smoking 'dependence' could not account for high relapse rates weeks or months after smoking had stopped, nor for the fact that altering nicotine levels experimentally (e.g. by reducing nicotine content in cigarettes or by providing nicotine chewing gum) did not result in the degree of alteration of smoking rate that should be expected, nor that smoking appeared to be responsive to changes in emotional states, environmental cues, and stress. Leventhal and Cleary went on to develop a 'multiple regulation model' which combined the nicotine factor and psychological elements. Their model goes some considerable way towards explaining both the strength and the complexity of the development of excessive appetitive behaviour, and at the same time offers a partial explanation for excessive involvement in non-drug activities such as gambling.

They believed that emotional regulation was the key to smoking, which was stimulated by departures from emotional homeostasis. The reason that heavy smokers behaved to regulate nicotine level was because certain emotional states had become conditioned to a drop in plasma nicotine level. Hence, a drop in nicotine level stimulated 'craving', although other external stimuli could also generate this reaction. Leventhal and Cleary suggested two possible mechanisms to explain how an unpleasant feeling state ('craving') came to be linked to a fall in nicotine level. One, following opponent-process theory (Solomon and Corbit, 1973, 1974; Solomon, 1980), suggests that nicotine gives rise automatically to a secondary, negative, response following the initial positive reaction, and that the former becomes stronger as the latter becomes weaker with increased experience of smoking. Because Solomon and Corbit have elaborated a theory of 'addiction' specifically, it is worth pausing here to consider their ideas a little more closely.

Solomon and Corbit's theory of 'addiction' is part of their general theory of acquired motivation based on the assumption that there exist brain mechanisms which function automatically to neutralize '. . . all excursions from hedonic neutrality, whether those excursions be appetitive or aversive, pleasant or unpleasant' (1973, p.158). Affect-arousing stimulations, such as free-fall parachuting which produces terror in the novice, or opiate use which produces euphoria in the relatively new user, or love which gives rise to ecstacy in the newly-attached, are followed, when the stimulation ceases, by an 'opponent process' of opposite hedonic quality (relief, withdrawal, loneliness). With repeated stimulation of the same kind, the primary affective response (State A) diminishes in strength (less terror, euphoria, or ecstasy—examples of adaptation), but the opponent process (State B) is strengthened (exhilaration, intense craving, and separation grief, respectively). It is this enhanced opponent process which is responsible, in Solomon and Corbit's view, for the development of 'addiction'. In cases where the A state is hedonically positive, the B or opponent state is aversive and increasingly so with repetition, and can be removed by reinstating the primary or A state:

> Because the B process is the opponent of A, the best way of getting rid of the B state is to use the substance which produces the A state. Thus behaviour involved in the use of the A-arousing substance will be strongly reinforced as an operant, because it produces A and it terminates B. The addictive cycle will lead to further strengthening of the B process. Therefore, amounts of the substance will have to be increased . . . (1973, p.169).

If such a mechanism exists, we should expect not only 'addiction' to drugs which initially provide an hedonically very positive experience, but also 'addiction' to the objects of people's loves and to all activities which at first provide an intense positive affective experience of sudden and clearly marked onset. Gambling and sex are two examples, not mentioned by Solomon and Corbit, which clearly fit the bill. Theirs is a general theory of addictive behaviour, in no way limited to drugs, and is therefore of considerable interest to us here. What is unique about it, setting it apart from operant or social learning theories, and from psychoanalytic or other personality theories, for example, is the automatic nature of the postulated mechanism involved. No conditioning process or susceptible personality type is necessary to explain 'addiction' according to their view, although without such additions to the theory it is difficult to see why 'addiction' to a wide variety of substances and activities is not universal.

Leventhal and Cleary's second possible mechanism for explaining how craving becomes linked to a fall in nicotine level does involve conditioning. If people used smoking to control their reactions to stress, then anxiety would reappear when smoking stops, and hence anxiety would be conditioned to a fall in nicotine level. Complexity is added to the model by assuming that several emotional processes may operate simultaneously; that changes in nicotine level generate a variety of bodily sensations that may themselves become conditioned to emotional states; that smoking itself can directly aid emotional control (for example by increasing alertness, by reducing feelings of social insecurity, or by enhancing relaxation); and particularly that people will form a strong emotional memory of this complex action of smoking. It is this 'memory schema' that was responsible for provoking desire, or as they called it 'craving':

> What it does is provide a mechanism for integrating and sustaining the combination of external stimulus cues (social events, work, nothing to do, taste, etc.), internal stimulus cues (sensations from drops in plasma nicotine levels), and a variety of reactions including subjective emotional experience and expressive motor and autonomic reactions associated with the hedonic experience and with smoking. The elicitation of any of the components can provoke the remaining components of this memory schema. Hence it is the schema that makes possible the re-experiencing of craving when one sees someone else smoke and it is the schema through which nicotine loss stimulates craving because the sensory features of nicotine loss elicit the other affective components of the schema (p.393).

A key point here, of importance for developing a *general* theory of excessive behaviour, is that the sensations generated by a drop in nicotine level do not themselves constitute 'craving', but become 'craving' only after they are conditioned to environmentally stimulated negative feelings. Emotional regulation is the core of the model, not titration of nicotine level itself, even for heavy smokers. The use of nicotine across a broad range of life situations helps, they suggested, to develop broad emotional smoking schema which may be particularly difficult to break. This is the process of generalization of appetitive behaviour which is probably of such crucial importance in the development of excess.

Like ideas on craving, the original, with hindsight, over-simple, concept of loss of control over alcohol intake amongst 'alcoholics', has also been revised in an important contribution by Keller (1972) in a way that makes a link between different excessive appetites much more possible. Although he, like others, believed that loss of control was central, he pointed out how the concept adopted by the medical world was based almost entirely on the writings of Alcoholics Anonymous and a misunderstanding of the work of E. M. Jellinek. Indeed, Keller recalled how he pointed out to Jellinek that a World Health Organization Report to which the latter had contributed was misleading on the subject, and did little justice to Jellinek's own complex view of the phenomenon, when it stated, 'As soon as any small quantity of alcohol enters the organism a demand for more alcohol is set up which is felt as a physical demand by the drinker but could possibly be a conversion phenomenon. This demand lasts until the drinker is too intoxicated or too sick to ingest more alcohol' (Jellinek, 1952, p.33).

For the simple loss of control concept, Keller would substitute the more complex view that an 'alcoholic' does not always have the choice of whether she will take the first drink or not. She *can never be sure* that she will be able to stop. Keller's ideas on how this loss of choice came about placed great emphasis on learning, on social context, and particularly on cue or stimulus generalization. Indeed, there is nothing in these ideas which need confine the process to the consumption of alcohol or indeed to the consumption of drugs at all:

> His disease consists precisely in this, that at some time, under the impulsion of some cue or stimulus which may well be outside his conscious awareness, he will drink. No rational consideration of consequences can prevent him . . . Addiction in this conception is thought of as a form of learned or conditioned response. In that most complex organism, man, addiction is a far more complex learned behaviour that the conditioned salivating of a dog in response to a bell. Nevertheless, people who have had a suitable background of rearing, or misrearing, with a suitable history of timely benefit from large amounts of alcohol and who are acted upon by and react to a sufficiently permissive or directive community, can and do learn to respond to individually significant cues by drinking to drunkenness. The possibility that some genetic factors make some people especially liable to this sort of development is not excluded . . .
>
> It has been convenient to speak of a cue or signal, in the singular. For any alcoholic there may be several or a whole battery of critical cues or signals. By the rule of generalisation, any critical cue can spread like the tentacles of a vine over a whole range of analogues, and this may account for the growing frequency of bouts, or for the development of a pattern of continuous inebriation (pp.160–1).

Keller added that an important element in this generalized spread of conditioning was that alcohol itself, or perhaps a particular blood alcohol level, might become a significant cue for further drinking. Or, he might have added, for further appetitive behaviour of other sorts: many people who are troubled by gambling or eating to excess report being more likely to indulge excessively after taking alcohol.

This issue of loss of control has led to widespread confusion amongst the general public, and in law, as Keller illustrated by reference to the famous Powell case in which Mr Powell's claim to be suffering from the disease of 'alcoholism' which forced him to drink was rejected by a U.S. Supreme Court of Justice. It was pointed out that on his way to his original trial he had stopped in a bar and had one drink only. According to a simple loss of control model, Powell could not therefore have been suffering from 'alcoholism'. Keller's model, on the other hand, allows for the possibility of this behaviour in someone who cannot always choose whether to control his drinking and is therefore suffering from 'alcoholism' in his terms. Fingarette (1981) pointed out what a dilemma this poses for the law. If 'addiction' impairs control generally but does not remove the capacity to voluntarily refrain from consumption or from excess on some occasions, then only a very permissive legal definition of 'involuntary' would excuse a criminal act or misconduct relevant to a civil case.

'Narrowing of behavioural repertoire' is another common, but only quite recently labelled, theme in the development of excessive appetites. It occupies a prominent position in the formulation of the alcohol dependence syndrome. Its inclusion was based upon clinical observation of the way in which some people with drinking problems developed a stereotyped, repetitive pattern of daily drinking which appeared to ensure, '. . . the maintenance of a relatively high blood-alcohol level throughout the waking period and the avoidance of withdrawal' (Edwards *et al.*, 1977, pp.12–13). There are strong hints of something very similar in McKennell and Thomas's (1967) description of adolescent and young adulthood developments in cigarette-smoking that occur within a few years of starting to smoke. If it is supposed that use of the drug comes progressively more and more under the control of the reinforcement which it provides by virtue of the relief of withdrawal symptoms, and if the symptoms mainly arise within a few hours of the previous ingestion of the drug, then it must be expected that drug use will become more regular, timing being determined more by time of deprivation since last administration than by social factors such as company or accompanying activities. In this sense drug use may become less flexible, less an activity with a social meaning, and more something done for its own sake.

Medically prescribed drugs are a special case. Although there seems to be a world of difference between the use of a 'minor' tranquillizer drug, for example, which has been taken on a regular daily schedule for a number of years, and use of the same drug taken less regularly, when required, the method of obtaining medically prescribed drugs reduces any social meaning which they might otherwise have had, and because of the way in which they are prescribed use may be highly regular and inflexible from the outset. The pattern of usage is therefore quite different from a recreational drug such as alcohol, and any progression towards 'biochemical dependence' may be obscured.

Nor should it be thought that this 'narrowing of repertoire' which has been observed in excessive drinkers and smokers, for example, is solely a consequence of the biological changes responsible for tolerance and withdrawal symptoms. There are clear parallels here with the increasingly stereotyped betting patterns which Dickerson (1974) observed amongst the more regular gamblers in betting shops. The supposed mechanism is different, behavioural shaping by a combination of fixed interval and variable ratio reinforcement schedules in Dickerson's opinion, but the results are not dissimilar—an increasingly stereotyped response pattern less reactive to controls other than those of biology or conditioning. It is this reduced responsiveness—the experience of family members, for example, who become increasingly baffled by repeatedly using to no avail the kinds of informal and usually mild forms of control which are normally effective in influencing other people and in other areas of conduct—that best illustrates the change that can come about in appetitive behaviour. In Edwards' (1974a) terms, behaviour has been robbed of some, but not all, of that normal 'plasticity' which we expect of social behaviour; it has become less mouldable, more independent of other people's reactions.

The argument of this chapter has been that repeated experience with an appetitive activity can produce changes that increase the attraction that activity holds for a person. This increased attachment, which is best thought of as a 'strong appetite', has at least three components: affective attachment to the object of the appetite, behavioural intention to consume or approach the object, and cognitive commitment to the object and its approach or consumption. The development of a strong appetite can be attributed to the relative weight of incentives for appetitive behaviour, or functions served by it, over the disincentives or restraints operating at each stage, plus the increasingly influential increment in attraction brought about by the powerful and complex learning and cognitive processes discussed in this and the previous chapter, helped on by biological changes in the case of some drugs.

The position adopted in this chapter has therefore been firmly within the 'exposure' orientation (Alexander and Hadaway, 1982): the contention is that excessive appetites cannot be understood solely in terms of the adaptive functions they serve or originally served. However, just because it has been felt important to stress the developmental aspects of appetitive behaviour in this chapter, this should not be taken to mean that the adaptive functions served at earlier stages, discussed in Chapter 8, are thought to have ceased to be of any importance by the time behaviour has become excessive. Far from it. Drinking to try to control depression, gambling to relieve boredom, smoking to boost social confidence, taking heroin to suppress pain, eating to express rebellion, having sex to increase feelings of masculinity—all may have been of crucial importance to certain people at some stage in the development of a strong appetite (although they are likely to have been overshadowed by peer group pressure at the very early stages). These functions may continue to be of the utmost importance later and this is especially likely to be the case when appetitive behaviour has become excessive very rapidly or almost immediately, as can very often happen. Two points must be borne in mind nevertheless. One is that functions are likely to change and multiply as appetite becomes stronger: other things being equal, appetitive behaviour *acquires* greater capacity to relieve tensions of all kinds as it gets stronger, and as we shall see in the following chapter, excess can bring about life changes that provide new and extra possibilities for the functional value of the appetite. The second point is that the developmental process can result in repetitive behaviour that is to a degree 'autonomous' of the functions it has served. Although I believe it very rarely provides a full account of an excessive appetite, even at a late stage of development, there is such a thing as 'habitual' or 'automatic' behaviour.

Thus, psychological functions are of major importance, but the development of excess is a dynamic, multi-stage, often very lengthy process affected by factors of many kinds, social and biological as well as psychological, and the outcome, as well as being highly uncertain, may bear little relationship to its origins.

CHAPTER ELEVEN

The Nature of Excess

> The diary records a ceaseless battle between the id and the superego, between Pepys's powerful appetites and his nagging, puritanical, bourgeois conscience . . . (Stone, 1979, p.350).

> . . . [binge eaters] commonly engage in severe self-criticisms, self-condemnation, and self-punishment following a binge eating episode. Common themes of resentment and self-contempt over being overweight and having no self-control are combined with disgust, shame or guilt at having *failed* and 'blown the diet' (Loro and Orleans, 1981, p.161).

In the earlier chapters it has been argued that excessive drinking, gambling, smoking, drug-taking, eating, and sexuality cannot fully be understood without taking into account the social context in which such appetitive behaviour was initiated, the personality functions which it serves, dynamic learning processes which can strengthen attachment to the appetitive activity, and the evolution of a person's life which may bring about changes in social context and personal needs at different stages. A comprehensive model must attend to social and cultural context, psychological functions, and development. To understand *excessive* forms of these behaviours, however, and particularly to begin to appreciate how and why people give up behaving excessively (the subject of Chapters 12–14), we must look closely at the conflict and ambivalence and social reaction associated with excess. These should be, in this writer's view, at the very centre of a psychological understanding of the natural history of excessive appetitive behaviours, although their importance has rarely been fully acknowledged in the past.

To try to do justice to these crucial aspects of our phenomena, we must return to the social learning theory model of behaviour which was introduced in Chapter 9 to help make sense of the findings of youthful appetitive behaviour and the appetitive consumption distribution curve.

EXCESS AS COSTLY BEHAVIOUR

The point made in Chapter 9 was that appetitive behaviour, or indeed perhaps any social behaviour, could not be understood without appreciating the importance of the balance struck between inclination and restraint, or, to put it another way, the balance between the positive and negative outcomes expected from behaviour at a particular stage of life. Both factors are subject to individual differences of multiple origin and both are subject to developmental changes. Hence, the resultant is difficult to predict for any one person at any given time. The importance of the development of increasing strength of appetite lies in the way this balance is altered as a result. The final effect is highly uncertain, for as inclination increases with appetite development, so too does the probability that increased 'costs' will operate as potential restraints upon further behaviour. A relatively strong investment in gambling, for example, carries greater risks of incurring financial 'costs' and an increased attachment to drinking, physical 'costs'.

There are at least two ways in which the operation of increased costs is highly variable: first their operation is highly relative; and second, as each comes into play, it may further alter the individual's circumstances and hence shift behavioural inclination in a direction and to a degree which it is difficult to anticipate. The first of these points should require little elaboration. People's circumstances are different, and so too are the cultural, social and familial attitudes and values which govern their own reactions to behaviour and those of the people they mix with. Tolerance levels vary, and hence what counts as inappropriate behaviour is not a constant. What constitutes excessive sexual behaviour is not the same on the west coast of Ireland and in Mangaia in the South Pacific (Marshall and Suggs, 1971), and what counts as excessive drinking is not the same in France and in Utah, U.S.A. Hence, what is felt as a cost of appetitive behaviour, and what leads to pressure for restraint, will vary from place to place, from time to time, and from person to person. This applies with greatest force to social costs generated by others, but as conscience is formed out of the milieu in which a person was socialized it applies with almost as much force to many of the self-generated sources of restraint.

The second point also requires relatively little elaboration. Increased costs may make for more effective restraint, but instead, or in addition, may serve to increase the functional value of the appetitive behaviour. For instance, the increased nagging of a family member in response to eating that is seen as inappropriate or excessive may prove a source of restraint which is effective either temporarily or permanently. Alternatively, it may act to increase the over-eater's anxiety or level of frustration, or to strengthen cognitive tactics which bolster sentiments supporting current behaviour. Relatively extreme costs, such as marital breakdown or imprisonment, may act as brutal shocks which bring about self-restraint (or bring the gambler or drinker to his personal 'rock-bottom' to use an AA and GA expression), but alternatively may deprive the individual of the very social supports and resources which constituted the main sources of pre-existing restraint upon further excess.

The uncertainty of predicting which way the balance of inclination and restraint will tip is yet further increased by the influence of increased appetite upon degree of responsiveness to restraint and control. One effect of the state of attachment which constitutes strong appetite is to make behaviour less vulnerable to, or less easily restrained by, the ordinary everyday personal and social incentives and disincentives which act as sufficient governors of behaviour in which there is less investment. At the same time as costs are being incurred, behaviour may be losing its 'plasticity' (Edwards, 1974a) and becoming more immune to the restraining influence of this harm associated with it.

A view of excessive behaviour as harmful or 'costly' social behaviour, or as deviance, is difficult to reconcile with a medical or disease view, as many authorities have pointed out. The former supposes that behaviour becomes noteworthy, and a cause for concern and attempts at help-seeking and modification, the more it is seen to be creating harm, and the further it crosses the boundary between behaviour defined as normal and that thought to be excessive. The boundary is wide and unclearly marked and its position is highly socially and culturally relative. The latter, on the other hand, supposes that there are signs and symptoms, albeit often difficult to detect and clustering in different ways for different people, of a diagnosable entity. The difficulty of applying this latter approach is obvious in the case of excessive sexuality (although Chapter 6 tried to make it clear that there have been many attempts to diagnose 'hypersexuality'), and perhaps in the case of excessive gambling also. Work on excessive drinking and eating illustrates the difficulties further.

Blaxter (1978), for example, has used 'alcoholism' as an example of the difficulties of applying the medical diagnostic method to conditions that are as much a matter of social behaviour as of altered psychobiological state. She was critical of the fact that in such classifications as the ICD (International Classification of Diseases, Injuries and Causes of Death):

> Social disorders which are not uniformly defined by all physicians (and probably cannot be precisely defined) appear side by side with disease categories as if they were the same sort of phenomenon and could be used in the same way (p.11).

Many would agree that the deciding factor in making a diagnosis in this kind of area is not whether a clearly specifiable disease exists, but rather whether the condition is considered to be one which medicine should investigate or treat. The question is not, 'Is this a disease?', but really rather, 'Should this person be under medical care?':

> If the prescribed action is impossible and known to be useless, there will be reluctance to make the diagnosis. If the action is defined as the business of someone other than the doctor, then the diagnosis will

> be avoided or used only in circumstances where structures exist for formal 'referral' to someone else. If the action is not considered to be appropriate for a doctor's particular skills, then the diagnosis may be translated into another and more properly 'medical' category. If the signs and symptoms of the disease are not ones which doctors feel themselves competent to identify and measure, then relatively crude or idiosyncratic stereotypes of the syndrome indicants or of the typical patient may take over (p.13).

Much of this thesis is borne out by the findings of Chafetz and his colleagues (1970) in the United States and of Shaw *et al.* (1978) in Britain. Chafetz found evidence that doctors failed to make diagnoses of 'alcoholism' when physical diagnoses could easily be made, and Blaxter, in her studies of diagnostic records from general hospitals in Scotland, found that even when diagnoses of 'alcoholism' were made these were usually secondary to primary physical diagnoses. Shaw *et al.* concluded their own studies of recognition of drinking problems by various medical and non-medical agencies by pin-pointing the confidence and 'role security' of agency personnel in handling drinking problems. Where these crucial ingredients were lacking, staff were reluctant to recognize the existence of drinking problems or to make them the focus of the treatment. Chafetz also found that diagnoses of 'alcoholism' were made much less frequently, even when closer examination showed drinking problems to exist, when patients were socially of better standing as indicated by smarter dress, having employment, and being married.

Reactions to appetitive behaviour such as drinking will vary from community to community as well as from one social position to another within a community. This is well illustrated by Cahalan and Room (1974) in their analysis of attitudes and rates of problem drinking in different regions of the United States. Of the nine regions into which they divided the country, attitudes in general were 'driest', or least permissive, in the East–South–Central region (Kentucky, Tennessee, Mississippi, and Alabama) and 'wettest', or most permissive, in the Middle Atlantic region (New York, New Jersey, and Pennsylvania). For example, according to one poll 41 per cent in the former region and only 19 per cent in the latter were in favour of retaining prohibition in 1932, and 61 per cent of the former and only 24 per cent of people in the latter region claimed that there was, 'nothing good about drinking', in the course of a survey carried out in 1964. These differences seem bound to have an influence upon the way in which drinking problems are responded to in communities within those regions. Indeed, from Cahalan and Room's findings there is support for O'Connor's hypothesis that when abstinence or non-permissive norms break down, or are overcome by individuals deviating from them, then the risk of problems relating to drinking are greater. In their national survey, East–South–Central Region produced the highest rate of people with 'high consequences' of drinking (20 per cent) as well as the highest number of abstainers (29 per cent). Although there are clearly other explanations, Cahalan and Room were aware that one is:

> . . . that the tangible consequences of drinking were not to be viewed simply as behavioural characteristics of the individual respondent but rather as properties of the interaction between the respondent's behaviour and the reactions of those in his environment. . . . The combination of individual heavy drinking behaviour and general community disapproval . . . yields quite a strong prediction of individual tangible consequences of drinking . . . (p.192).

McKirnan (1977, 1978) has more recently examined norms relating to the recognition of drinking problems in three contrasting areas in Montreal in Canada—a lower income area, a solidly middle income area, and an affluent suburban community. Respondents were asked to say how much they thought they themselves, a 'social drinker', a 'problem drinker', and an 'alcoholic', would be likely to drink (on average, maximum, and minimum) in four different circumstances (lunchtime on a workday, in the evening with family, at a social event, while alone). Analysis revealed a significant main effect of type of community, with the overall anticipated alcohol consumption decreasing steadily from the low to middle to high socio-economic status area. The more interesting results, however, concerned the range given by respondents between maximum and minimum expected consumption. Ranges were consistently greatest for the low income area and least for the high status community. The effect of these differences in range was to make the drinking norms for different categories of drinker much less distinct in the lowest income area. Whereas in the affluent suburban community, respondents generally saw no overlap at all between their own drinking or the drinking of a typical social drinker and that of problem drinkers or 'alcoholics', there was more overlap in the middle income group, and a great deal of overlap for the lowest status community (McKirnan, 1977). Although the hypothesis remains to be tested, the implication seems clear that tolerance of drinking considered deviant in some other communities would be highest in the lower income community and labelling as 'problem drinker' or 'alcoholic' would not be made so readily there, at least on the basis of drinking quantity alone. McKirnan speculated that in such communities the *how* and *where* of drinking may be more important than how much.

McKirnan's later report (1978) touched, amongst other things, upon the all-important question of perceived responsibility for behaviour. When the same respondents were asked for their perceptions of self, social drinker, 'alcoholic', and 'ex-alcoholic', one dimension which emerged, but only clearly for the lowest income community, contrasted people perceived as having 'internal problems' ('. . . such as emotional or personality problems . . .') with people perceived as having 'external problems' or 'problems not their own fault'. 'Alcoholics' and social drinkers tended to be seen towards the former end of this dimension, and 'ex-alcoholics' and the self tending to be perceived towards the latter end. McKirnan suggested that the lower income community had a more complex and better articulated perception of alcohol abuse than members of the other communities. An alternative interpretation is that members of the lower status group may have viewed 'internal problems' in a more negative light than others.

The question of imputed responsibility for behaviour and its effect on attitudes of acceptance or rejection is taken up by Orcutt and Cairl (1979) in their analysis of data from a public survey conducted in Florida in 1974. They reported a complex 'path analysis' in an attempt to tease out the factors that make people relatively tolerant or intolerant of 'the alcoholic'. Three types of variable were considered: demographic variables such as age, occupation, and education; 'ideological world views' of which there were two—the moral, based on notions of 'weak will', 'moral weakness', and 'willpower', and the medical; and perceptual variables—the degree to which 'alcoholics' were seen as unpredictable, a threat, and responsible for their own behaviour.

Although the highest zero-order correlation appearing in their matrix was 0.48, some highly suggestive patterns emerged. For example, intolerance was moderately positively correlated with perceiving 'alcoholics' as responsible for their behaviour. This perception was positively correlated with adopting a moral world view which itself was more common amongst older people and those with lower status occupations. Those who took more of a medical world view, which was somewhat more likely amongst those with more education and with higher status occupations, were *less* likely to perceive 'alcoholics' as responsible for their behaviour. Adopting a medical as opposed to a moral view was therefore linked with greater tolerance. On the other hand, perceiving the 'alcoholic' as a threat was positively correlated with both world views (slightly more strongly with the moral than the medical), and, as might be expected, threat was positively correlated with intolerance. Adopting a medical view, therefore, did not much reduce the perception of threat posed by deviant drinking. Overall there was only a modest positive correlation between moral world view and intolerance (0.29), and a near-zero correlation between medical view and intolerance (0.02). The authors of this report conclude:

> These results suggest that responses of stigma and social rejection persist among those who label the alcoholic as a 'sick person', a pattern that has been noted in earlier work (Orcutt, 1976; Roman and Trice, 1968) (p.295).

They are careful to point out, however, that a previous very similar survey conducted by Ries (1977) did not find this effect.

The importance of social factors in the process of identifying and labelling deviance of the excessively appetitive type is nowhere better illustrated than in the literature on over-eating and obesity. In their paper entitled, 'The Social Psychology of Dieting', Dwyer *et al.* (1970) reviewed the evidence existing at that time which related the prevalence of concern about weight and dieting behaviour to such variables as age, sex, social class, and ethnicity. In summary, the evidence showed a strong association between weight concern and dieting and age, with adolescents more frequently being concerned about their weight and more frequently attempting dieting than adults, and also with sex, with women much more frequently than men showing concern and dieting behaviour. For example, Dwyer *et al.* (1969) found that 16 per cent of high school senior girls and 19 per cent of the boys could be classified as obese on the basis of triceps skinfold thickness, but that over 80 per cent of the girls, in contrast with less than 20 per cent of the boys, expressed a wish to weigh less than they did, and 60 per cent of the girls but only 24 per cent of all boys had ever dieted. Almost all girls, other than the leanest, wished to weigh less than they did, whilst most boys at all weight levels wished to be heavier than they were. Dwyer *et al.* cited Huenemann *et al.* (1966) who reported racial as well as sex differences, with white girls wanting to lose more weight than black or oriental girls, despite the fact that black girls were heavier.

These results suggest the crucial importance of self-image. Dwyer *et al.* suggested that boys on the whole wished to gain weight and to be larger in almost all dimensions, especially those that might indicate strength or athletic prowess, whilst girls wished to be smaller in almost all dimensions except those such as busts which are important for sexual attraction. They went on to suggest that girls and women tend to attribute over-weight to over-fatness, even in cases when weight should more correctly be attributed to body build, whilst boys and men are liable to attribute weight to aspects of build other than fat. They even cited one report in which men undergoing weight reduction had been observed to be obsessed with the thought that weight loss was causing them physical disintegration by sapping strength and virility. When males do diet, they added, they are particularly attracted to high protein diets in combination with increased physical activity.

Ashwell and Etchell (1974) and Silverstone (1968) have since confirmed this sex difference in their studies in London (see pp.83–84, above). Dwyer *et al.* (1970) offered a number of possible explanations for these very consistent and considerable differences. They considered the possibility that over-weight may represent more of a social liability for women than for men, with over-weight inhibiting relationships with members of both sexes and inhibiting social mobility. Secondly, they asked whether weight-related aspects of appearance may not be more intertwined with the self-concept in women than in men, a view strongly supported by Orbach who has argued that, *Fat is a Feminist Issue* (1978). They cited studies showing that girls are more likely to know their weights accurately than are boys, and weigh themselves more frequently. The third possibility was that extra weight might be more visible in women because of the different distribution of fat on their bodies, and the fourth possibility was, as already noted, that women might over-emphasize fat deposits, and men body-build, as a component of over-weight. Fashion constituted their fifth suggested explanation, fashions being dictated, they argued, more by appeal to the establishment of status hierarchy and utility in men, and more by considerations of sexual attraction and seduction in women.

Amongst factors motivating people to diet, whether women or men, Dwyer *et al.* considered fear of poor health and questions of appearance. In addition, however, they reviewed at some length the evidence suggesting that people may be motivated to diet because of pervasive negative attitudes towards obesity. They reviewed studies showing both that people do tend to blame the obese for being fat whilst excusing those with other physical handicaps from blame, and that fat people are less liked. They cited a study by Staffieri (1967) which appeared to show that stereotypes were well established even by the age of seven years, with such descriptions as, 'fights', 'cheats', 'mean', and 'lazy', being attributed significantly more often to people of endomorphic body build than to those of other body types (ectomorphs tended to be seen as, 'sneaky', 'afraid', 'quiet', etc. and mesomorphs as 'strong', 'best friend', 'clean', etc.) At least one study has revealed that a negative characterization of fat people extends to doctors' attitudes as well (Maddox and Liederman, 1969), and Blaxter (1978) hints at a more negative view of obesity (also of smoking) than of 'alcoholism' on the part of doctors in Scotland. Other research reviewed by Dwyer *et al.* suggested that obese girls had fewer dates and fewer other social activities, and that they had lower acceptance rates into relatively high ranking colleges despite previous academic performance which was equal to that of other girls. Obese children and adolescents, and those of predominantly endomorphic body build, had lower self-regard than others, and there was some evidence that obesity beginning in childhood was more detrimental to self-image than that of adult onset.

The importance of perceived responsibility for behaviour is illustrated by a study by de Jong (1980). Adolescent girls were asked to make various ratings of a girl depicted in a photograph who might be obese or non-obese, and whose accompanying description might or might not include the 'excuse' of thyroid disorder, and might or might not contain the information that the girl had recently been successful in achieving a 25 pound weight reduction. The conclusion was:

> . . . the results of these . . . experiments demonstrate that derogation of the obese results from the presumption that such persons are responsible for their physical deviance. Unless the obese can provide an 'excuse' for their weight, such as a thyroid condition, or can offer evidence of successful weight loss, their character will be impuned (p.85).

These studies of drinking and eating illustrate the point that the recognition of excess is not simply a matter of making a correct 'diagnosis'. What is 'excessive' is personally or socially defined and depends upon a person's age, sex, socio-economic status, social network, responsibilities, and a host of other factors. Equally relevant are characteristics of those such as family or general medical practitioner who know a person well enough to be in a position to make their own influential judgements as to whether behaviour is excessive or not. The more important question is not whether Jill is or is not suffering from 'bulimia' or whether John is or is not 'an alcoholic', but whether they and others who have influence with them think their eating and drinking is excessive and should be controlled.

The view espoused here is that strong appetites can produce any of a whole range of effects, at least some of which are harmful or may be perceived to be dangerous or potentially damaging. Some of these effects are physical, others are social. Some are immediately felt, others are anticipations. These negative effects may add to the forces naturally restraining or disinclining a person from such behaviour. Elsewhere (Orford, 1971a) I have put forward the view that contrary pressures deriving from awareness of the harmful consequences of drug use are not only important for an understanding of 'drug dependence', but are actually definitive of it. It is not just that 'addiction' is not apparent until a person wishes to give up drug use or until other people put pressure upon him or her to do so, but rather that the very notion of drug 'dependence' has no meaning until such circumstances pertain. I argued then, '. . . that drug dependence can only be seen to exist to the degree that pressure is put upon the individual, or some incentive offered him, to reduce his drug-taking' (1971a, pp.131–2), and the argument applies in my view with equal force to non-drug forms of strong appetite such as excessive heterosexuality, excessive gambling, and over-eating.

Pressures contrary to continued excessive behaviour or, to put it another way, pressures to conform to norms of moderation or abstinence, may be categorized in countless different ways. They might for example be listed under the three headings of *cost* (of resources spent in acquiring and consuming), *interference* (with other activities of the individual or of others), or *risk* (of future harm or discomfort). Alternatively they might be classified as *self*-generated pressures or pressures generated by significant *others*. The exact sources and extent of pressures felt by an individual towards the modification of appetitive behaviour will clearly depend much upon social role, including whether the person has a family or not, what his or her occupation is, and upon the values and goals of the peer group. It will also depend, equally clearly, upon the particular form of appetitive behaviour involved. As Reinert (1968) has pointed out, heavy alcohol consumption may produce contrary pressures as a result of interference with other activities on account of the drug's pharmacological depressant effect. By contrast, pressure to modify smoking behaviour seems more likely to derive from the perception of risk of future bodily damage, and from awareness of continuing financial outlay. Heterosexual behaviour which is excessive may give rise to contrary pressures on account of social disapproval, or the risk of it, conscience, and risk of physical infection. If sexual appetite is of the order that Walter claims his to have been (Chapter 6), then effort, financial loss, and interference with other activities may also constitute important sources of disincentive. Cornish (1978) has outlined in his review a not dissimilar picture of the pros and cons that may determine an individual's gambling behaviour.

Pressures to restrict forms of drug use such as opiate-taking and cannabis use must have varied hugely in quite recent historical times as a result of changes in the law, public attitudes, and the availability of newly synthesized drugs and newly available methods of self-administration (Brecher, 1972; see also Chapter 4). Studies of illicit drug users in Britain in recent times have shown clearly that the social significance of drug-taking, and the general life-style that goes with it, vary so greatly that no general statement can easily be made about the harmful effects of 'drug-taking' or about the contrary pressures likely to arise. Both Plant's (1975) study of drug-takers in an English provincial town, recruited informally rather than through medical or other official channels, and Stimson's (1973) and Ogborne's (1974) study of opiate users being prescribed heroin at London drug clinics, demonstrated the variation to be found in factors such as the number of drugs being used and the frequency of use, the regularity of a person's employment, the stability and style of accommodation, involvement in crime, and the degree to which the person associated with other drug users.

Plant showed variation in the degree of commitment to a drug-centred way of life, varying from incidental and occasional drug use to regular drug use and exclusive association with other heavy drug users. Although Stimson and Ogborne were concerned with a narrower range of the drug-using population, they demonstrated variation along the same dimensions. Stimson (1973) described four types of addict to be found within the clinic population. 'Stables' he described as employed, in relatively little contact with other addicts, and engaged in few criminal activities other than possession of drugs. Their income and support came principally from their own earnings. The second group, 'junkies', were opposite to stables in almost all respects. 'Loners' were unemployed like 'junkies', but unlike the latter had relatively little contact with other addicts, reported little criminal activity, and were dependent upon Social Security payments. Finally, the 'two-worlders' were stably employed with income mainly from their own earnings, but also participated in the 'drug scene', having a relatively higher degree of contact with other addicts and reporting a relatively high degree of criminal activity.

The point is that, even for a group of people recruited from a single source and liable to be treated as an homogeneous group (clinic 'drug addicts'), the variation in the exact form of appetitive behaviour and variation in social circumstances means that the disincentives for continued drug use are highly variable. Types of harm, or potential harm, include life-threatening overdose, serious illness as a result of unsterile drug administration practices, the consequences of detected law-breaking, disapproval by family or friends, financial loss, interference with other activities such as work, and a serious mismatch between behaviour and ideals. Which of these constitutes pressure towards modifying drug use in a particular case, and how strong this pressure becomes, depends upon the exact form of drug use, the exact nature of a person's social circumstances, the person's attitudes and values, and the complex interaction between all these.

The earlier discussion of over-weight illustrates this point well. The importance of sex differences here gives us important insight into the nature of strong appetite. The relationship between a young woman and her eating, if she perceives herself to be becoming heavy, who views herself as ugly when over-weight, who increasingly wishes to hide herself from social gaze particularly that of men, and who is struggling unsuccessfully to modify her eating, is fundamentally different from the relationship between a young man and his eating where there is happy oblivion regarding the putting on of weight, and a perception of weight being associated with toughness, sporting ability, and perhaps with a capacity for holding drink. The relationship between these two hypothetical people and their eating would be quite different even if pound for pound they had been eating equal amounts, and even if it was the case that they would experience an equal degree of struggle if they had equal motivation to reduce weight.

It may reasonably be argued that strength of appetite or degree of 'dependence' is equal in these two cases. On the other hand, the psychology of someone who is subject to strong pressures towards reducing appetitive behaviour, but who finds these pressures met by equally strong inclination towards continued appetitive behaviour, is quite different from that of someone who does not experience such pressures. Indeed, excessive appetite can hardly be shown to exist without such contrary pressures. It is to underline this point that the adjective 'excessive' has been used throughout this book. It will be argued by some that 'excessive drinking', 'excessive gambling', and 'excessive heterosexual behaviour', are inadequate terms because they cannot be defined; they depend upon individual attitudes, social circumstances, and cultural mores. This is exactly the point, however. It is just because definitions of what constitutes 'alcoholism', 'compulsive gambling', 'hypersexuality', drug 'abuse', and over-eating are individually, socially, and culturally relative that the word 'excessive' is so appropriate. The word offers no pretence that these things constitute entities that can be precisely defined and counted and compared across different social and cultural groups. As Cohen (1971) put it in his book, *Images of Deviance*, '. . . a problem can only be a problem to somebody. So, whenever we see terms such as deviance and social problems, we must ask: "Says who?" ' (p.17). Similarly, if we say that appetitive behaviour is excessive, we must ask: 'Exceeds whose definition of normal or moderate?'

EXCESS AS DEVIANCE

Cohen was writing from the general perspective of deviancy theory, an approach which has been applied to a wide range of social behaviours and which offers one of the major alternative perspectives to a disease view of appetitive behaviour. Deviance, according to this perspective, is the breaking of rules, whether written or unwritten, and it can therefore only be understood by consideration both of the rules and of the behaviour which breaks them. This model therefore parts company with the disease view, and with most psychological perspectives which are concerned with maladaptive behaviour, in its major concern with the rules themselves, and with those that make them and enforce them.

As Rubington and Weinberg (1968) put it in their book, *Deviance, the Interactionist Perspective*:

> For deviance to become a social fact, somebody must perceive . . . departure from social norms, must categorise that perception, must report the perception to others, must get them to accept this definition of the situation, and must obtain a response that conforms to this definition. Unless all these requirements are met, deviance as a social fact does not come into being (Introduction, p.v).

This implies a fairly radical departure from the disease perspective. At its most succinct, the deviancy view is that, like beauty, '. . . deviance is in the eyes of the beholder' (Rubington and Weinberg, Introduction, p.v).

It is at this point that deviancy theory is most liable to be misunderstood. Does this statement imply that there is nothing to deviance other than the reaction to it, or that appetitive behaviour is only excessive when someone says it is excessive? Probably not. One of the more useful statements of the deviancy position for present purposes is, in my view, the relatively early statement by Lemert (1951). He described his theory of 'sociopathic behaviour' as, '. . . one of social differentiation, deviation, and individuation . . .'. By this he meant that social differences emerged between people, some appearing to become more deviant than others in certain ways, and that this process of differentiation had a variety of sources. He clearly recognized that in many instances a major source of social difference was some primary deviation which existed quite independently of social reaction and which could indeed be genetic and present at birth. Congenital blindness or physical handicap are examples. Even in such instances, however, he stressed the importance of societal reaction.

It was Lemert's conclusion that societal reaction was much more likely to be 'out of proportion' in its formal rather than informal responses, especially where, '. . . the close organic relation between the deviation and attitudinal responses to it is mediated by a chain of formal relationships . . .' (p.55). In informally organized groups and communities, on the other hand, there would be, '. . . a direct and spontaneous quality in the societal reaction which tends to be immediately relevant to the deviation' (p.54). In the case of excessive appetitive behaviours at least, the distinction is unlikely to be clear cut. For one thing it ignores the element of secrecy and lack of trust which often develops between those whose appetites are excessive and those, such as close family members, who are most likely to react informally, and which makes direct and spontaneous reaction difficult. Secondly, it takes no account of the quasi-medical or other labels or constructions which husbands and wives, parents and children, and others may have incorporated from the prevailing wisdom on the subject and which may distort their informal reaction just as much as they distort societies' more formal responses.

Very often the effect of the reaction may be an amplifying one. Wilkins' (1964) statement of the principle of 'deviance amplification', in his book, *Social Deviance: Social Policy, Action and Research*, drew, for an example, upon studies of juvenile gang behaviour. Behaviour that may be seen by a youth as play, adventure, fun, excitement, or mischief, may be seen by others as evil, a nuisance, or delinquent. These reactions are almost bound to lead to a degree of exclusion and make the formation of groups of like-minded youths more probable. Entry to a gang, the learning of its values, the spreading of behaviour within the gang by a contagion-like process, all make negative reactions including rejection by others even more likely, may strengthen the need to belong to a gang, and cut off gang members from influence by the outside system of values and controls. The mechanism is like a positive feedback one with the relationship between youthful behaviour and reaction to it similar in some ways to the relationship between confidence and prices on the stock market.

The principle that reaction creates, or at least amplifies, original deviance has become a central tenet of the deviance perspective. As Rubington and Weinberg put it, 'Seen in this light deviance becomes a matter of social definition. And this definition often produces the deviant acts' (1968, p.4). However, it is again necessary to go back to Lemert (1951) for a more general view:

> . . . we start with the idea that persons and groups are differentiated in various ways, some of which result in social penalties, rejection, and segregation. These penalties and segregative reactions of society or the community are dynamic factors which increase, decrease and condition the form which the initial differentiation or deviation takes (p.22).

In other words, societal reaction always occurs, but it is not always rejecting and segregating, and when it is it has an effect which need not always be an amplifying one. Thus, self-help groups, Alcoholics Anonymous, Gamblers Anonymous, and Weight Watchers amongst them, are good examples of segregation which purports to be deviance *reducing*. Becoming a fully functioning member of one of these organizations demands not only attendance at an exclusive club, but also a vigorous mental segregation involving 'recognizing', 'admitting', and declaring oneself to be 'different from other people'. The argument is that only by recognizing oneself to be in a special class of 'alcoholic' or 'compulsive gambler', for example, can the member realize the impossibility of drinking or gambling like most other people, and only by this means can he obtain the motivation to *give up* his deviance.

Despite this more moderate, general statement of the deviance model, it is the case that the greatest champions of the deviance perspective (Rubington and Weinberg, Cohen, and others) have been particularly concerned with forms of behaviour whose 'deviance' or 'problem' aspects can most readily be understood as almost pure social creations. There are modern examples, of which perhaps homosexual behaviour and marijuana use are amongst the clearest, where a strong argument can be made out for saying that virtually all the problematic aspects of these behaviours are the result of social reaction. It is with behaviour of this sort that deviancy theorists appear most in their element and where the deviance model has strongest claims to have exclusive territorial rights.

They have shown rather less interest in some of the forms of behaviour which are central to this book, such as excessive drinking, gambling, and eating. This is not because a general deviancy perspective, as put forward by Lemert, is not highly relevant to excessive appetitive behaviour, indeed I believe it is, but because the more radical, exclusive, deviance model is most relevant to behaviour about which fairly clear 'rules' exist and which is to a degree 'outlawed' if not by the law itself, at least by public morality. As was pointed out in the first, introductory chapter, excessive drinking, gambling, and heterosexuality with an adult partner shade off imperceptibly into almost fully acceptable moderation. This in itself does not represent an insurmountable impediment to the application of the deviancy model but it makes its application more difficult. In addition, there are features of excessive appetitive behaviour which are relatively ignored by, or which are at least peripheral to, a deviance model but which are, according to the present view, central to this rather special category of excessive appetitive behaviours. Principal amongst these are the developmental processes responsible for the formation of powerful habits which are then difficult to break.

The neglect of excessive appetitive behaviour by deviancy theorists does not hold, however, in the case of forms of drug-taking other than alcohol and tobacco use. A firm deviancy view of drug-taking is held, for example, by Young (1971) and by Brecher (1972). In addition, as noted in Chapter 6, many of those who have written on the subject of heterosexual behaviour, including Kinsey *et al.* (1948), have frowned upon any idea of 'hypersexuality', taking the view that this is a 'condition' created entirely by social reaction. Explicit deviancy and labelling theory explanations of other kinds of excessive appetitive behaviour are relatively rare, but Sargent (1979) is one author who has presented a power relations theory of drinking and 'alcoholism', in this case in Australia. Her view was that 'alcoholism' is used by those of high status in society as a means of social control of those of low status:

> An 'alcoholic' is a person who has been subjected to social control processes, which both discredit him and assign to him a particular role which may prove irreversible; 'alcoholic' is also a stigmatising label applied by the most powerful to the less powerful in order to justify exercising social control (p.92).

In the context in which she was writing, it was the aborigines who were of lower status, and Sargent cited figures for rates of imprisonment as sentences for drunkenness in 1973 which certainly show a sharp differential between towns with high concentration of aborigines (48 per cent receiving custodial sentences), other rural areas (13 per cent), and the major urban area, Sydney (1.4 per cent). She drew a parallel with labelling of political dissidents as 'mentally ill' in the U.S.S.R., and cited high rates of labelling Navaho Indians as 'alcoholics' by Anglo-Americans, and the council provision of beer gardens in white former-Rhodesia (studied by Wolcott, 1974), as further examples of the use of 'alcoholism' as a means of social control and repression.

The view taken here is that such an extreme deviancy perspective cannot provide a total account of excessive forms of appetitive behaviour, even when these are of a type such as illicit drug use or sexual behaviour which breaks social conventions, or when those of high power or status are very ready to label as excessive the behaviour of those of lower status. Each of these behaviours has the capacity for developing into a strong appetite. The processes of acquiring strong appetites are, at least in part, those described in Chapters 9 and 10, and best summed up as learning processes within a social context.

Although a thoroughgoing deviancy view of excessive appetites such as Sargent's or Brecher's has rarely been taken and cannot in this writer's view provide a complete understanding, there have been a number of theoretical statements which make good use of a social reaction perspective. For instance, there have been few better attempts to construct a social view of the process of developing an excessive appetite than Bacon's (1973) description of 'the process of addiction to alcohol'. He was concerned to explain the progression from 'impulsive' drinking towards 'compulsive' drinking. The former was, '. . . relatively careless, capricious, whimsical, perhaps spur-of-the-moment; nor did it occur on every or almost every occasion . . .' (p.4), whilst the latter was '. . . more commanding, more frequent, more demanding, less individually and more automatically determined . . .' (p.4). The progression appeared to involve a, '. . . strengthening of the tendency to use alcohol for reasons other than merely those attached to the drinking custom' (p.4). These are the changes attributed to the generalization of a learned habit in Chapter 10.

In addition, however, this progression was, he thought, aided by what he termed 'dissocialization'. An individual would show marked changes in terms of the groups to which he or she belonged, the movement being towards groups which tolerated more drinking and more drinking effects, but which in other respects were less demanding. This part of the process Bacon considered to be of vital importance on account of the behavioural control function of the groups of which a person is a member.

In fact Bacon was particularly at pains to correct what he saw as the undue emphasis usually placed upon the individual excessive user in the process. He pointed out that control processes are not learned by individuals alone, nor are they expected to be maintained without the collaboration of others. Losing control in his view was a phenomenon involving the actor and others. The 'symptoms' of 'alcoholism' were such because they were offensive or insulting to others. 'Alcoholism' could not in his view exist without the reactions of others, with the interaction revolving, '. . . around the individual's unusual and unacceptable use of alcohol . . .' (p.17). In particular, Bacon introduced the notion of 'disjunction in labelling'. The process of moving towards compulsive use was, he suggested, accompanied by increasing irritation, annoyance, distress, and criticism from others, but particularly in the early stages this, often mild, negative social reaction was either not received at all by the drinker or could be lessened in its impact by misinterpretation or in other ways. Meanwhile, critics might be coming to label the excessive user as a problem drinker or 'alcoholic' to the point that others will speak of drinking as excessive even if the person has only had one drink or has not touched a drop for days. If this process proceeds to the point where the excessive drinker starts to be excluded from social groups, then the relationship between the drinker and, '. . . the carriers, signallers and enforcers of social control has been manifestly weakened' (p.20). This is an example of the out-of-proportion response of which Lemert wrote, acting in a way that threatens to amplify excess.

Zinberg (1975, 1981) writing about drug 'addiction' and from the psychoanalytic tradition, one very different to that from which Bacon was writing, put the same matter in different terms. Ego autonomy, he argued, needed a constant 'supply' of input both from inner drives and from the environment. The superego in particular was dependent on consistent 'stimulus nutriment'. 'Junkies' had lost various sources of input which bolstered the superego; they were alienated or had lost previous social relationships and had been declared deviant by the larger society. They had become isolated from, '. . . those views of the world which permit a coherent and integrated sense of self' (1981, p.183).

To illustrate this process, and the apparent personality change that might occur, Zinberg described a man he had interviewed twice with a gap of six years between. The first time he had been active, with a wide circle of friends, in close touch with family despite some disagreements. On the second occasion he was in the process of being detoxified from heroin for the third time, had not seen or heard from his family for two years, was functioning poorly cognitively, was preoccupied with drugs, and was on probation for two offences with another charge pending. 'He gave every evidence of being an impulsive, poorly controlled person. Physically it was hard to recognise him as the same man, and he too said, "I am not the same person you talked to then" ' (1981, p.185). Zinberg was critical of the tendency to assume that all stems from severe personality maladjustment. This assumption of a pre-addictive personality was based in his view on 'retrospective falsification'. In the case of the man described, there was some hint that he had experienced conflict over responsibility, self-sufficiency, and rebellion, but it was the apparent *change* in personality that struck Zinberg most forcibly. A similar dynamic combination of predisposition and change in determining the personality of excessive drinkers was studied by Kammeier *et al.* (1973). As we shall see shortly, there are a number of good psychological reasons why 'personality' might appear to 'deteriorate' as appetitive behaviour becomes more excessive.

Each of the forms of behaviour with which this book is concerned breaks social rules if it crosses certain, usually fairly indistinct, bounds between normality or moderation and excess or abuse. Social reaction is therefore a vitally important part of the necessary total account of excessive behaviour. Lemert's secondary deviance is undoubtedly a reality to some degree or other for anyone whose drinking, gambling, sexual behaviour, smoking, eating, or drug-taking becomes 'excessive' by their own definition or by the definition of any one or any group important to them, and Bacon's 'dissocialization' and Zinberg's alienation certainly becomes a reality for some. It must be said, however, that Lemert's distinction between primary and secondary deviance may be difficult to uphold. It suggests that primary deviance comes first, meets with social reaction, and that secondary deviance then ensues. Enough has been said already about the origins of different forms of appetitive behaviour to make it abundantly clear that pre-existing attitudes may affect behaviour very early, certainly before much of the learning process responsible for strong appetite has had a chance to occur. Ambivalence about drinking amongst Anglo-Irish youngsters in London, or amongst citizens of Alabama, is part of the social climate within which drinking behaviour develops, and is not just a reaction to the development of strong appetites on the part of a minority. The same can be said of the ambivalent attitudes to sex to which Boswell and Walter and generations since have been exposed during their upbringing, and of attitudes to gambling. Indeed, it might be said to be a chief characteristic of this whole range of appetitive behaviours that their use is attended by ambivalence. This is displayed by the concern that individuals and governments have shown in trying to draw distinctions between moderation and excess, by the need of legislators to create controls upon these behaviours, particularly upon behaviour of the young, and by the inconsistency which has been shown in the way these behaviours are defined and controlled from time to time and from place to place. However, we are concerned here principally with the development of a model to account for excessive appetitive behaviour in individuals, and hence it is with ambivalence and conflict at the *individual* level that the remainder of this chapter will be concerned.

EXCESS AS MORAL DILEMMA

It is an important part of the present thesis that, amongst the costs incurred as a result of excessive behaviour, self-generated costs have received less attention than they deserve. It is well known to clinicians that matters of morality, conscience, and values weigh heavily for many people who seek help on account of the excessiveness of their appetites. Such 'costs', generated as a result of an awareness of mis-match between actual and ideal behaviour, are intertwined with the individual's awareness of more tangible physical and social harm, and with pressures put upon the individual by others who may be affected by the behaviour. It is a difficult task for the individual, or those who attempt to help him or her, to sort out which is which. Nevertheless, it is the case that, amongst the stated reasons for dissatisfaction, the need to restore 'self-respect', the desire to prove to oneself that one is in control of one's own behaviour, or the need simply to do the right thing or to set a 'good example' for one's children (e.g. Premack, 1970, with regard to smoking), have a very important place.

Moral dilemmas can arise in relation to each of the appetitive behaviours discussed, but are perhaps particularly evident in the case of sexual behaviour. Proscriptions on sexual behaviour in medieval Christianity (Bullough, 1977), and continuing through the centuries, and reflected most clearly now in the evangelical movement in the United States and the attitudes of the National Viewers and Listeners' Association in Britain (Morrison and Tracey, 1980) have left a legacy of ambivalence and guilt surrounding sexual activities. The same may be said to differing degrees about indulgence in gambling, drinking, some other forms of drug-taking, and even of over-indulgence in eating. Hardy (1964) used a Lewinian model of driving and restraining forces (Lewin, 1947), similar to the model of inclination and restraint employed here, in describing, '. . . the approach–avoidance dynamics involved in sexual conflict and the management of sex appetite' (p.12). Principal amongst the sources of 'negative affective expectations' surrounding sexual behaviour which Hardy outlined was guilt arising out of, '. . . moral compunctions against various expressions of sexuality' (p.11).

The relationship between conduct and conscience has been considered at length, especially in its developmental aspects, by Aronfreed (1968). He pointed out that the idea of conscience as an, '. . . internal agency of control and sanction that commands, warns, and chastises in terms which refer to strong affective states' (p.2), goes back at least as far as Saint Augustine. It was the emotional power of conscience that impressed Aronfreed most. He defined conscience as pertaining to, '. . . conduct where social experience has attached substantial affective value to . . . cognitive representation and evaluation of . . . behaviour' (p.6). Again he stated: '. . . powerful affective components of conscience are reflected in the sense of essential unanalysable rightness or impelling obligation . . .' (p.13). He found evidence in children's behaviour that acts transgressing the dictates of conscience tended to lead to certain reactions. These reactions to transgression included self-criticism (including remorse, and commitment to modify future behaviour), reparation, confession, and reactions oriented towards external punishment (seeking out punishment or alternatively avoiding or escaping punishment by withdrawing from the vicinity of socializing agents or hiding the consequences of one's acts). He devoted a whole chapter to a discussion of fear, guilt, and shame—three varieties of aversive affective state associated with behavioural transgression.

These, then, are some of the further consequences we should expect from the development of strong and excessive appetite. In this light it comes as no surprise that in their study of a large number of excessive drinkers, Horn and Wanberg (1969) found guilt and shame to be the only 'symptoms' almost invariably present. Suicide is perhaps the ultimate response to chronic, unresolved dissonance created by the rift between actual and ideal behaviour: the rate of suicide is known to be exceptionally high amongst excessive drinkers (e.g. Kessel, 1965) and is believed to be similarly high amongst excessive gamblers. Rushing (1969) summarized studies of the link between excessive drinking and suicide. His review revealed that between 7 and 21 per cent of 'alcoholics' eventually committed suicide, and that between 6 and 31 per cent of suicide victims were adjudged to have an 'alcoholism' problem. Rushing put these findings in the context of the view of suicide that it is linked to social isolation and to loss and disruption of, or friction with, family and other close associates, but neglected to add that this 'loss' is usually confounded by an awareness that it has been brought about, at least partly, by the person's own strong appetitive behaviour over which he or she feels powerless.

Hiding the behavioural acts or their consequences is a common sign of excessive appetitive behaviour on an individual level, and Ryan (1973) provided a good example of mass secret consumption when he described the efforts of a whole small town community in the United States to give up cigarette-smoking together. The greatest changes in behaviour were not towards massive reduction is consumption, but rather towards more secretive consumption on a large scale.

The evidence from experimental studies with adults which bear on the question of the psychological effects of immoral action has been comprehensively reviewed by Klass (1978) and is of sufficient relevance to summarize here. The work reviewed included experiments where people had been induced to perform such acts as lying, cheating, and harming other people, for example by delivering electric shocks believed to be painful. There appears to be fairly conclusive evidence that such acts produce discomfort about one's behaviour, a higher rate of compliance with direct requests for help (even if the help does not in any way ameliorate previous harm), and that when lying is involved the transgressor is afterwards more likely to believe the lie he or she has told. Although Klass found the experimental data too sparse to draw definite conclusions about some other effects, there was at least suggestive evidence that guilt was increased, that actions that are not relatively distinct tended to be forgotten, and that given the opportunity to do so, transgressors were likely to punish themselves. Although subjects of such experiments showed discomfort about their behaviour afterwards, there was no evidence that self-esteem changed in a negative direction. An interesting set of findings concerned liking for the victim following an immoral action. The regular finding was that transgressions toward the victim resulted in increased *dislike* of that person, and this was particularly the case if the victim had few resources with which to retaliate.

Klass concluded by outlining a number of theories which might integrate these findings. They include the theory that post-transgression behaviour is motivated by the desire to reduce guilt, or the more general theory that such behaviour functions to relieve a generalized negative mood state of which that induced by immoral actions is merely one instance. An alternative, of particular relevance to the interpersonal events surrounding immoral actions, is that of equity theory (Walster *et al.*, 1970):

> Harm doing of all sorts is seen as producing inequity between actor and victim, and this distressing state of affairs is alleviated by restoring equity either 'psychologically'—through derogation of the victim, denial of responsibility, or minimization of harm—or 'actually'—by means of compensation or self-punishment (Klass, 1978, p.766).

Increased dislike for a victim, for example, may be rooted in a kind of justice motive. It may be comforting to immoral actors to perceive their victims as deserving their fates. Klass suggested that devaluation of a victim might also be interpreted as arising from the feeling that the victim serves as an unpleasant reminder that one has broken a moral rule and hence is disliked. Ghinger and Grant (1982) have pointed out that such interpersonal moral dynamics occurring in families where one member transgresses on account of excessive behaviour such as over-drinking have been well known to novelists and playwrights for a very long time (Thomas Hardy's, *The Mayor of Casterbridge*, provides a good example). Klass's review was completed by cognitive dissonance theory which has been one of the most influential in attempting to explain the effects of attitude-discrepant behaviour.

In classical dissonance theory, well described for example by Kelman and Baron (1974, pp.558–9), action discrepant with attitudes—the conflicted or dissonant smoker, for example, may be said to be performing an attitude-discrepant act whenever he or she smokes—produces a drive state that will motivate efforts to reduce the inconsistency. A key postulate of the theory is that dissonance will be lower, and hence the motive to restore consistency will be less, the greater the justification for the discrepant act. In the kinds of experiments that have been performed to test the theory, justification was provided in the form of financial inducement, the threat of punishment for not acting, or an attractive person who induces the subject to act in an attitude-discrepant fashion. Kelman and Baron (1974) preferred to view inconsistency as a 'signal' to the individual that coping mechanisms were not functioning effectively. The nature of the signal and the types of behaviour used to try and restore consistency would, they suggested, be different in the case of 'moral dissonance', where action had violated a moral precept or value, than in other cases:

> The violation of an important moral precept or the negation of an important value carries direct implications for central aspects of the person's self-image. That is, such an inconsistency affects both a person's basic sense of worth and his beliefs as to his defining attributes. In this kind of situation we expect that the inconsistency will arouse a guilt reaction, manifesting itself in a concern over the goodness or badness, the rightness or wrongness of his behaviour (p.561).

Baron (1968) has also considered the effects of moral dilemmas from a dissonance viewpoint. To the list of effects already discussed, he added one which may have particular application in the field of excessive appetites. He suggested that if a moral dilemma is created and a person evaluates his actions as bad or wrong, this will preclude increased interest in or enjoyment of the immoral action. Indeed, he suggested it is likely that people experiencing such a dilemma would tend to emphasize the negative attributes of their situation. People who seek help on account of excessive drinking, gambling, or eating, and people whose accounts of excessive heterosexuality have appeared in the literature, frequently disclaim any positive pleasure accruing from their present behaviour, although they will usually admit that similar behaviour brought pleasure formerly. There are of course a number of explanations for this phenomenon, but the possibility that it is at least in part an effect of perceived moral transgression must be included amongst them.

Work such as that reviewed by Klass on the effects of immoral actions concerns general processes and there are only hints of individual differences which must be assumed to be important. One study is mentioned in which subjects who initially expressed higher guilt about aggression, reported more negative feelings about shocking someone than were experienced by lower-guilt subjects (Okel and Mosher, 1968, cited by Klass, 1978). Mosher (1972) has also reported a study in which sex guilt (assessed by means of a sentence completion test. For example, 'Masturbation . . .', 'If in the future I committed adultery . . .', and 'When I have sexual desire . . .') was associated with heightened perceptual defense for sexually taboo words in complex fashion. Those whose responses to the test indicated relatively high sex guilt displayed moderate levels of perceptual defense whether looking at 'pin-ups' during the experiment was construed as reprehensible or normal, whilst subjects low on sex guilt were much more affected by these conditions, showing even higher perceptual defense than the high sex guilt subjects when viewing the 'pin-ups' was said to be bad. Mosher presented these complex results in the context of a social learning theory account of the inhibition of unacceptable behaviour which distinguishes between fear of external punishment, and guilt based on internalization of moral standards as motives. The important point for us here, however, is that reactions to transgressions will doubtless vary from individual to individual, but the ways in which they vary are likely to be complex and are certainly poorly understood at present.

Kelman and Baron (1974), however, made an interesting and potentially very important suggestion concerning individual differences when they wrote that the nature of the subsequent behaviour employed in an effort to restore consistency would depend upon self-esteem. If this was high, attempts at justification should be expected; if low, then there might follow a reassessment of one's own worth rather than of the object of the morally discrepant action or of those who have been harmed, and self-evaluation might be lowered further still. One of the changes that often occurs in the course of the development of an excessive appetite is a decline in self-esteem. If Kelman and Baron were correct, therefore, this change must alter a person's reaction to his own behaviour. Whether or not this makes further excessive behaviour more or less likely will depend on other factors (it might bring about helpful self-appraisal, but alternatively might instil a sense of hopelessness), but once again we have identified a process of *development*, that changes the picture from what it was.

Besides self-esteem there may be other important differences between people in the degree to which dissonance is generated, or in the degree to which discomfort is felt on account of inconsistency between behaviour and attitude. Ways of coping with dissonance, once generated, may also be subject to much individual variation. For example, people high on authoritarianism and ethnocentrism may be more likely than other people to handle ambivalence by rigidly adhering to one form of behaviour (continued excess or abstinence) at a time. This may require repression of attitudes and knowledge supporting alternative behaviour. People who characteristically use intellectualizing defences, on the other hand, may be more able to express, at the same time, sentiments which support alternative behaviours (Minkowich *et al.*, 1966; Nalven, 1967). Davidson (1964) reported that better educated smokers were more likely to use defiance, while less well educated subjects were more likely to employ denial rationalizations.

An effort has been made to establish the importance of personal reactions to one's own excessive appetitive behaviour, and to show the relevance of the psychology of cognitive dissonance and immoral action, because this aspect of the development of excess is easily neglected. On the one hand it has been proposed in the past that at least some excessive appetites are diseases and that the most important processes at work are psychobiological. On the other hand it has been argued that the harmful effects of some forms of excess are due almost entirely to negative social reactions and the effects of labelling.

It should not be thought that deviancy theory is unconcerned with the individual's moral conflict and its consequences, however. Quite the reverse is true in fact. It is an important tenet of deviancy theory that labelling can become 'internalized' by the person (Staats, 1978) or, to put it another way, that, 'The deviant individuals must react symbolically to their own behaviour aberrations and fix them in their sociopsychological patterns' (Lemert, 1951, p.75). The way the individual reacts to his or her own deviance is as important as, if not more important than, reactions by others. Lemert had a great deal to say about behaviour and social roles. He was aware that much deviant behaviour could exist without a shift in a person's major roles, that, '. . . normal and pathological behaviours remain strange and somewhat tensional bedfellows in the same person' (p.75). Amongst those with excessive appetites, he would probably have accepted Walter or Samuel Pepys as good examples, as well as those urban opiate users described as 'two-worlders' because they participated in crime and mixed with other 'addicts' whilst continuing to engage in the conventional world of work (Brotman *et al.*, 1965, cited by Kurland, 1978; Stimson, 1973). Walter's adult life-long double life suggests an answer to Lemert's question: How far and how long can people go in dissociating in this way?

Some of the excessive appetites we have considered, and tobacco-smoking in most present-day societies is probably the clearest example, require little or no role adjustment because the behaviour concerned is publicly condoned and no clear distinction is made between moderate use and excess. Even here, however, there may be stages, such as adolescence, or settings, such as hospitals, or circumstances, such as family disapproval or chronic ill-health acknowledged to be due to smoking, in which smoking may take on the characteristics of deviant behaviour and some adjustment to continuing with deviance whilst continuing with other roles may be necessary. Furthermore, smokers are as liable to incorporate others' attitudes of disapproval as are those who indulge in other kinds of excess, as Meyer *et al.*'s (1973) study of conflict experienced by cigarette smokers showed. Amongst their sample of over 200 smokers, 23 per cent showed 'minimal', 44 per cent 'moderate', and 10 per cent 'great' conflict. The latter group especially expressed much self-doubt and self-blame over their smoking and appeared to Meyer *et al.* to be engaged in a constant struggle to manage the guilt they felt about smoking and to achieve some degree of control or else to justify the absence of control. Some cut down, some denied they were 'real smokers', some claimed lack of will-power, some made vague promises or planned to quit in the future, and others stressed the 'costs' of stopping: loss of pleasure, less easy social interaction, the prospect of gaining weight. Meyer *et al.* also identified amongst conflicted smokers a cycle of events and associated feelings which has obvious parallels in other forms of appetitive behaviour. They called this cycle 'postponement and plunge' because it consisted of repeated alternations between delaying smoking because of feeling out of control and shameful, followed by increasing tension and 'relapse' into smoking. Each phase, delay or renewed smoking, brought its own rewards (a feeling of pride and control in the delay phase, release and relief at the renewed smoking phase), but each led to a fresh building up of feelings (tension or guilt) that promoted the next phase. This cycle they viewed as a very brief abstinence–relapse cycle in which there was no serious intention to quit. Other smokers were true 'oscillators' showing longer periods of abstinence before return to smoking. Meyer *et al.* saw this pattern as one method of reducing conflict because it provided an illusion of self-management, and certainly the oscillators in their sample showed less regret about smoking than others.

This pattern of oscillation, or vacillation, is at least a reflection of conflict and is very characteristic of appetitive behaviour that has reached the point of excess and great personal concern. Repeated attempts to control or to abstain from appetitive action are common amongst excessive gamblers, drinkers, eaters, and drug-takers, and amongst those who have written of their excessive sexual behaviour. Associated with this behavioural cycle may be a characteristic cycle of affects of the kind Meyer *et al.* described. The recently described 'abstinence violation effect' (Cummings *et al.*, 1980) refers to the behaviour and associated affect experienced with that part of the cycle where abstinence is broken and relapse occurs.

Meyer *et al.* also described interpersonal conflicts over smoking within the family. Many couples were of course 'united' on the matter, either both partners smoking or both not smoking. Other families were 'divided' and here they described attempts by the non-smoking spouse to get the smoking spouse to stop, and counter-measures by the latter, including rebelliously smoking more, charging the partner with nagging, and generally appealing to the right to manage one's own life. Nor, of course, are conflicts over smoking confined to husbands and wives, as Meyer *et al.* pointed out. Parents were often at pains to control their children's smoking, and smoking parents were often 'bugged' by their children to stop smoking especially since the latter were far more likely to have been exposed to anti-smoking education from an early age.

Many of the other forms of excessive appetitive behaviour, including some kinds of excessive drinking, gambling, and drug-taking, are associated not just with self-doubt and conflict within the family, but with far-reaching changes and losses of role which can act like a positive feedback servo mechanism and create circumstances which make excessive behaviour even more likely (Golüke *et al.*, 1981). Changes in identity or commitment to a new role and to those others who share it or support it may be evident in such things as clothes, speech, posture, and mannerisms (Lemert, 1951, p.76) as well as in the company one keeps (Wilkins, 1964), and in the use of, '. . . deviant behaviour or a role based upon it as a means of defense, attack, or adjustment to the overt and covert problems created by the . . . social reaction to him . . .' (Lemert, p.78).

Changes in social role are not to be thought of, however, as simply determined by the development of a certain type of excessive appetite or as being purely consequent upon excess. People have certain roles ascribed to them and acquire others throughout life as part of the normal developmental process. Appetitive behaviour is just one of the many factors involved in this dynamic process. As we have seen, drinking and drug-taking are both antecedents and consequences of change (Jessor and Jessor, 1977; and Chapter 7), and there is nothing inevitable about the social roles arrived at even by those whose drug-taking comes to the notice of the authorities (Stimson, 1973).

Lemert put one aspect of this complex process into the framework of incentives and constraints which is being adopted here, when he wrote of the limits imposed upon roles by virtue of age, sex, physical characteristics, geography, mobility, and economic factors:

> . . . there is a definable set of alternative roles which are subjectively congenial to him in terms of his covert symbolic processes and perhaps in terms of his unverbalised responses. . . . Aspirations to status and roles arise within the scope of the internal limits; likewise social pressures upon the individual to accept certain roles and status which fall beyond the internal limits will be resisted, circumvented, selected out, and rejected (p.86).

In other words, there are psychological barriers for some people which stand in the way of adopting certain roles which are consistent with some forms of appetitive behaviour. One person may be constrained from moving towards the role of 'junkie' (Stimson, 1973), for example, because of features of his personality or attitudes, another because of her social circumstances, another because of both. The important point is that the factors in play are not just the incentive or 'pulling' factors of 'appetite' but also the restraining or 'holding' factors of person and environment.

CONFLICT AND ITS CONSEQUENCES

The point has been made a number of times that appetitive behaviour cannot be understood without appreciating the importance of the balance struck between inclination and restraint. The development of a strong appetite alters this balance in a fundamental way. What characterizes an 'ism' or a 'mania', or a strong and troublesome appetite, as distinct from relatively trouble-free, restrained, moderate, or normal appetitive behaviour, is the upgrading of a state of balance into one of conflict. The difference is between behaviour which is mostly kept within moderate limits by a variety of discriminations and restraints, the influence of which may scarcely be consciously realized, and behaviour which relatively frequently gives rise to information that behaviour is 'in excess' or should be brought under a greater degree of control. This 'information' may be conveyed by other people, by a mis-match between awareness of one's own behaviour and some idea about proper or ideal behaviour, or through bodily state, or by some other means. At one end of a continuum lies unremarkable behaviour characterized by relatively little inclination and requiring little obvious restraint to keep it within bounds. At the other end lies behaviour that excites much emotion and arouses much comment, which seems to be characterized by a powerful drive, and which calls for relatively vigorous efforts at control. Either the person herself, or others, or both, are dissatisfied with the person's conduct. Behaviour is 'dissonant', to use the term which McKennell and Thomas (1967) used to describe some tobacco smokers. Either the person or others would like him to do less of it, or to do it less often or at different times, in different places, or with different people, or else would like him to give it up altogether.

There have in fact been a number of previous attempts to conceive of habitual appetitive behaviour in terms of balance or conflict. It is surprising that none of these has been incorporated into current thinking about excessive drug-taking, despite the fact that one (Heilizer, 1964) was put forward in the context of a discussion about alcohol, another (Astin, 1962) of 'bad habits' with special reference to drug addiction, and the third (Janis and Mann, 1968) of tobacco-smoking. That these valuable contributions to theoretical discussion about excessive behaviour have been ignored can be partly attributed to the insulation of the specialist fields of alcohol and 'addiction' studies from the wider discipline of psychology (for Janis and Mann's work, at least, is fairly well known in psychology), and partly to the general resistance there has been to viewing an 'addiction' such as 'alcoholism' as an example of habitual behaviour.

Both Astin and Heilizer based their ideas on the model of approach–avoidance competition put forward by Miller (1944) and studied by him and others using laboratory animals trained to approach food and to avoid shock in the same place. Miller explained the experimental findings in terms of two gradients, one for the approach tendency (inclination towards appetitive indulgence in present terms) and the other for the avoidance tendency (restraint) with the strength of both tendencies increasing with nearness to the goal (the act of 'consumption'). It was a crucial part of the theory that the avoidance gradient was the steeper of the two (i.e. that restraint became *relatively* stronger the nearer the animal or person to the consumptive act). Of particular interest in the present context was the suggestion that the degree of conflict was proportional to the height of the two gradients above the horizontal axis at the point of their intersection. This enabled a diagrammatic representation to be made of the contrast between a relatively low level 'normal' balance of motives which excited relatively little subjective distress and, on the other hand, a relatively intense conflict of two strong motives which was accompanied by marked ambivalence and distress (Figure 9).

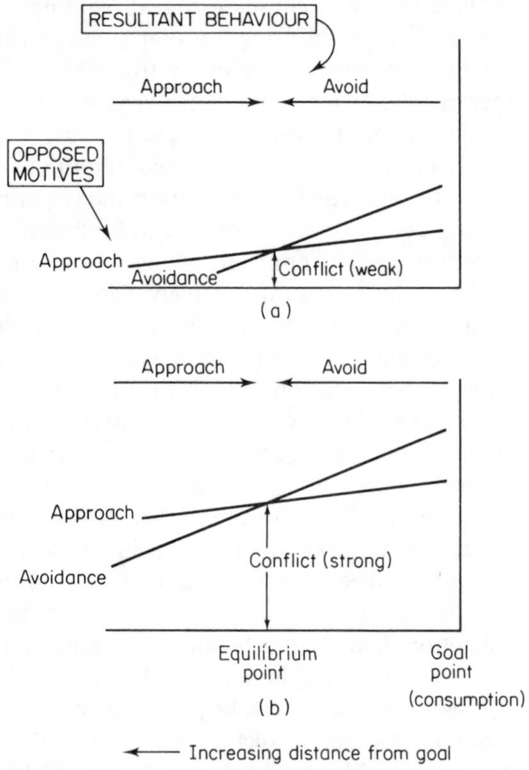

Figure 9 Approach–avoidance conflict: (a) Stable equilibrium, weak conflict (Miller); (b) stable equilibrium, strong conflict (Miller)

What is particularly intriguing about Astin's and Heilizer's theoretical contributions is their independent criticism of Miller's assumption that avoidance gradients are steeper than approach gradients. They argued that when drinking behaviour, drug-taking, or 'bad habits' in general are involved, then the appetitive approach inclination may well become relatively *stronger* as the goal (the consumptive act) becomes closer. Interestingly, they reached this conclusion from different principles. Astin argued from the principle of *temporal contiguity* of behaviour and reinforcement. If the rewarding consequences of drug-taking, for example, followed relatively soon upon consumption, whilst the punishing consequences were delayed (assuming a fairly immediate drug effect but delayed social harm), then the approach inclination would rise more steeply than the inclination to retreat from consumption as the goal was advanced upon. Heilizer's argument, more convincing to the present author, was that the relative steepness of appetitive and restraining inclinations (approach and avoidance motives) depended upon the relative importance of *internal and external cues*. In the case of habitual appetitive behaviour appetite may be strongly cued by external stimuli (the sights and sounds of people and places associated with gambling, for instance, or the sights and odours accompanying favourite foods) which become more and more prominent as the act of placing a bet or eating food is approached, whilst restraining cues may be largely internal cognitive representations of past and likely but not totally certain future events (what one's husband or wife will say or what one will look like next week, or how much money one will have tomorrow, for example), the force of which is likely to remain relatively constant as the act of consumption gets nearer. Hence, both authors, for different reasons, considered that the circumstances of the habitual drinker or drug-taker might be that represented in Figure 10.

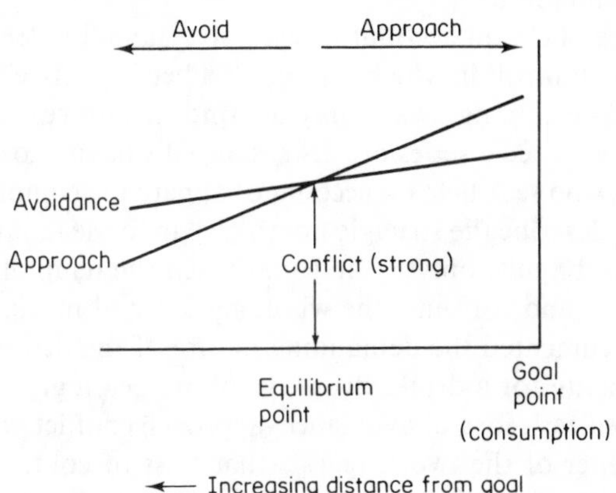

Figure 10 Avoidance–approach conflict: unstable equilibrium, strong conflict (Heilizer; Astin).

There is an important difference between the two types of conflict. The rat in approach–avoidance conflict (Figure 9) is in a sort of 'stable equilibrium'. At any one point the net resultant of inclining and restraining motives is such as to direct it towards the equilibrium point of intersection of the two gradients. In contrast, the dissonant smoker attempting to refrain, who may experience avoidance–approach conflict (Figure 10), is in a state of 'unstable equilibrium' with the resultant of motives being such as to remove him further from the point of intersection of gradients. Further *from* the goal than the intersection point, he should retreat still further from the goal, but between the intersection point and the goal he would be expected to experience an increasingly strong resultant inclination to smoke. Behavioural self-control should be relatively easily exercised well away from the goal, but would be expected to be lost relatively easily if the smoker found himself, for whatever reason, beyond the danger point of no return.

These useful ideas provide one possible psychological explanation for the experience of 'loss of control'. The subjective experience of having an inclination so strong that self-control is severely diminished is a reality for people who experience strong and troublesome appetites, and whose personal accounts are replete with references to the controlling influence of their desires and to the personal tactics and strategies which are adopted, some successfully some unsuccessfully, to try to reinstate self-control. One excessive gambler described giving his wife his week's wages for safe keeping and trying to ensure that he never went out with more than a pound in his pocket; another was driven to spend all day sitting in church to escape the temptation of betting. An excessive eater banned all cakes and other fattening food from her kitchen, and an excessive drinker forswore spirits and deliberately set out for the pub late in the evening to restrict his intake. One excessive heterosexual tore up his list of contacts, and another, like Walter, masturbated before going out in an effort to reduce his inclination.

People who seek help on account of excessive gambling frequently describe a form of 'loss of control' in which they enter a betting office intent on placing one bet only before coming away, only to 'find themselves' still there several hours later having placed a series of bets and usually having lost a lot of money. Similarly, people who seek help on account of apparently compulsive over-eating not infrequently describe the struggle not to give in to the temptation of eating, let us say a sweet biscuit, only to find that when the temptation is yielded to they 'lose control' and consume the whole packet and more. The chapters in Part I amply documented the demanding nature of the drives experienced by those whose appetite for a drink, drugs, gambling, eating, or sex is excessive.

Astin's and Heilizer's idea of avoidance–approach conflict, with the approach gradient the steeper of the two, suggests that 'loss of control' is an expected consequence of the kind of unstable equilibrium which this kind of conflict produces. People with appetites of this sort are constantly trying to keep away from sources of temptation, but if they put themselves, or perhaps accidently find themselves, in the way of temptation (the equivalent of being 'near' to the 'goal' in the animal experiments) then inclination becomes relatively stronger and stronger and resolve becomes more and more difficult to maintain.

Thus, the element of conflict, introduced once appetitive behaviour becomes at all excessive by the standards to which the person concerned refers or is subject, changes the very nature of that behaviour in fundamental ways. Another feature which is likely to come into operation, or at least to increase, has been termed 'anticipatory anxiety'. Even if it was before, the mere possibility of appetitive indulgence is now no longer affectively neutral but has become itself arousal-producing and is likely to be thought of as 'temptation'. For someone who is conscious of fighting the urge to succumb to enter a betting shop or to buy an item of fattening food, the very prospect can produce a state of near-panic. This of course produces a new dimension in the person's motivational state. Rachman and Teasdale (1969) suggested that anticipatory anxiety might increase the 'incentive value' of the appetitive act. Another way of looking at it is to say that the anticipation of action makes acute the conflict that exists for the person over this particular kind of behaviour, and that indulgence is one way of temporarily resolving this aversive state.

In a sense someone experiencing avoidance–approach conflict over gambling, drug-taking, or sexual behaviour is 'restrained' in the same way as a 'restrained eater' (see Chapter 5) and would be expected to indulge their appetite in compulsive binges similar in form to those of the 'binge eater'. In their discussion of binge eating, Wardle and Beinart (1981) put forward a very similar conflict view based on the idea of restrained eating. Some obese individuals, under much social and medical pressure to reduce weight, plus diet-conscious people of moderate or even underweight, were they suggested in an approach–avoidance conflict in relation to food. In their view this conflict led to 'externality'—eating largely being determined by external cues such as the smell, sight, and taste of food, the sight of others eating, and the passage of time—rather than to obesity *per se*. This proposed link between conflict and externality would lend support to Heilizer's particular model of avoidance–approach conflict and excessive appetitive behaviours which stressed the increasing importance of external cues associated with the appetitive object as the 'goal' or consummatory act was approached.

Wardle and Beinart reviewed studies, such as that by Spencer and Fremouw (1979), which are remarkably similar to those carried out by Marlatt *et al.* (1973) and Hodgson *et al.* (1979b) on the 'loss of control' phenomenon amongst excessive drinkers. As in the alcohol studies, a relatively large amount of food, or what the subject *believed* to be food of relatively great calorific content, was sufficient to trigger relatively larger amounts of eating amongst those who were usually restrained in their eating. If it can be accepted that the 'highly dependent' excessive drinkers, who showed the triggering effect in the studies by Hodgson and his colleagues, were relatively highly 'restrained' in their drinking (i.e. like dieters they are under pressure to keep their drinking below a particular threshold), then the comparison is complete.

Wardle and Beinart suggested that an eating binge was a 'kind of capitulation' in the light of the belief that the decision to diet has already been broken. They point out that this is analogous to the response of an excessive drinker who attempts abstinence, but after one drink gives up and goes on a binge—the 'abstinence violation effect' (AVE). A recent statement about the AVE (Cummings *et al.*, 1980) has in fact broadened out the concept in a way that makes it much more compatible with the general view of excessive appetites being developed here. First put forward in the context of excessive alcohol use, it has now been expanded to include, '. . . any violation of a self-imposed rule governing consummatory behaviour' (Cummings *et al.*, p.297). Cummings *et al.* described two components to the AVE: cognitive dissonance about the 'relapse' which is greater the longer the preceding period of abstinence and the greater the degree of private and public commitment to abstinence; and self-attributions of blame, personal weakness, and failure which, as Eiser *et al.* (1978) have suggested, may provide the justification for and prediction of continuing excessive behaviour. It may be also that attributing 'addiction' to oneself provides an explanation for failing to stop or modify an excessive appetite, and perhaps a partial justification for continuing as before despite the costs. Eiser *et al.* took this view on the basis of their findings that smokers who saw themselves as more addicted viewed giving up as more difficult, were more likely to be 'dissonant' about their smoking, and were more likely to have recently failed in an attempt to give up or reduce.

Janis and Mann's (1968, 1977) formulation was different from, but complementary to, those of Astin and Heilizer. It had nothing to say about variation in motive strength at different times and places (the central concern of Astin's and Heilizer's conflict models) but rather filled out the picture in terms of the different sources of incentive and disincentive for appetitive behaviour. Janis and Mann's original contribution (1968) was concerned with 'addictive' smoking and their core idea was that of a 'balance sheet' of the pros and cons associated with each of several ways of resolving the smoker's 'decisional dilemma' (see Table 8 for a condensed version of their balance sheet). The present author has suggested a very similar 'pay-off matrix' formulation of 'alcoholic' conflict (Orford, 1971a, 1976). The similarity between the kind of social learning theory (Akers *et al.*, 1979) which proved useful in making sense of the results of surveys of youthful appetitive behaviour, and the 'balance sheet' and 'pay-off matrix' models which turn out to be useful in summarizing the dilemmas faced by people whose appetitive behaviour has become excessive, is obvious and important. That the same kind of forces-in-opposition model should be of value in ordering what we know about appetitive behaviour in two such different settings—the University Students' Union on the one hand and the doctor's surgery or psychiatrist's consulting room on the other—makes it clear that although a process of development may have intervened, and appetite may be stronger and even personality and social position may be changed as a result, the fundamental psychological dilemma is the same in both settings. The stakes may be higher in the latter case, and the dilemma more obvious, but appetitive behaviour constitutes a 'decisional conflict' in both. In their later, more comprehensive, work Janis and Mann (1977) put conflict over excessive eating, drinking, drug-taking, and smoking into the wider context of health-related decisions and important life decisions in general. This provides a valuable and much-needed link between the theory of excessive appetites and a major theme in general psychology.

The attraction of the terms 'addiction' and 'dependence' can be appreciated in the light of the conflict model of excessive behaviour being developed here. A process of increasing affective–behavioural–cognitive attachment to a particular form of behaviour produces an inclination sufficiently strong that behaviour is unresponsive to some of the normal restraints. Behaviour is apparently self-defeating and often as mysterious to the individual as to those around her. 'Dependence' or 'addiction' appears to provide an explanation of such behaviour. It represents an attempt to create a psychosocial disease out of excessive habitual behaviour, but in fact it explains nothing. In the terms used here, it merely signifies conflict brought about by a combination of strong inclination and strong restraint concerning a particular activity. The terms 'dependence' and 'addiction' are only used when both inclination and restraint are above a certain threshold. Until behaviour becomes harmful, or is subject to criticism or attempts at control, behaviour is never seriously referred to as 'dependent' or 'addictive'.

It is, according to this view, the sense of conflict attending the development of strong appetitive behaviour which accounts for much of the behaviour seen by others as characteristic of those with an 'ism' or 'addiction', and which at an individual level is responsible for most secondary deviance. Many of these characteristic, secondarily deviant, features of behaviour might well be termed the 'consequences of dissonance'. Continued appetitive behaviour in the face of social reaction and awareness of 'costs' may lead to the types of reaction to transgression outlined by Aronfreed (1968) and others, including deviousness and secrecy. Other consequences of behavioural conflict include ambivalence, vacillation, and inconsistency, all characteristics that make people with excessive appetites awkward to 'treat' and unreliable as 'patients'. Subject to opposing motives of great strength it is difficult to know one's own mind let alone to behave with any consistency. Different elements in the balance sheet may be relatively salient at different times, depending upon such things as time elapsed since last consumption, nearness to the appetitive 'goal', and the presence of different 'audiences'. Shortly after an episode of consumption, when the full force of the harmful consequences has been felt and whilst they are still freshly in mind, in the safety of a clinic or hospital, and in the presence of the staunchest advocates of reform (e.g. 'therapist' and husband or wife), sources of restraint may be most salient and may come most readily to mind and be most easily verbalized. At contrasting times, and in quite other company, other elements of the balance sheet may be more salient. Oscillating between periods of abstinence and periods of excessive drinking becomes the pattern for many excessive drinkers who have reached a stage of undeniable conflict about drinking, as does oscillation between periods of smoking and giving up smoking for many dissonant tobacco users, and between periods of dieting and 'bingeing' for many over-eaters.

Furthermore, continued commitment to a form of behaviour which is harmful or troublesome calls for *dissonance reduction* in the interests of consistency. It is the central tenet of dissonance theory in social psychology that the uncomfortable state of 'dissonance' arising from an awareness of behaviour being out of line with ideals, norms, or expectations gives rise to motivation to reduce that state of discomfort. Thus, on theoretical grounds, if it is right to

Table 8 Hypothetical balance sheet for a smoker challenged by publicity about smoking and lung cancer (reprinted with permission of Academic Press, Inc. from Janis and Mann, 1968)

		Type of cognition			
		Anticipated utilitarian consequences		Anticipated approval or disapproval	
Alternative courses of action		For self	For significant others	From self	From significant others
1. Original policy (continue smoking about one pack per day) Judged unsatisfactory	+	Provides daily pleasure; sometimes relieves emotional tension	Helps me to get along better with my family and fellow workers	I pride myself on not scaring easily	My statistician friend will be pleased I do not accept correlation as proving causation
	–	Possibility of lung cancer; respiratory illness more serious; costs money	Family would suffer if I had cancer	I would feel untrustworthy and weak; I'd feel guilty for having ignored medical evidence if I became ill	Would lose respect since I told friends I was going to change my habits; doctor and other friends will continue to disapprove
2. New recommended policy (stop smoking) Judged mixed	+	Chances of cancer greatly reduced; respiratory illness less troublesome; money put to good use	Family will feel more secure; good influence on children's smoking	Feeling of satisfaction; acting on evidence shows one is mature, realistic, and intelligent	Friends will see I am living up to my commitment; doctor and friends will strongly approve
	–	Unpleasant craving; more irritable and angry; possibly anxiety symptoms and overweight	Increased irritation and tension could strain the marriage	Might lose my temper more often, which would make me feel like a heel	My statistician friend will think I am stupid

3. Alternative compromise policy (smoke about one-half a pack per day) Judged most satisfactory	+ Same as no. 1 to a milder degree, risk of cancer greatly reduced	Same as no.2 to a milder degree	Same as no. 2 to a milder degree	Same as no. 2 to a milder degree
	– Same as no. 2 to a milder degree; no overweight; slight risk of lung cancer	Same as no. 2 to a milder degree	Going only part way may show a lack of self control	Doctor and some friends will not approve of this compromise
4. Alternative non-recommended policy (switch to filter cigarettes, one pack per day) Judged Satisfactory	+ Same as no. 2 to a milder degree, but no money saved; cancer risk reduced?	Same as no. 2 to a milder degree	Same as no. 2 to a milder degree	Same as no. 2 to a milder degree
	– Same as no. 2 to a much milder degree; same drawbacks as no. 1 to a milder degree	Same as no. 2 to a milder degree	Same as no. 3 to a stronger degree	Doctor and several friends will not approve

think of someone whose appetitive behaviour is excessive as essentially someone who faces a dilemma or conflict of a behavioural, conduct, or even moral kind, we should expect such a person to experience discomfort and to be motivated to escape from it much as people wish to escape from pain or anxiety. Indeed this 'dissonance' should not be thought of as just theoretical, but as something very real, experienced as tension, depression, confusion, or even panic.

It is therefore only to be expected that people with an excessive appetite who continue to indulge that appetite will attempt to justify the behaviour, either to themselves or to others. Such justification-promoting behaviour is probably to be seen as an integral part of excessive appetitive behaviour, even though it may appear quite transparent to the onlooker, and is yet another consequence of dissonance which makes its perpetrator yet more unpopular. The use of 'rationalizations' for behaviour is one way in which actions can be 'justified'. Davidson (1964), for example, asked continuing smokers for their reasons for continuing and called the replies that he received 'rationalizations'. These he classified as 'denials' (e.g. 'you can prove anything by statistics'), 'demurring' (e.g. 'I have already cut down on my smoking'), 'diversions' (e.g. 'polluted air is more dangerous'), 'defiance' (e.g. 'I would rather enjoy life even if it is a bit shorter'), 'gospels of moderation' (e.g. 'moderation is desirable in all things'), 'doctrines of the lesser evil' (e.g. 'going without smoking makes me anxious, irritable, nervous and impossible to live with'), and 'comments based on misinformation' (e.g. 'there is no cancer in my family, so I don't have to worry'). Boswell showed great inventiveness in rationalizing his sexual excess when he appealed for support to the polygamy of the Old Testament patriarchs (Stone, 1979; see Chapter 6).

In the language of Janis and Mann's (1968, 1977) 'conflict theory of decision making', the excessive drug-taker, gambler, or eater has begun to fall short of the ideals of 'vigilant information processing'. More will be said of this in Chapter 13, when we consider the ways in which excessive appetites are successfully brought under control, but here we can usefully borrow from Janis and Mann's theory some ideas about the ways in which successful resolutions are avoided and how the conflict engendered by excessive behaviour and its consequences is perpetuated and in many cases worsened.

First of all, the kinds of issues with which people whose behaviour is excessive are concerned are likely to be particularly 'ego-involving' because of the degree of affective–behavioural–cognitive attachment that is likely to have built up towards the object of behaviour. This need not necessarily be the case, of course; indeed, it is the earnest hope of health educators that people will take health-enhancing decisions about appetitive behaviours at an 'early stage' before attachment is too strong. Almost certainly, as we shall see in Chapter 12, many people do in fact reduce their involvement in appetitive behaviour of one kind or another at various stages, and at various levels of attachment. What concerns us here, however, is why many do not, despite mounting evidence, apparent at least to others, that the behaviour in question is harmful. To the degree to which attachment has formed to the behaviour, a significant 'loss' will be anticipated at the prospect of reducing one's involvement. The individual is in a sense 'committed' to appetitive behaviour which has become excessive. These are the circumstances for decisional conflict according to Janis and Mann (1977). Emotions are involved: the ideas in play are 'hot cognitions' to use Abelson's (1963) vivid phrase. The stress associated with conflict is likely to produce in the '. . . harassed decision maker . . .', a '. . . further decline in cognitive functioning as a result of the anxiety generated by their awareness of the stressful situation' (Janis and Mann, p.17). In plain language, it is difficult to think straight. Once again, then, we have a clear statement, this time from the perspective of the theory of decision-making, that conflict itself has consequences; that whatever led up to conflict, once conflict exists the psychological situation is no longer the same.

Besides 'vigilance' (scanning alternative solutions objectively) the main alternative styles of coping with decisional conflict according to Janis and Mann's model are 'unconflicted inertia', 'hypervigilance', and 'defensive avoidance'. The first is likely when there is very little conflict, low stress, and little motivation to change behaviour: it corresponds to a low level of approach and avoidance motivation in the Astin and Heilizer models.

'Hypervigilance' is likely, according to Janis and Mann, when conflict is severe but time to make a decision is short and the kind of scanning and weighing of alternatives that 'vigilance' involves are not possible. At its most extreme it resembles a kind of panic; thought processes are disrupted, memory span is reduced and thinking becomes simplistic. Although it is in the context of reactions to disaster warnings, or business decisions that have to be taken quickly, that 'hypervigilance' is most apparent, there may be parallels with excessive appetitive behaviour. Certainly I have talked to excessive gamblers who have reached a stage of near panic as the culmination of increasingly out-of-control gambling, mounting debts which are becoming quite beyond their capacity to cope with, and escalating social pressure and self-neglect. Cognitive functioning, in the sense of the ability for calm reflection and appraisal, is quite obviously impaired. The same could certainly be said of some excessive drinkers and no doubt of others with other forms of excessive behaviour.

It is 'defensive avoidance', however, which has the clearest application to the decisional conflict faced by those with excessive appetites. As Lewin (1935) noted, there is a strong tendency for people to withdraw from making a decision at all if all the options that are open seem to involve major 'losses' or 'costs'. Cognitive dissonance theorists have stressed that there is loss involved in all decisions, and that all decisions are followed by some dissonance, but decisions about excessive appetites are probably particularly good examples involving as they do either continued social and other losses from continued excessive behaviour or the loss of a form of action that has served valued functions for the individual. Amongst tactics under the heading of 'defensive avoidance', Janis and Mann list selective inattention to relevant informal or mass media communications, distracting self, buck-passing, 'bolstering' by rationalizing the disadvantages of the least objectionable solution, and recourse to alcohol or drugs! That Janis and Mann should recognize that excessive appetitive behaviour can provide a major alternative to dealing with decisional conflict, of which excessive appetites are themselves good examples, is an excellent illustration of the thesis being propounded here; namely that excessive appetitive behaviour can take on additional dimensions as a result of the conflict it produces. Here is a prime example of such a process: further excessive behaviour (Janis and Mann could have added over-eating, gambling, and excessive sexual behaviour as behaviours to which reluctant decision-makers have recourse) is itself one way of coping with the dilemma created by excessive behaviour. The 'vicious circle' is plain.

Signs of 'bolstering' recorded by Janis and Mann include over-simplifying, distorting, evading, omitting major considerations, exaggerating favourable consequences, minimizing unfavourable consequences, denying negative feelings about consequences, exaggerating the remoteness of any action required, minimizing the social surveillance of new action ('no one will know if I don't live up to it'), and minimizing personal responsibility.

Before concluding this chapter, a few words are in order about how some of the changes that accompany excessive appetites, and which have been attributed here to conflict and its consequences, have been misconstrued in the past. The kind of mental face-saving or attempted justification which, it is being argued, follows from the conflict in which excessive appetite places an individual is not merely unpopular with other people but often gives rise to charges that the person concerned has not just a fault in their behaviour but, more fundamentally, a fault in their character. Nor is this just a layman's error. Indeed, psychiatric texts have often reflected considerable confusion about the link between forms of excessive appetitive behaviour such as 'alcoholism' and 'drug dependence' on the one hand, and aspects of character or personality on the other. Indeed, in some psychiatric systems of classification, these forms of behaviour were actually listed as 'personality disorders' and it has been known for psychometric tests of 'psychopathy' or 'personality disorder' to be validated against criterion groups including 'drug addicts' and 'alcoholics' amongst the supposedly 'personality disordered' criterion group (Miller, P. 1980). This is probably because many of the consequences of dissonance outlined above are behaviours that might be seen, depending upon the perspective of the observer, as defects of character. Attribution theory in social psychology may provide a useful perspective here. Jones and Davis (1965) asked themselves how it was that an observer perceived a *disposition* in the person they were observing on the basis of the latter's behaviour: in short, how did they move, 'From acts to dispositions'—the title of Jones and Davis's chapter. Their theory was that of 'correspondent inferences'. Correspondence they defined as, '. . . the extent that the act and the underlying characteristic or attribute were similarly described by the inference' (p.223). For example, if an individual is observed to be devious about his or her gambling or sexual behaviour, under what conditions will the inference be made that the individual is a devious *person*?

The answer Jones and Davis gave was that correspondent inferences would be made when the observer saw that the observed person had a reason for acting as he or she did (the intention), had knowledge that the act would produce the effect it did, and had the ability to bring the act and its effects about. In so far as appetitive behaviour is seen to be motivated by desire for pleasure or gain of some kind, and to the extent that the person is seen to have known what they were doing and to have had the ability to do it and to foresee the consequences, then the correspondent inference will be drawn. One variation on cognitive dissonance theory (Bem, 1967) in fact proposes that the actor herself draws inferences about her own behaviour in much the same way. This helps explain how it is that people with excessive appetites often wrongly draw the conclusion that their basic personalities or characters must be badly at fault to enable them to behave in a way so damaging to others. It is not only other people who stand in judgement on the excessive drug-taker, over-eater, excessive gambler, or drinker, failing to understand the psychological processes involved; the man or woman involved is often his or her own sternest critic.

The importance of perception of responsibility for behaviour which came up earlier in this chapter arises again here, and the implications of this type of attribution theory for the legal handling of people whose excessive behaviour may be said to be due to a disease condition are quite clear. Herein, of course, lies one of the principal values of a disease model of excessive appetitive behaviour. It has been the intention of much of this and previous chapters to develop the view that people may develop strong appetites for drugs, gambling, eating, or sex. To the extent that such appetites render behaviour less responsive to normal restraints or controls, then responsibility for action may truly be said to be somewhat diminished. To say that such a person is suffering from a disease may therefore have some positive consequences. If it enables family members, for example, to appreciate that there is something special in the relationship between the individual and the object of their appetite, and that choice and responsibility have become reduced, then this may help produce a more sympathetic view and possibly a more functional response. Similarly, if it enables government and other policy planners, and providers of care facilities of all sorts, to re-direct individuals away from the criminal justice system and towards the health-care system (witness the recent attempts to decriminalize public drunkenness by allowing the police to take people to 'detoxification centres' rather than to police cells and thence to court and perhaps prison), and in so far as this achieves the desired objectives, then calling a strong appetite a disease may be said to have achieved something.

CHAPTER TWELVE

The Place of Expert Help

> It does appear that the generally accepted professional and public impression that nicotine addiction, heroin addiction, and obesity are almost hopelessly difficult conditions to correct is flatly wrong. People can and do cure themselves of smoking, obesity and heroin addiction. They do so in large numbers and for long periods of time, in many cases apparently permanently (Schachter, 1982, p.442).

> The treatment setting of prime significance for recovery from alcoholism is not a hospital, a clinic, a doctor's or minister's office, a social agency or a jail, or any other specialized institution or place. The prime setting of significance is the social, interpersonal setting of the daily life most appropriate and probable for the particular individual. And, equally important, it is that setting through time (Bacon, 1973, p.25).

In the previous chapter it was argued that excessive appetitive behaviour could not be properly understood without taking full account of conflict, ambivalence, and dissonance over behaviour. Such behaviour cannot be comprehended unless cognizance is taken of the restraints and pressures which oppose it. Excessive appetitive behaviour is not just repetitive behaviour, but is repetitive behaviour which comes into conflict with other needs of the person or with those of other people in his or her life. Amongst the consequences of dissonance which were considered in the previous chapter are guilt, inconsistency, and a variety of behaviours the effect of which is to prevent objective appraisal of behaviour, and which in extreme form may appear to others to constitute 'personality change'.

The present chapter and the following two, which are concerned with reaching a tentative psychological understanding of the processes that occur when people attempt to regain control over such behaviours, will pursue this line of argument by presenting a model based upon the resolution of conflicts. According to this way of understanding the problem, the task facing a person who has developed a strong and troublesome appetite is that of coping with the dissonance created between actual behaviour (e.g. gambling incurring heavy losses, sexual behaviour which runs counter to the person's moral standards, heavy drinking which threatens the stability of marriage) and sensible behaviour or right conduct (saving money, being monogamous, drinking socially and moderately). One set of options for the reduction of dissonance consists of actions and attitudes which will be construed by those who advocate change (family members, the person's medical practitioner, the next door neighbour) as 'defensive'. It includes the frequent rehearsal and public use of 'rationalizations', the under-reporting of the frequency or severity of the behaviour and its harmful consequences, and the use of the 'defence mechanisms' of projection, intellectualization, and outright denial. Another set of options consists of modifying appetitive behaviour to make it compatible with other needs, with other values or attitudes, or with the desires of other significant figures such as husband, wife, and other family members. It is in fact the principal argument of these next two chapters that change, in the direction of moderation or abstinence, is a *natural* consequence of the development of strong appetite. To put it another way, it should be expected on theoretical grounds that adopting a new, reduced level of appetitive behaviour will be part of the natural history of strongly appetitive behaviour, following *in some cases* upon the development of distressing conflict as a result of the processes outlined in Chapters 9–11. A major problem in viewing change as a spontaneous, or naturally occurring process, is the qualification that it occurs as part of natural history in only a proportion of people whose appetitive behaviour develops to the strong and troublesome stage. Our ability to predict when such changes will occur and when not is, admittedly, rather poor.

EXPERT TREATMENT

We will begin, however, by considering in this chapter the nature of the treatments that have been professionally prescribed for excessive appetitive behaviours. The most striking fact when treatments were considered in the opening chapters in Part I was the great range and diversity of techniques which had been employed. It is not possible here to mention more than a proportion of them. Almost without exception they have been backed up by impressive rationales, and although some have passed out of fashion, it is probably true to say that the majority still find favour somewhere. All that can be done here is to point out a number of facts regarding this impressive array of treatments.

One is that drug treatments have occupied an important place. Sometimes the rationale for medication has been the suppression of appetite, for example the use of amphetamines as suppressants of the appetite for food (see Chapter 5), and anti-androgenic drugs to suppress sexual appetite (see Chapter 6). Others, such as cyclazocine, have been used as antagonist drugs to block the action of a drug of 'addiction', whilst disulfiram (Antabuse) has held a popular and unique place as a 'deterrent' drug which, when taken with alcohol, produces a highly noxious effect. Of particular interest is the fact that drugs with 'dependence potential' themselves, either known at the time or discovered later, have been widely used in an attempt to control strong drug-seeking behaviour: it was mentioned in Chapter 4, for example, that both morphine and heroin have in their day been used in the treatment of opiate 'dependence' in the mistaken belief that they themselves were not 'addictive'. Up to the present time, drugs such as barbiturates and minor tranquillizers have been prescribed for people with excessive appetites either to reduce anxiety or to combat symptoms of withdrawal from alcohol, tobacco, or other drugs.

Drug treatments have sometimes been used quite explicitly as replacements for a drug used excessively. Best known is Methadone (physeptone) pioneered by Dole and Nyswander (1965) as a treatment for heroin 'addiction'. The controversial rationale for its use is that, being a synthetic opiate, it relieves the craving set up by withdrawal of opiates, but, being a much longer-acting agent, it requires to be taken less often and is less 'addictive'. Lobeline sulphate has been popular in the treatment of excessive smoking and has a similar rationale (see Chapter 4). Finally, there is the intriguing fact that in the case of heroin and nicotine at least, maintenance on prescribed doses of the drug has been used as a treatment. The prescribing of nicotine as gum or intravenously for smokers has been reported to have met with considerable success (Pechacek, 1979), the argument being that tar and other constituents of tobacco smoke are more harmful than nicotine itself. The argument for maintenance heroin treatment is rather different; namely that the harmful effects of regular heroin use lie more in the circumstances of its procurement and administration—involvement in criminal activity, use of unsterile apparatus, the risk of overdose—than in the fact of regular consumption itself. A further advantage claimed for maintenance heroin, or the 'British system' as it is often known, is that regular attendance for prescriptions at a recognized treatment centre provides practitioners with the maximum opportunity to persuade users to come off heroin altogether.

That there has from time to time been felt to be a need for very radical treatment is illustrated by the use of surgical treatments which have included the implanting of Antabuse as a deterrent to drinking (Wilson *et al.*, 1978), intestinal by-pass surgery and jaw-wiring in the treatment of obesity (Chapter 5), brain surgery in a case of 'compulsive gambling' (Chapter 3), and quite recently in Czechoslovakia, brain surgery in a number of cases of 'chronic alcoholism'—the rationale in this case being that 'alcoholism' indicated 'compulsive hedonism' or a pathological desire for pleasure due to an abnormality in the hypothalamus (Patoprsta *et al.*, 1976).

Psychological treatments have been even more diverse, covering individual, group, and milieu approaches. Different psychological treatments have been in vogue for different types of behaviour at different times. Amongst behavioural therapies, aversion therapy, for example, which at some time or another has been tried for all types of behavioural excess, was until quite recently frequently prescribed in cases of excessive drinking, smoking, and gambling. 'Rapid smoking' in which smokers were required to puff at a series of cigarettes much more rapidly than usual appeared to hold great promise as a treatment for cigarette smokers but has lost ground more recently (Lichtenstein and Rodrigues, 1977; Paxton, 1980), and 'self-control' procedures including 'self-monitoring', 'stimulus control', 'self-reward', and 'self-punishment' most recently found favour in the treatment of excessive drinking, smoking, and eating (Miller W., 1980). Others include 'covert sensitization' (a kind of aversion therapy in fantasy), video-tape confrontation for excessive drinking (being made to watch oneself intoxicated on video), and the use of 'deposit contracts' (depositing money at the onset of treatment which is returned in stages dependent upon appropriately moderate or abstemious behaviour). Non-behavioural treatments include just about the whole panoply of available techniques including individual non-directive psychotherapy, transactional analysis, hypnosis, marital therapy, family therapy, and perhaps most consistently popular of all, various kinds of group psychotherapy.

This energetic search for successful treatments tells its own story. Each new treatment has its rationale and is pursued vigorously and optimistically by its initiators (Vaillant, 1980), but quickly turns out, when used routinely, to meet with much the same moderate level of success as did previous therapies. There is in fact a remarkable consistency in the conclusions reached by those who have reviewed studies of the effectiveness of treatment for different forms of excessive appetitive behaviour. Reviewers of such work on obesity (e.g. Leon, 1976; Ley, 1978), smoking (e.g. Raw, 1977; Leventhal and Cleary, 1980), alcohol problems (e.g. Emrick, 1975; Orford and Edwards, 1977), and other forms of excessive drug use (e.g. Kurland, 1978) have reached essentially the same conclusions, which may be stated as follows:

(1) Follow-up success rates at 6–12 months after treatment mostly lie within the range 20–45 per cent, averaging around one-third.

(2) When those receiving treatment have been randomly assigned to different forms of treatment, or when groups receiving different treatments have been carefully matched, the large majority of findings have been uniform, i.e. different treatments tend to produce very similar results.

Such conclusions have often led researchers and practitioners to view the whole treatment enterprise, wrongly in this writer's view, in a negative light. This has particularly been the case when a new form of treatment has excited much positive expectation which has then been dashed by the finding that results are little or no better than those achieved with earlier methods. This has been true, for example, in the treatment of excessive eaters. The general conclusion about behavioural techniques seems to be that although the 'self-control' procedures are the most promising (Ley, 1980), results in terms of weight loss are disappointingly modest (Leon, 1976; Stunkard, 1978). In the case of groups such as Weight Watchers, Ashwell (1978) concluded, 'There is no doubt that commercial groups achieve weight losses from their members which are comparable with other groups treated either in general practice or hospital out-patient clinics', but, '. . . the results concerning the maintenance of weight loss are as poor for commercial groups as they are for the medical profession' (p.275). Elliott (1977) also concluded from her review of treatments for excessive eating that no studies of more than a very few people had demonstrated, 'clinically significant losses in a significant proportion of the sample' (p.2), and that there was no evidence from 'self-control' or other treatments to refute earlier negative conclusions such as that of Stunkard and McLaren-Hume (1959). She also noted how similar this conclusion was to that drawn from reviews of the smoking treatment literature.

Leventhal and Cleary's (1980) conclusion on the basis of their review of smoking intervention studies was:

> . . . the evidence suggests that all methods have failed to produce sustained change; neither public health programs nor face-to-face therapies have proven effective in achieving long-term reductions in smoking when compared with control cases or with the rates of spontaneous quitting in the population at large (p.371).

The same pessimism is to be found in reviews of treatment for excessive use of drugs other than alcohol or tobacco, although Kurland (1978, p.52) for one believes this interpretation of the findings of evaluative research to be unnecessarily negative, partly because of the inappropriately stringent criteria adopted in much of this research, whereby any use of an opiate is counted as a total 'failure'. The same, of course, has been true of the alcohol treatment field, dominated until quite recently by a total abstinence philosophy (Pattison *et al.*, 1977).

There are other reasons too why the modest results of treatment for those who seek help for excessive appetites should not be interpreted too negatively: in particular there is the finding that very large numbers of people do well without the kind of specialist help which has usually been the subject of research, and sometimes without any formal help at all. Nor should the very broad conclusions about treatment outcome stated above be interpreted, as I hope to make clear later in this chapter, to mean that treatment never works. Nevertheless, they do have important implications for theory: it is what these conclusions may tell us about the nature of the processes underlying change which is of most interest here. Only if we can understand how and why some people give up excessive appetitive behaviour whilst others do not, shall we be able to design more effective responses. Increased understanding of the change process may also add to our comprehension of the nature of excess itself.

Many reviewers have argued from the uniform treatment results that when treatments work they must be doing so because of the operation of 'non-specific' factors, or factors which are common to a variety of treatments despite their different theoretical bases and superficial appearances. Studies which particularly lend themselves to this type of interpretation are those that have involved a comparison of treatments with and without theoretical rationale, the latter sometimes even contravening theoretically derived principles. For example, a number of studies of treatment for cigarette-smoking have shown that conditions as supposedly different as support, contingent aversion therapy (aversive stimulation being delivered contingent upon smoking as dictated by theory), and non-contingent aversion (contrary to theory), have no differential effects on outcome (Carlin and Armstrong, 1968; Russell *et al.*, 1976). Similarly, Keutzer (1968) found that placebo capsules or tablets given under circumstances in which the, '. . . characteristics of the . . . treatment setting and verbal and non-verbal communication of therapeutic intent [were] preserved', thus imparting an, 'illusion of authenticity', produced as much success in comparison with a no-treatment control group, as was produced by 'coverant control', 'breath-holding', or 'negative practice'. Almost incidentally Keutzer added the very significant statement that common to all treatments was, as he put it, '. . . the collection of smoking data, the dispensation of resolution rearmamentation . . . and discussion . . .'. It is just these elements which, according to the view of treatment to be offered here, constitute the effective ingredients.

Another example of a study using a counter-theoretical treatment was one of a series of dieting experiments carried out by Ley (Ley *et al.*, 1974, cited by Ley, 1980). They used a 'will-power' control group who were recommended the opposite of the behavioural self-control procedures recommended to the main treatment-proper group. They were told, for instance, to shop only when hungry and to be sure to leave tempting foods around. No significant differences in weight loss were obtained although, as Ley (1980) points out, all participants in this study received a lecture on weight control, and were monitoring their diet and their weight regularly.

Equally intriguing are the results of those studies which have compared the effectiveness of treatments that differ markedly in intensity—and therefore usually in financial cost also. For example, in the alcohol problems treatment literature there exist a number of studies demonstrating that little difference results when long-term in-patient treatment is compared with short-term in-patient treatment (e.g. Willems *et al.*, 1973), when in-patient treatment is compared with out-patient treatment (Edwards and Guthrie, 1967), when long-term out-patient treatment is compared with short-term out-patient treatment (e.g. Armor *et al.*, 1978), or when relatively costly treatments such as 'self-control' training are compared with relatively inexpensive therapies such as 'bibliotherapy'—the provision of books, pamphlets, and instructional manuals (Miller and Taylor, 1980).

Particularly germane to the present argument are the results of those few studies that have examined the effects of 'unaided quitting' in comparison with 'treatment', controlling for the effect of expectation of future help. Bernstein (1970) reported the results of such a study of smoking. In comparison with 'treated' subjects, those asked to quit on their own displayed as much change, but only if future aid was not expected. Bernstein stressed the need to inform subjects that determination was the key to quitting and that no one else could help them in their attempt.

The present author and colleagues have reported an essentially similar study of excessive drinkers (Orford and Edwards, 1977; Edwards *et al.*, 1977). One hundred patients (all married men) were assessed and randomly assigned either to conventional hospital out-patient 'treatment' (with additional in-patient treatment for some) or to simple advice confined to a single session. Great care was taken to convey to subjects in the advice group that the decision to change was theirs and that only they could take it and carry it through, and that for this reason no further help would be offered by the hospital. Monthly research follow-ups were conducted with the patients' wives for a period of a year, after which time the results for the two groups were found to be identical.

Results of a smoking study by McFall and Hammen (1971) led them to conclude that non-specific factors were operative in smoking reduction. Volunteer college students who smoked at least one pack of cigarettes a day, and who wanted to stop smoking, met as groups and were told:

> . . . that they were to stop smoking 'cold turkey'; only in this way would they develop real self-control; and in the long run self-control was necessary to achieving continued abstinence. Thus the function of the Smoking Clinic was not to provide 'gimmicks' or 'crutches', since none of these was really effective, rather it was merely to provide a convenient structure—a starting point and end point—within which each S was to try on his own to stop smoking (p.82).

For the next three weeks volunteers were to hand in completed records of their smoking twice a week to the clinic office. Here they were dealt with by a 'low status' experimental assistant from whom students were instructed to buy any cigarettes that they needed. These interactions lasted approximately 3 minutes and:

> No advice giving or treatment occurred during these interactions, which were carried out in a clerical, matter-of-fact manner. However, in the process of conducting this business, Es routinely told Ss to keep striving for abstinence. . . . over the course of treatment, Ss met with a succession of Es, who were for the most part blind as to Ss' conditions and impassive about their individual problems (p.83).

Results were comparable to those obtained in other smoking reduction studies, with smoking rates reduced to approximately 20–30 per cent at the end of the 3-week treatment period, being restored to 45–75 per cent at 6-weeks follow-up, and to between 70 and 80 per cent for three of the four sub-groups (which differed in the type of self-monitoring required) at 6-months follow-up. McFall and Hammen concluded that success depends on a combination of client motivation to quit, the provision of some treatment structure, and the requirement of self-monitoring of behaviour.

Edwards (1970) has rendered a valuable service in pointing out that, 'The essence of treatment [for alcohol and other drug problems] as practised today is remarkably similar to that practised by Thomas Trotter (1804)' (p.9). Trotter's prescriptions were largely 'non-specific' and left little room for the paraphernalia of specific pharmacological or psychological treatment. For example, he taught that, 'The relationship is the essential tool', that, 'Within the setting of that relationship confrontation can be used—Particular opportunities are therefore to be taken to hold a mirror as it were, that he may see the deformity of his conduct and represent the incurable maladies which flow from perseverence in the course of intemperence', that, 'Confrontations be joined with offer of hope—At the conclusion of every visit, something consummatory must be left for amusement, and as food for his recollection', and finally in the list cited by Edwards, that, 'The wife's behaviour bears on the chances of recovery—The good sense and management of an amiable wife, we know, can often accomplish wonders (cited by Edwards, 1970, pp.9–10).

CHANGE WITHOUT TREATMENT

The finding that some people troubled by excessive appetites moderate or give up altogether their offending behaviour relatively unaided or with minimal treatment, raises the possibility that there may be a substantial rate of spontaneous remission from excessive appetitive behaviour in the general non-clinical population. Eysenck and Beech (1971) were of the view that spontaneous remission rates for appetitive disorders such as 'alcoholism' or drug 'addiction' would be negligible or small in comparison with those for problems such as phobias, obsessions, and anxiety states. Research carried out since that time has tended to prove them wrong.

Roizen *et al.* (1978) concluded from their review of the literature concerned with those with drinking problems who had either been refused treatment or had refused it themselves, as follows:

> In spite of the climate of opinion in which spontaneous improvements are often regarded as rare, what literature exists on the subject suggests that remission in the sense of six months of abstinence can be expected in 15 per cent of the cases, and remission in the sense of some improvements in about 40 per cent (p.201).

They continued by discussing the results of their own longitudinal study of a sample of 21–59-year-old men in San Francisco. They were interviewed twice, with an interval of approximately four years between, and remission rates for drinking problems between time one and time two were calculated. Roizen *et al.* made much of the point that in such a non-clinical population the exact answer to the question, 'What is the rate of spontaneous remission?' depends upon the definition of a drinking problem and of its remission. Their strictest criterion—a drop from a high problem drinking scale score at time one to having 'no problem' at time two—yielded a rate of around 12 per cent, whilst the most lenient definition—a drop of one or more points on the scale between time one and time two—yielded a rate of between 55 and 70 per cent. Whatever figure is chosen between these two extremes in order to represent the best estimate, it seems fair to agree with them that:

> . . . the general trend of the figures is clear, and it supports . . . much of the earlier literature: By most criteria, there was a substantial amount of spontaneous remission of drinking problems in a population in which the overall trend in drinking problems was stable or even increasing. This suggests that the conventional clinical picture of drinking problems as relatively stable and lasting phenomena may need changing. Instead we might picture a great deal of episodic and situational flux in a relatively large fraction of the population that ever drinks enough to risk drinking problems (p.214).

Saunders and Kershaw (1979) have added an important report to this literature. They interviewed 19 people who, from all available evidence, had been 'definitely alcoholics' in the past but who had been located in a survey in Clydeside, Scotland, as having no drinking problem currently. They also interviewed a further 41 former 'problem drinkers', again without current drinking problems, two-thirds of whom had been under 30 at the time of their drinking problem. The latter group nominated getting married (more likely for those who had been under 30 at the time), changing job, and having a physical illness (more common for those over 30 at the time) as the three most common causes of giving up a drinking problem. Family advice, financial factors, general practitioner advice (three cases only), and ageing, were other causes stated by more than one respondent. This group made no mention of specialized treatment for 'alcoholism' at all. Even for the smaller group of 'definite alcoholics', getting married and changing job still headed the list of stated causes of change. Treatment, in the form of Councils on Alcoholism, special hospital treatment, and Alcoholics Anonymous, was however mentioned by seven members of this group, with general practitioner advice mentioned by one other. Even here, then, the majority claimed to have given up a severe drinking problem without the aid of formal treatment.

In Texas, U.S.A., Tuchfeld (1981) carefully screened people who responded to advertisements requesting interviews with people who had given up drinking problems without formal treatment, and finally concentrated on 51 people who reported having had social, psychological, and/or physical problems associated with their alcohol use, but who had lost their drinking problem with, at most, intervention by friends, family, untrained or lay ministers, or diagnostic medical warnings from a doctor. Like Saunders and Kershaw, the general conclusion was that, '. . . several types of problem drinkers, including "alcoholic persons", sustained a continuing state of resolution without the aid of treatment'.

Tuchfeld was concerned to investigate the processes of change amongst these untreated excessive drinkers. He was struck, first, by the resistance of many to being labelled 'alcoholic' and their negative attitudes towards institutional forms of intervention. Many were adamant that they had helped themselves without the aid of others. As one respondent put it:

> The one thing I could never do is to go into formal rehab. For me to have to ask somebody else to help with a self-made problem, I'd rather drink myself to death (p.631).

Amongst factors associated with the problem resolution, Tuchfeld, like Premack (1970) in his analysis of the reasons for quitting smoking, which will be mentioned later, put 'humiliating events' first in the list. For example, he cited instances of a pregnant woman drinking and feeling her baby quiver and concluding she could be harming her unborn child; the person who stopped drinking when his father died having concluded that his own drinking was one of the causes of his death; and a third lying in hospital and coming to the realization that drinking had been a major cause of health and other problems. A second factor was the role played by 'negative role models' such as Skid Row drinkers who shocked people into considering change. Loved ones, particularly family, were stated to play a major role, particularly when they were seen to have provided persistent support. For example:

> I knew it was hurting my family, her [his wife] especially. But she never fussed at me. If she had fussed at me I would still be drinking (p.634).

Religion and religious conversion were mentioned as critical factors by some, but although a few cases seemed like, '. . . classic cases of sudden religious conversion', most reflected, '. . . an incremental process of commitment'. Advice from friends or concerned strangers, as well as unexpected critical events, also received mention.

Like several others who have commented on the process of resolving the problem of excessive appetitive behaviour, Tuchfeld wrote of two stages, initial commitment and longer-term maintenance. Amongst factors assisting maintenance, Tuchfeld's subjects reported significant alterations in social and leisure activities in the direction of situations and circumstances serving as effective informal social controls over drinking, positive changes in self-concept, 'commitment mechanisms' including religion, and 'justifying rhetorics' which helped to explain the person's former excessive drinking, as well as financial stability, good health, and employment.

In summary, Tuchfeld came to the following conclusion about the essentially social nature of the change process:

> Few, if any, cases in this study could be characterized as 'spontaneous' (i.e. developing without apparent external influence . . .).

> The observations suggested that internal, psychological commitment is usually activated by social phenomena in the external environment. Further, recognition and commitment appeared to require reinforcement by socially based maintenance factors if disengagement from problem drinking status was to lead to sustained resolution. In general, these maintenance factors were characterized by significant alterations in social and leisure activities (p.638).

Bacon (1973) had arrived at the same conclusion about the everyday social nature of the recovery process some time before most of the recent studies of unaided change had appeared. His statement is consistent with what is known about the effectiveness of formal treatment, and what is beginning to be known about the process of change without formal treatment, and is an excellent statement of the position being adopted here:

> The recovery personnel of prime significance are the associates, the significant others. Perhaps medical or welfare or religious or law-enforcement personnel are essential at this or that stage, are necessary requirements for the treatment process even to begin, but the crucial persons for recovery are the daily life associates through time, not the specialists during formal 'treatment' periods.
>
> The treatment methods crucial for recovery . . . are those processes and structures and interrelationships and attitudes and behaviours of the person and of the relevant surrounding others which rebuild control . . . recovery itself comprises the moulding of such changes into a pattern of life, life through time, life with meaningful others, life more satisfying to the person, to his associates, and to the community. It is that moulding through time, persons, and society which is the core of treatment (pp.25–6).

If it is the case that many excessive drinkers change without the aid of expert help, there can be little doubting the ability of many dissonant smokers to do the same. Horn (1972) reported some results of a study of 2,000 cigarette smokers in the United States interviewed first in 1966 and again in 1970. Of the men, 26 per cent had stopped successfully for a year or more, of the women 17 per cent. On this basis Horn estimated that 13 million adults must have become ex-smokers in the United States in that interval of time, of whom he guessed that 99 per cent had done so without any treatment or formal help:

> The level of change in smoking habits in the United States has been quite massive and I regard it as a change in health behaviour that is largely dependent on individual decision (p.61).

Much larger numbers still had shown evidence of 'dissonance' over their smoking by thinking seriously about giving up (87 per cent of men smokers,

84 per cent of women). Of this number 71 per cent had made an actual attempt, and of those who had attempted it 72.5 per cent of men and 58.5 per cent of women had been successful at least for a month. A large part of Horn's report dealt with the apparent determinants of moving through this four-stage process of thinking about change, attempting it, succeeding in the short term, and staying stopped. Some of the results were surprising. For example, although valuing health and believing it would be improved by stopping smoking contributed to thinking about and trying to stop, it made no contribution to success in stopping. Similarly, being motivated to be a good example to someone else influenced thinking about stopping, but little else. The same was true of the aesthetic motivation to stop, and the mastery motive—the importance of being able to control yourself and make your own decisions—which made little contribution to any step of the process. A factor that was related both to attempting and being successful, however, was having confidence in the ability to stop. There were differences too depending upon the reported motives *for* smoking. Smokers high on tension reduction, habit, and 'addiction', were less likely to be successful at stopping.

Horn reported, in addition, some interesting sex differences which invite speculation about the connection with both over-eating and the use of other drugs such as the 'minor tranquillizers'. Horn found that many more women than men reported using cigarettes, '. . . as a kind of tranquillizer . . .' (p.64), for tension reduction. Another difference was that personal relevance of the health or other threat from smoking interfered with stopping smoking, but only for women. Finally, dose had a much stronger influence at all stages of the process for women, so much so that there were very few instances recorded of women who smoked more than 40 a day subsequently stopping.

Schachter (1982) is another who has stated his opinion that although '. . . there is probably overwhelming professional consensus that addictive-appetitive behaviours are markedly resistant to long-term modification' (p.436), this may give a quite false impression because people who cure themselves may not be those that go to therapists, and most of the treatment studies are based on single attempts, whereas people who achieve success may often do so after *multiple* attempts.

In order to study the natural history of attempts at self-cure of smoking and over-weight, Schachter interviewed 161 people who represented substantial majorities of two selected populations, the staff of a university psychology department and those who worked in shops and businesses on a particular stretch of the main street of one small town. Between them, these two groups covered a good range of social groups. With regard to smoking, 64 per cent of those who reported attempting to quit had succeeded at the time of the interview. Eighty-eight per cent of these had been non-smokers for a year or more, and the average time since giving up was seven years. Comparing these reports to those of formal treatment, Schachter concluded that, '. . . those who attempted to quit were at least two to three times more successful than were those self-selected subjects who in other studies went for professional help' (p.439). Nearly half of those who had been heavy smokers (smoking at least 17 and an average of 33 cigarettes a day) reported major difficulties on giving up, such as marked irritability, sleeplessness, cravings, fevers, and cold sweats, and another quarter of this group reported minor difficulties of this kind. Although the very large majority of former light smokers (smoking 12 or fewer cigarettes a day and an average of 7) reported no such difficulties, they were no more successful at quitting than the heavy smokers had been.

Forty-six people had at some time been obese (15 per cent or more over-weight) and of these 40 had made an active attempt to lose weight. Of this number over 60 per cent had succeeded in losing substantial amounts of weight and were no longer fat. Amongst the men 67 per cent had lost an average of 39 lb and an average of 13 years had elapsed after beginning to reduce, and amongst women 58 per cent had lost an average of 29 lb an average of eight years after starting. Even amongst the most obese, ranging from over 30 per cent to over 70 per cent over-weight, over 60 per cent were classified as 'cured'. Success rates seemed to be markedly in excess of those reported in the literature on therapeutic outcome.

Although self-selection may be the most obvious explanation for the disparity—only the most difficult cases seek formal help—the fact that treatment outcome evaluations are based on studies of *single* attempts to give up excessive appetites may be equally at fault. From such results, Schachter pointed out, '. . . nothing can or should be inferred about the probable success of a lifetime of effort to quit smoking or lose weight' (p.443). Of his sample two had at some time sought help for smoking and 12 for obesity. Of this number 43 per cent were categorized as either 'cured fat' or 'cured smoker', a much higher success rate than those reported in the literature.

An alternative approach to the question of spontaneous change was adopted by Drew (1968) who pointed out that the decreasing prevalence of 'alcoholism' after middle age (shown by age distribution curves for people seeking help on account of drinking problems in many different parts of the world) could not be explained in terms of mortality or treatment success alone, and must in large part have been due to spontaneous recovery. If 'alcoholism' was a disease at all, it was for many people, he argued, a self-limiting one. Recovery might be attributable to factors such as increasing maturity and responsibility, decreased drive, and changed social pressures with age. Winick had earlier (1962) advanced an essentially similar theory of the 'maturing out' of excessive drug use with increasing age. From his examination of records held by the Federal Bureau of Narcotics, he found evidence that the average length of drug 'addiction' was in the region of 8–10 years, and that the majority of 'addicts' appeared to have given up using drugs in their late twenties or early thirties. The 'spontaneous' giving up of heroin use by Vietnam veterans on return to the United States which was referred to in an earlier chapter (Robins *et al.* 1977), adds to the conclusion that spontaneous 'recovery' from excessive drug use is possible.

Long-term follow-ups of users, for example a recent follow-up of heroin 'addicts' known to have attended London 'drug dependence clinics' seven to eight years earlier (Thorley *et al.*, 1977; Stimson *et al.*, 1978), have also shown a substantial proportion giving up drug use over such a period of time. In the London follow-up studies, abstinence from opiates had been achieved by at least 40 people out of the original cohort of 128. Of these 40, 21 had achieved withdrawal voluntarily without hospitalization or other institutionalization, most of this number reduced their drug use over 12 months or more, and for 8 abstinence was preceded by a period of occasional use. The large majority had no treatment after withdrawal. Abstinence was associated with social and work stability: for those withdrawing voluntarily in the community this stability seemed most often to have preceded withdrawal, for others it most often followed withdrawal (Wille, 1978). Besides these successes we are told that 48 per cent of the sample were still using opiates at follow-up and 23 per cent appeared to have used heroin without interruption since first attending one of the clinics. It is important to realize, therefore, that both in the case of opiate use and excessive drinking, remission, often without treatment, occurs with considerable frequency but that it is equally true that drug use continues for many years in very many, perhaps the majority, of cases. The outcome of an excessive appetite is very difficult to predict, as a comparison of the history of O'Neill's and Fitzgerald's excessive drinking (Chapter 2) and of Pepys' and Boswell's excessive sexuality (Chapter 6) makes clear.

Follow-up studies in the United States, such as Vaillant's (1973), also show that a proportion of 'addicts' achieve stable abstinence over a period of years, although Vaillant has challenged the notion of 'maturing out' and has concluded rather that compulsory community supervision is necessary (Kurland, 1978, p.45). On the other hand, there are a variety of 'pushes' and 'pulls' which might be expected to operate with increasing age and time 'addicted' (Brill *et al.*, 1972, cited by Kurland, 1978) and which could be responsible for 'spontaneous' cures:

> The pushes for getting off the drug have been traced to the negative self-image; the bad life, resulting from arrests, imprisonments, and hospitalizations; the narrow escapes or dramatic happenings confronting the individual with the possibility of some serious hazard or punishment; the exhaustion of resources; and the fading of the glamour associated with the activities of the drug subculture. The pulls have their origins in the legitimate aspirations of the individual; the assistance provided by treatment facilities; personal relationships that may be constructive; and the opportunity to think about one's self as the ageing process takes place (Kurland, p.49).

In one of the series of reports by Zinberg and his colleagues on controlled drug use, Zinberg and Jacobson (1976) described five cases illustrating 'controlled' or 'stable' *opiate* use. These were amongst 54 located, admittedly with some difficulty, through newspaper advertising and by contacting community agencies and professionals. The patterns of drug use represented by these five were diverse, some confining use to weekends, two taking opiates more often, with some variability in two cases. In four of the cases it appears that present level of use represented a reduction from a previous level, and in two of the cases the reduction appeared to have been associated with getting married as was the case for a large number of Saunders and Kershaw's (1979) former problem drinkers. In at least one case opiates were admittedly being used to control tension associated with life stress, and in at least one other case drug use was prone to increase depending upon company. What united these people, however, was the apparent lack of major interference with their lives due to their current, relatively 'controlled' drug use.

There is much evidence, therefore, that people with excessive appetites can rid themselves of them without formal external assistance, or as some have termed it, 'spontaneously'. This term 'spontaneous remission' is really a misnomer of course. As Roizen *et al.* (1978) pointed out it is a term derived from medical practice to refer to changes that occurred apparently spontaneously or without clinical intervention. Thus, the assumption that conditions are involved which generally require treatment of some kind underlies the use of the word 'spontaneous' here. It is implied that what goes on in treatment is substantial and important, and that what occurs elsewhere is of secondary importance. Hence, any positive changes that occur without treatment are deemed 'spontaneous' and by implication therefore surprising and of unfathomable origin. The view towards which the studies of treatment and unaided quitting considered in this chapter lead, reverses these assumptions, as indeed does the whole model of excessive appetitive behaviour being developed here.

RELAPSE

A further line of work which is helpful in gaining understanding of what is happening when a person overcomes an excessive appetite is that on relapse following treatment. It is part of clinical experience that it is relatively easy to bring about a short-term change in eating, gambling, or drug-using behaviour. Maintaining cessation or reduction of behaviour is the problem. Many individuals who have struggled to control their own habitual behaviour can testify to the same. To quote Hunt and Matarazzo (1973)—'As the late W. C. Field observed about drinking, it is easy to stop. He had done it thousands of times!' (p.111). Those who have examined treatment research results report the same thing. For example, Litman (1976) concerning excessive drinking and Leventhal and Cleary (1980) for smoking have noticed the high rates of success produced during or immediately after treatment in comparison with the relatively modest rates of success recorded at follow-up.

Hunt and his colleagues (e.g. Hunt and Matarazzo, 1973; Hunt and Bespalec, 1974) have written a number of papers on the topic of relapse following treatment for drug problems, and these reports are important for at least two reasons. First, Hunt noticed that there were certain aspects of the relapse process which were similar for smoking, drinking problems, and heroin 'addiction'. Secondly, potentially important conclusions were drawn about the nature of the change process itself.

Hunt's observation was that the 'relapse curves' following treatment for one or other of these problems, or the 'cumulative survival curves' as they should more correctly be termed (Litman *et al.*, 1979b; Sutton, 1979), took similar negatively accelerated forms. These curves showed a rapid fall in the number of people remaining un-relapsed during the first few weeks after the termination of treatment, but showed a fairly abrupt break around 3–6 months after treatment after which the curve reached an asymptote around 25 per cent, this being the proportion of treated individuals who appeared to have made a longer-term change.

Hunt and his colleagues could well have included over-eating in their analysis, even though 'relapse' may appear to be harder to define in this case. Ley (1980) noted the high rates of relapse of the over-weight after treatment and acknowledged that the maintenance of weight losses was a major problem for treatment. His review suggested that overall about one patient in five would maintain a substantial weight loss for a year or more after treatment, an estimate remarkably similar to Hunt and colleagues' estimate of the number of excessive drinkers, smokers, and drug users who make changes that lasted for more than 3–6 months.

A number of criticisms can be made of Hunt's analysis. One concerns the limitations of their definition of relapse, namely any departure from total abstinence. When such a strict criterion is used, at least for former excessive drinkers (Vallance, 1965; Orford *et al.*, 1976), relapse does not stop after a few months leaving a substantial proportion unrelapsed, but rather continues until all individuals, with some very rare exceptions, have broken total abstinence. Nevertheless, Orford *et al.* (1976) were able to show that if a more reasonable and lenient criterion of relapse is adopted—we used a total accumulation of 10 problem drinking days as criterion—then approximately 25 per cent of our sample of male excessive drinkers remained 'unrelapsed' as long as 2 years after first consultation.

Litman *et al.* (1979b) and Sutton (1979) have criticized Hunt and his colleagues for placing too much emphasis on the shape of such curves when drawing conclusions about the process of relapse. Litman *et al.* pointed out that very similar negatively accelerated curves of this kind can be generated even when the ways in which the probability of survival changes in the months after treatment are very different. For example, they showed that if the probability of survival during the first month after treatment is 0.8 and *falls* to 0.5 in the twelfth month after treatment (i.e. if a person has survived unrelapsed for 11 months the probability of surviving one further month is 0.5), then the resulting relapse curve is very little different from the curve that results from an initial monthly survival probability of 0.6 which *rises* to 0.8 in the twelfth month. Both are negatively accelerated curves and look rather similar to those drawn by Hunt. Sutton (1979) made the additional point that such curves can be derived from many different kinds of data. For example, the survival of infants in the first four years of life (Sutton used the data for England and Wales for 1931) shows such a form. Sutton also pointed out that such curves are due to the operation of two very general processes, namely the progressive selection of individuals as time proceeds—once an individual has 'relapsed' then he/she does not enter into the calculations for later months which are thus based upon an increasingly selected sub-populaton—as well as the changing probability of survival with time. Since it is impossible to know how relatively important each of these processes is in any particular set of data, he argued that few conclusions about relapse processes can be drawn.

Litman *et al.* (1979b) made a major additional point, the force of which will be recognized by those who have undertaken treatment outcome research (e.g. Yates and Norris, 1981, who made a very similar critique of much outcome research). They used month-by-month follow-up data from our study (Orford *et al.*, 1976) to illustrate the point that group data mask individual differences in the course of behaviour following treatment. Hunt's analysis assumed that group data were sufficiently meaningful to be interpreted, and furthermore contained the assumption that relapse is a single discrete event which marks a clear transition from a pre-relapse state to a post-relapse state. Litman *et al.*'s reanalysis of our data showed how variable was the course of events for many individuals over a year's follow-up period with many individuals showing a relatively erratic course.

Despite these valid criticisms, Hunt's analyses of the relapse process have been valuable in pointing to the likely similarities in this respect between different forms of appetitive behaviour, and in generating valuable hypotheses about the change process. Litman *et al.*'s and Sutton's criticisms overlook two features of Hunt's observations. First, they thought they observed a quite abrupt turn in relapse curves after approximately 3–6 months. A related and second observation was that the curve descended rapidly at first 'as if' it would eventually reach zero but in fact levelled out to reach an asymptote around 25 per cent. Although similar in overall shape, these curves are thus quite unlike the infant survival curve drawn by Sutton (only a very small percentage of infants failed to survive) or the hypothetical curves drawn by Litman *et al.* which fall off to zero. Hunt and colleagues' interpretation of their relapse curves was that they represented two distinct processes, the first being a process of extinction or forgetting of the new learning that had taken place during treatment. This was responsible for the negatively accelerated form of the curve. They argued that because what was being dealt with was habitual behaviour, repeated in the past many times and thus 'over-learned', decay of what had been 'learnt' during treatment was often rapid and early relapse was frequent.

Hunt was concerned to account, in addition, for the fact that a substantial minority of formerly excessive drug users seemed to arrive, nevertheless, at a favourable resolution of their problem which surmounted this decay process and lasted for at least several months and possibly permanently. Indeed, the longer-term follow-up studies referred to above show that a sizeable minority of any group of people who admit to appetitive problems or who seek help on account of them make changes which are very long-lasting, measured in terms of years rather than months. It is this second process which is most intriguing and which the critiques of Hunt's work fail to address. The more interesting question is not why does relapse occur in the majority of cases, for what we know about the nature of strongly appetitive behaviour would lead us to expect relapse, but rather how do many individuals overcome the forces that lead most to relapse, and make dramatic changes in their behaviour? Hunt's guess was that what is operating is:

> . . . some kind of decision-making process or encoding, which isolates the response in question from the usual mechanisms of reinforcement and establishes the permanence of the behaviour outside the influence of reinforcement (Hunt and General, 1973, cited by Hunt and Bespalec, 1974 p.87).

Elsewhere, Hunt and Matarazzo (1973) cited H. F. Hunt (1968) as follows:

> People do become persuaded, do see themselves and others differently, do come to view the world in new ways, and so on. These ideas and insights may be thought of as verbal or symbolic responses, however covert, with consequences . . . that affect overt behaviours over a broad range . . . in a unitary fashion. . . . such that the change is hard to explain in terms of piecemeal, response-by-response alteration . . . In effect a new strategy appears to have been adopted, with the specific elements of the new behaviour representing tactical implementation of the strategy, as determined opportunistically by the present situation and by previous learning (Hunt and Matarazzo, p.113).

Thus, Hunt's formulation of change relies heavily upon cognitive, symbolic processes rather than upon notions of stimulus and response. The former are recognized to be of 'higher order' than the latter because they influence behaviour over a greater range of circumstances rather than in piecemeal fashion. These are processes that lend themselves to description in terms of expressions such as 'decision-making' and 'strategy'.

Once again there are clear parallels with excessive eating. Kingsley and Wilson (1977), for example, reported a study in which behaviour therapy produced good short-term results in terms of weight loss, but group methods (whether behavioural or not) resulted in the better maintenance. They drew a conclusion, not dissimilar to that drawn by Hunt and colleagues, namely that the process of losing weight and maintaining this gain is a two-stage process, the first requiring the mastering of techniques for losing weight, the second resting upon the 'commitment and motivation' necessary to go on applying those techniques for more than a few weeks beyond the period of treatment itself.

It is on the basis of concepts such as commitment, motivation, decision-making, and strategy that the most adequate explanation of our current knowledge about how people give up excessive appetitive behaviour can be offered. Such an explanation does a number of things which we should expect of it. It serves to unite knowledge about the different kinds of excessive behaviour which might otherwise be held distinct: to view the giving up of excessive drinking in terms of 'treatment' and the giving up of excessive smoking in terms of 'decision-making' is less helpful. It also unites clinical work carried out largely by professional clinicians working with patients in hospitals and clinics, with work done by epidemiologists and sociologists in the community. Finally, and possibly of most significance, it unifies our understanding of how excessive appetitive behaviour is taken up and given up in terms of one model of appetitive motivation. In the following chapter a decision-making model of giving up excess will be presented which suggests that the processes at work are in essence the same as those affecting the behaviour of the Jessors' students faced with choices about the extent of their involvement in a variety of appetitive acts.

DOES FORMAL TREATMENT WORK?

This will take us a long way from the clinical preoccupations of 'treatment', but before leaving the subject of treatment for excessive appetites we should look more critically, and in greater detail, at the question of whether treatment works at all. It is at least a tenable argument, on the basis of existing evidence, that to all intents and purposes treatment has negligible effect. Relapse rates following treatment are sufficiently high, and the rate of successful change without treatment is sufficiently great, that it is difficult to establish worthwhile differences between rates of positive change with treatment and without it (Orford and Edwards, 1977). This conclusion is reminiscent of an earlier debate about whether psychotherapy works for psychological problems in general. Spurred on by Eysenck's (1952) charge that it did not, a flurry of research activity was devoted to addressing this question which many have argued since is an absurdly over-simple one. Some (e.g. Bannister, 1975) have taken the view that it is illogical to question whether psychotherapy is effective or not; as a significant interpersonal experience it is bound to have some effect. The question is what effect it has, not whether there is an effect. Others (e.g. Bergin and Lambert, 1978) have suggested that this single question should be replaced by a set of questions, asking for Whom Psychotherapy does What under Which Conditions? To answer such a complex set of questions clearly requires a complex research response.

In research on treatment for excessive appetitive behaviour, we should be content with nothing less, and must be wary of drawing premature and over-simplified conclusions. Sorting out to what extent the outcome following treatment is due to the nature and intensity of that treatment, turns out to be a highly complex problem as recent studies of treatment outcome and excessive drinking have shown. Costello's (1980) analysis of 35 previously published reports is one of these. Such 'meta-analyses' have shortcomings and are controversial (Wilson, G., 1982) but Costello's analysis did suggest that extensity of treatment (three components: a co-ordinated complex of treatments available;

Antabuse available; a 'collateral' involved, such as family member, friend, pastor, employer, or probation officer) and vigorousness of follow-through (maintaining contact via regular telephone calls, home visits, reminders, homework assignments, provision of transport to aid participation in treatment, etc.) did make a difference to success rates (accounting between them for between 26 and 37 per cent of the variance in outcome rates depending upon whether shared influence due to correlation with client characteristics is included or not). Client social stability (marriage and employment) was far more influential, however (accounting for between 49 and 60 per cent of the variance).

One of the shortcomings of combining reports from different studies in the way Costello has done is that a unitary and undoubtedly over-simple criterion of success has to be employed. For one thing it is uncertain how much weight should be given to aspects of the appetitive behaviour itself in comparison with other aspects of psychological functioning or well-being. Not only has account now to be taken of the fact that some people appear to have a good outcome whilst continuing to drink, though more moderately than before (Pattison *et al.*, 1977), a fact which much complicates the issue in the case of drinking (the question has obviously always been a complex one in the case of sexual behaviour and eating), but there are also other and possibly more valid criteria altogether. Particularly if, as has been suggested, the hallmark of *excessive* appetitive behaviour is its interference with the individual's other needs or the needs of other people, then it may be more important to establish whether this harm or interference has lessened rather than to assess the details of the appetitive behaviour itself.

Some light is thrown on this, and other treatment evaluation issues, by a study of over 400 patients treated in one of five contrasting treatment programmes (a Salvation Army programme, a public hospital, a half-way house, a private programme using aversion therapy, and a private group and family therapy programme), analysed and reported in a series of papers by Moos and his colleagues. For example, Finney *et al.* (1980) reported the intercorrelations of six different outcome measures for a sub-sample of these clients for whom such measures were available at both 6 months and 2 years after treatment. In general, this analysis showed how very modest were the correlations between such outcome measures, and how much room this left for outcome to be favourable in one particular but not in another. For example, social functioning (participation in social, sports, cultural, and community activities) and occupational functioning (having worked at any time in the previous 6 months) were virtually independent of each other and of drinking outcome criteria.

Cronkite and Moos' (1978) analysis of data from the same study was also able to enlarge upon Costello's results by showing that the relative contributions of treatment and person being treated depended upon the outcome criterion. With alcohol consumption at follow-up as the criterion, programme type and treatment experiences together accounted for more of the explained variance in the criterion (38 per cent) than did social background and intake symptoms together (11 per cent). With each of the other outcome criteria, the latter two person variables accounted for over twice as much of the explained variance as did programme type and treatment experiences, and in the case of occupational functioning nearly five times as much. The matter is more complex still, however, on account of variance which cannot simply be attributed on the one hand to treatment, or on the other hand to the people entering it. Their data, like Costello's, demonstrated a large amount of variance shared between the two. They calculated that the combined contribution of social background and intake symptoms, counting the contributions that were unique to them as well as those shared with treatment variables, ranged from 12 to 61 per cent of the explained variance depending upon the criterion. In the case of the 'programme-related' variables the range was 16 to 62 per cent.

It does appear, however, that in their effort to be fair to treatment they may have over-stated the case by including the patients' *perception* of treatment as one of the 'programme-related' variables—the most influential one in fact. As Cronkite and Moos admit, a more favourable perception of treatment may reflect not only treatment quality but also the patient's motivation to recover, a more positive attitude toward the programme, better functioning within the programme, and a greater likelihood of participating in after-care.

Further complexity is added when we consider the range of people and problems for whom treatment has been prescribed and the possibility that to achieve greater success treatment needs to be tailored to suit the individual. A particular concern in the wider field of psychotherapy research has been the need for more homogeneous samples of clients (Bergin, 1971). Clients of psychotherapists are frequently extremely mixed, often covering between them a wide range of presenting problems and traditional psychiatric diagnoses. Indeed, it might be noted here that people with problems of excessive appetitive behaviour, such as excessive drinkers, drug-takers and gamblers, are often amongst the few types deliberately excluded, for the very sorts of reasons discussed in Chapter 11.

Even within the realm of one kind of excessive appetitive behaviour, the same comment is relevant. Glaser (1980), in particular, has proposed that the general negative findings in the treatment literature are due to a failure to appreciate, first, the differences, as opposed to the similarities, between people, and, second, the failure to match treatment and person. Indeed, a criticism voiced by several commentators (e.g. Tuchfeld, 1977; Hingson and Day, 1977) on our comparative study of 'treatment' and 'advice' for excessive drinkers and their wives (Edwards *et al.*, 1977; Orford and Edwards, 1977) was that we were unable to detect real differences that might have existed in outcome after these two contrasting approaches, because of the heterogeneity of our sample. As Glaser has put it:

> If the population being treated is in fact heterogenous, but is dealt with as if it were homogeneous, those variables which are critical for successful client–treatment interaction for both forms of intervention will tend to be uniformly distributed in the differing conditions of the experiment, and the results in each condition will be the same for that reason (Glaser, 1980, p.180).

Finally, there are two points to be made about treatment for excessive appetites which help to broaden out the picture and to put formal 'treatment' properly within the wider context of circumstances which aid personal change in behaviour. First there is the point that 'treatment' has often been viewed as a neat package as if it could be specified and applied in standard form by any competent therapist for many different clients (Athey and Coyne, 1979). There are a number of important respects in which this assumption is invalid in the case of psychological treatments. For one thing treatment techniques are rarely so well specified that they remain invariant: it is difficult to make certain that treatments are always given and 'taken' in the 'dosages' prescribed. In any case, psychological treatments are usually complex and we can rarely be certain which components are 'taken' and have impact. We know that patients frequently ignore their doctors' instructions to take particular drugs, or to take drugs in the dosages and at the frequencies prescribed (Ley *et al.*, 1976). Psychological treatments are more complex still and research reports rarely provide the detail necessary to know what really happened from the helper's perspective, let alone that of the client.

Neglect of the therapist variable, long recognized in psychotherapy research but remaining largely ignored in research on treatment for excessive appetites (Cartwright, 1981), is a further consequence of the assumption that treatment can be mechanically applied independently of personal qualities and preferences of the participants. It may be that some therapists are much more successful than others, independently of the type of programme or treatment techniques with which they are operating. Certainly some people are more interested in working with people with excessive appetites and specialize in this kind of work. Equally certainly there are many people in the helping professions who have relatively little experience of working with these groups of clients and who lack what Shaw *et al.* (1978) called 'role security' in working with them. On account of the nature of excessive appetitive behaviour, with its moral undertones and uncertain course and outcome, attitudes of potential helpers undoubtedly vary from those that are unsympathetic and rejecting to those that are more accepting, optimistic and sympathetic (Cartwright, 1980). Such attitudes seem likely candidates for discriminating more successful from less successful therapists in working with those with excessive appetitive behaviour. Whether it is possible to identify other differentiating characteristics *within* a sample of helpers equally sympathetic and committed to working in this area remains an interesting question. Edwards (1974b) has posed a number of questions, or dilemmas, for the intending therapist. He was writing about excessive drinking and its treatment, but his remarks could apply with equal force to any variety of excessive appetitive behaviour. Two of these questions are particularly pertinent, and arise from the very nature of excessive behaviour itself which invites attention, criticism and attempts at persuasion. He asked:

> What is the relative balance of attention which the professional is going to give (and expect his client to give), to the client's drinking

> problem as opposed to other aspects of that person's life? Leaning too far in one direction, the social worker then becomes so alcohol focussed as to miss the fact that an actual and whole human being is sitting in front of him, while in the other direction mistakes happen when this or that consequence of the drinking is patched up and the destructive importance of the underlying drinking is somehow forgotten. . . .
>
> What is to be the balance between the judgemental and the non-judgemental? If the helping person sets himself up in the role of moral judge, as the re-incarnation indeed of the most frowning sort of magistrate, not much therapeutic work is likely to be done. But to seek to portray the professional's role as that of a persistently indulgent parent whose child/patient can do no wrong, is equally anti-therapeutic (p.92).

It simply is not known whether there is a best answer to these questions, and whether some helpers consistently manage to strike the best balance between behaviour-focused and non-focused work, and between confrontation and non-directiveness, and thus consistently produce better results. The clinician's guess is likely to be that it depends upon the client, the circumstances, and the abilities and inclinations of the helper, and that there is no consistently 'right' approach.

The second and even more salient point on which to close this chapter is that expert treatment, the detailed examination of which has attracted an amount of research attention out of all proportion to its importance, is directed at people who are at the same time being influenced by a host of factors quite beyond the control of those responsible for treatment. Many of these factors, 'extraneous' when viewed from the treatment perspective, operate more intensively, for far longer, and hence seem likely to be by far the more influential. A point about the treatment studies that is easily missed is that the amount of outcome variance which can be explained at all is usually quite small. In the Cronkite and Moos study, for example, this proportion varied from 18 to 27 per cent depending upon outcome criterion. Although it is rarely done, some advance on these figures may be made by assessing the extent and quality of clients' environmental resources in the period during and following treatment. Bromet and Moos (1977) found not only that being married and having a job conferred a favourable prognosis, thus confirming some of the results of 'spontaneous' remission studies like Saunders and Kershaw's (1979), but furthermore that when such resources existed the perceived quality of these environments had predictive significance. The lower the degree of marital conflict, and, for unmarried clients, the greater the degree of job commitment and peer cohesion at work, the better the outcome for the drinking problem. The study of 'treatment' versus 'advice' produced a very similar finding, namely that higher levels of marital cohesion predicted a better outcome (Orford *et al.*, 1976). Clients who did well tended to attribute their success to improvements in their marriage or job circumstances, rather than to advice or treatment received (Orford and Edwards, 1977).

Once again, however, the complexity of the matter needs to be stressed:

> . . . the causal relationships . . . are likely to be dynamic and reciprocal, rather than simple and unidirectional . . . individual functioning . . . often fluctuates over time and may be associated with variation in social environment and other post-treatment factors through complex, reciprocal processes.
> . . . traditional input–program–outcome modes of . . . treatment and program evaluation are inadequate. Therapeutic efforts must go beyond the patient to deal with the contexts in which the patient functions after treatment . . . Similarly, evaluation research paradigms need to be expanded to include assessment of the multiple settings in which patients are located after treatment . . . (Finney *et al.*, 1980).

Even this catholic statement, however, relegates the extra-treatment world to the position of something that happens *after* treatment, something that has to be taken into account the better to understand how treatment has its effect. In Chapter 13 the argument will be pursued that the boot is really on the other foot: it is the individual's day-to-day world and the decisions he or she takes to accommodate to it or to change it that are primary, and it is within that framework that expert treatment plays its modest part.

CHAPTER THIRTEEN

Decisions and Self-control

> Like Lewin, we see man . . . not as a rational calculator always ready to work out the best solution, but as a reluctant decision maker—beset by conflict, doubts, and worry, struggling with incongruous longings, antipathies, and loyalties, and seeking relief by procrastinating, or denying responsibility for his own choices (Janis and Mann, 1977, p.15).

> . . . in the acquisition of a new habit, or the leaving off of an old one, we must take care to *launch ourselves with as strong and decided initiative as possible*. Accumulate all the possible circumstances which shall re-enforce the right motives; put yourself assiduously in conditions that encourage the new way; make engagements incompatible with the old; take a public pledge, if the case allows; in short, envelope your resolution with every aid you know . . . (Professor Bain on *Moral Habits*, quoted by William James, 1891, p.122).

Drug-taking, drinking, gambling, eating, and sex all have the capacity to beget both pleasure and pain, fulfilment and harm. Accordingly, most societies have been at least ambivalent towards these activities and have been at pains to control them and to instil conformity to moderate, discriminating indulgence in them. Each individual person is heir to that ambivalence and continually faces a set of choices about the extent of his appetitive activity, although the weight of formal and informal pressures for and against greater or lesser indulgence may be so constraining that most people may not be aware most of the time that they are 'choosing' at all. If, however, because of the circumstances that pertain at certain stages of a person's life, because of the functions that appetitive behaviour serves at those stages, and because of developmental processes of learning and biological adaptation, behaviour exceeds the limits of what is considered normal, sensible, or harmless, then the need to make a rational choice may become more salient. Paradoxically, of course, choice has then probably become more difficult.

In Chapter 11 it was argued that much of the behaviour of a person who experiences an *excessive* appetite can be understood as being a reflection of intensified conflict. Such a person shares the general ambivalence that people feel towards appetitive behaviour but experiences it to a heightened extent as a result of her increased attachment to it and the increased harm that it is causing her. This conflict, it was suggested, could be depicted in the form of a 'balance sheet' of pros and cons, of the type Janis and Mann (1968) drew for a hypothetical smoker facing a decision about his future smoking. It is part of the natural history, the argument continued, that people with excessive appetites should at some stage become aware of the need for change, or should at least be coerced by others into considering it. We should expect change towards reduced involvement to occur as part of the natural course of events. In Chapter 12, some work was then reviewed which supports that expectation. One way to read the research evidence is to conclude that a great deal of change takes place outside of formal treatment, and that the latter, although probably effective to a modest degree, constitutes only a small part of the picture. Understandably, in view of what we know of excessive appetites, relapse rates are high immediately following treatment. Impressive, however, is the fact that a substantial minority of people do make drastic changes towards reduced appetitive behaviour either following expert treatment or without it. The purpose of the present chapter is to propose a way to understand these changes.

CHANGE AS DECISION-MAKING

It is tempting to construe such changes in the language of decision-making. It seems intuitively correct to speak of someone with a strong appetite as facing a difficult 'decision'. Certainly the pay-off matrix and balance sheet formulations of conflict lend themselves to this construction. According to this view the individual faces a choice between behavioural options. The choice is a particularly difficult one, because good intentions are opposed by an attachment which may have grown to considerable strength and which the person may not understand. Like other major life choices and decisions, however, it is one for which the individual is responsible and it will be made personally. Equally, however, like most choices, it will be made with the help, encouragement, and manipulation of the most influential other people in a person's life.

It is interesting to note that this language comes readily to mind when speaking of smoking and eating (the decision to quit smoking or the decision to diet), but is less familiar in the context of 'alcoholism', 'drug addiction', 'compulsive gambling', or sexual 'manias' such as 'nymphomania'. The latter constructions on behaviour are themselves products of a process of medicalizing behaviour, a process that inevitably shifts the emphasis away from personal responsibility for decision-making and towards the acceptance of the existence of a disease or illness condition which requires treatment. However, just as there is evidence (pp.212–214) that the adoption of a medical view of excessive behaviour does not remove stigma and is not incompatible with holding simultaneously the view that a person is responsible for his or her own behaviour, so this chapter will review some evidence that medical and other forms of professional treatment for excessive appetitive behaviour are conducted partly, and sometimes largely, within a framework of personal responsibility and decision-making.

That successful change in appetitive behaviour is associated with some kind of higher-order mental process of this kind has been suggested by a number of writers including Hunt and his colleagues (e.g. Hunt and Matarazzo, 1973) who investigated relapse curves. The model of the change process which I have advocated (Orford, 1976; 1980) speaks of the making of decisions on the basis of an appraisal of the type of balance sheet or pay-off matrix proposed by Janis and Mann (1968). It assumes that the motivation for change derives from an accumulation of 'losses', 'costs', or harm resulting from behaviour, and that these have accumulated to the point at which they exceed 'gains', benefits, or pleasurable outcomes of appetitive behaviour to such a degree that the conflict between the desire to continue with the appetitive behaviour on the one hand, and other needs (to be a bread-winner, to be a family person, to enjoy life, to have a clear conscience, to have friends, to have self-respect, etc.) on the other hand, cannot be resolved by the defence mechanisms which have served up to that time. This is the core of the proposal, although it may be supposed that some crisis or triggering events in a person's life may be necessary in addition to dissatisfaction with the behavioural balance sheet, before change takes place (Orford, 1980).

Motivated by the unhealthy state of the balance sheet, and prompted by some crisis event, the individual becomes sensitized, so the model supposes, to the possibility of new solutions. Although some possible solutions to such behavioural dilemmas may be suggested by experts, such as mental health professionals or self-help groups, there seems no particular reason to suppose that these have any monopoly upon advice that may be useful under such circumstances. It is not so much that change may be 'spontaneous', but rather that sensitized to the need for change, an individual may receive advice or encouragement from any one or more than one of a variety of sources, or indeed may 'come to his senses' as a result of his or her own appraisal of the state of affairs:

> One way or another, with professional help or without, with friendly advice from uncle or neighbour or without it, with constant nagging from wife or husband or without it, the individual, sensitized to the need for a new solution, makes a decision. . . . Perhaps one could go so far as to argue that there is no such thing as 'treatment' as such, . . . [for excessive appetitive behaviour problems] . . . merely the possibility of advice or encouragement (Orford, 1980, pp.156, 158).

A very similar scheme for understanding change in drinking problems has been proposed by Armor *et al.* (1978) in the controversial Rand Report,

Alcoholism and Treatment, which summarized the results of a large evaluation study of the National Institute of Alcohol Abuse and Alcoholism treatment centres in the United States. They found, as have others, that successful change was not strongly related to the amount of treatment received, nor was it easily predictable on the basis of the kinds of social and psychological client variables which they examined:

> We suggest that [recovery] has to do with individual factors, among which individual decision making might be especially prominent. Decision making, in this sense, refers to what is probably a highly complex cognitive process involving at least three components: (1) experience of the 'costs' of alcoholism that outweigh short-run reasons for drinking; (2) a breakdown of psychological defenses (e.g. denial) enabling a recognition of the problem; and (3) a commitment to change (p.138).

The model of appetitive behaviour change developed and elaborated by Janis and his colleagues (Janis and Mann, 1968, 1977; Janis and Rodin, 1979) is also one of decision-making. In the earliest of these works, a five-stage decision process was posited through which it was suggested a heavy smoker might pass having decided to stop smoking after having been exposed to anti-smoking publicity (see Table 9). This scheme is very similar to Horn's (1972) discussed earlier, but places more emphasis on the existence of a specific recommendation for new behaviour, and the individual's evaluation of it and subsequent commitment to it. Again there is no suggestion here that the source of the recommendation need be expert or professional, although it may come from a prestigeful source such as a general medical practitioner (Russell *et al.*, 1979) or the Surgeon General's Report on Smoking and Lung Cancer.

In their 1977 book entitled *Decision-making: a Psychological Analysis of Conflict, Choice and Commitment* (as well as in the more recent chapter by Janis and Rodin), Janis and Mann have included decisions about behaviour such as smoking and drinking along with a whole range of important but difficult life decisions such as personal decisions about job moves, housing, marriage, and divorce, as well as political and executive decisions, and responses to warnings about impending disaster such as earthquakes, floods, or air-raids. In this later work, 'recommendations' have been broadened to include all relevant 'communications'—personal or mass media—and also significant 'events'. This recognition that a variety of everyday happenings may provide the stimulus for reconsidering behaviour makes it doubly clear that change is to be expected both with and without the intervention of experts.

Such decisions as those affecting smoking and drinking are included in a sub-class of decisions concerning the restoration of health and the avoidance of illness. Many such decisions involve, they argued, 'loss'. Examples include the physical discomfort of orthopaedic exercises, the side-effects of medicines, and the risks and discomforts of surgery. The greater the loss involved the greater

Table 9 The five stages in making a decision to adhere to a recommended policy (reproduced by permission of Rand McNally & Company, copyright holder)

Components of attitude change	Initial Attitude of Complacency	Stage 1 Positive Appraisal of Danger	Stage 2 Positive Appraisal of recommendation (R)	Stage 3 Selection of R as the best alternative	Stage 4 Commitment to decision to adopt R	Stage 5 Adherence to R despite negative attack
Overt behaviour						
1. Acts in accordance with R following major challenges to the new attitude?	No	No	No	No	(?)	Yes
2. Acts in accordance with R under normal circumstances?	No	No	No	No	Yes	Yes
Verbal evaluation of R						
3. Feels willing to act in accordance with R?	No	No	No	No	Yes	Yes
4. Believes R is best available means?	No	No	No	Yes	Yes	Yes
5. Believes R is a satisfactory means worth considering?	No	No	Yes	Yes	Yes	Yes
6. Accepts assertions that R is an effective means?	No	No	Yes	Yes	Yes	Yes
Verbal evaluation of threat						
7. Believes the threat is serious?	No	Yes	Yes	Yes	Yes	Yes
8. Accepts assertions that the threat is serious?	No	Yes	Yes	Yes	Yes	Yes

the conflict about taking health-promoting or illness-avoiding decisions. This wider perspective is helpful in considering the sort of decisions about excessive appetitive behaviour with which we are concerned here. If the social learning theory, pay-off matrix, or balance sheet perspective is at all apposite, and if the notion of conflict as crucial for an understanding of excess is at all accurate, then it follows that any inclination to reduce or control or abstain from appetitive behaviour will be opposed by the positive incentives for continuing with behaviour as before. The incentives for taking up appetitive behaviour which were considered in Chapters 7 and 8 have become the *dis*incentives for change, although this is true only in a general sense because the particular motives for drug use, eating, gambling, or sexual behaviour which pertained at the time of initial use may have changed markedly in the months, years, or even decades that have elapsed between initial use and a time of potential decision to reduce or abstain.

Janis and Mann's model of general decision-making contains, then, the idea of dilemma or conflict, the vital ingredient for a theory of excessive behaviour, and one which is missing from disease and other previous formulations. Another benefit which it was anticipated would accrue from viewing excessive appetitive behaviour and its change from the wider perspective of general decision-making was that it would help put the type of behaviour change required of someone who has developed an extremely excessive and troublesome appetite on a continuum with the type of decision faced by someone who is told that their present behaviour (smoking, excessive fat consumption, casual sexual behaviour, etc.) runs certain risks for *future* harm. Typically these have been seen in the past as involving quite separate processes: the latter a question of personal decision-making subject to the influence of mass media health education campaigns, and the former a question of engagement in 'treatment' in a clinical setting. Viewing these behavioural dilemmas as varieties of the same kind of decision or problem enables us to consider the possibility that 'early' decisions—i.e. decisions taken relatively early in life, relatively early on in an individual's appetitive 'career', or at a time when behaviour has produced relatively few or relatively slight harmful consequences—are no different in kind from relatively 'late' decisions. The difference in terms of the present model lies in the degree of conflict, or more precisely the 'height' of approach and avoidance gradients at their point of intersection—to use the language of approach–avoidance conflict introduced in Chapter 11. 'Early' decisions may be 'taken lightly', whilst 'late' decisions may be 'a matter of life or death', but our basic understanding of the processes involved may be the same.

Janis and Mann's stage model concerns reactions to one communication or event, and the time-scale of the processes suggested may be relatively short—a matter of weeks or months at most. However, if early and late decisions are to be considered as qualitatively similar within the same model, their scheme may be extended by hypothesizing the kind of appetitive career shown in Figure 11. The career consists of a number of *choice points,* which are the times when decisions to alter the course of appetitive behaviour are particularly likely to be taken. Perhaps these are times when the individual is presented with evidence that behaviour is harmful (a court sentence or the discovery of organ damage for example), times when life circumstances change and former behaviour may not be as appropriate as before (e.g. marriage or the birth of a child), times when specific recommendations are made by others (e.g. a girlfriend points out how unattractive smoking is or a work colleague gives a straight talk), or just times when there is contemplation on the course of life (e.g. a special holiday or a period in hospital.)

Armor *et al.* (1978) presented a very similar career or multi-stage model of the development and change of excessive drinking, and such a scheme also has affinities with stage models of the development and remission of drug-taking discussed in Chapter 7 (e.g. Kandel, 1978; Robins *et al.*, 1977). One of the

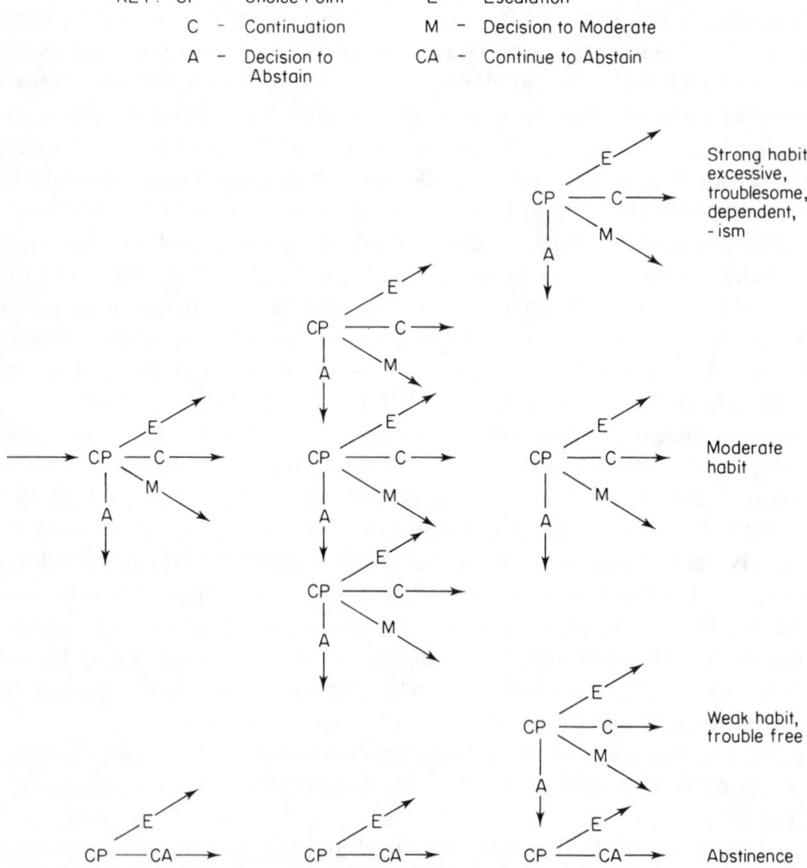

Figure 11 The appetitive career as a series of choice points.

implications of adopting such a view is that chronic excess is to be seen not as the inevitable result of a progressive disease process, but rather as the end-result of a succession of wrong or failed decisions. Hence, a dissonant smoker is someone who has not only developed a strong appetite for smoking, but is also someone who has not yet reacted to the dissonance involved by becoming an ex-smoker or by making a drastic reduction in consumption. This leads to one important conclusion, stated earlier but worth repeating, namely that prediction of whose behaviour will ultimately become so excessive that they seek help on account of it cannot be expected at the outset of a career. The model is not one of the unfolding of a process which was latent from the beginning and which could be predicted on the basis of personality or social factors, but rather one of uncertain movements upwards and downwards with the ever-present, although perhaps diminishing, possibility of removing oneself from the group at risk by making a decision to drastically reduce or perhaps abstain from use or activity.

Janis and Mann (1977) acknowledged that the first of their stages, in particular the necessary initial reappraisal, might occur slowly and gradually over a very long period of time—the 'slow burn' type of chronic reappraisal as they call it. Furthermore, by no means all decision-makers proceed smoothly through all five stages in the approved sequence, once stage one has occurred, according to Janis and Mann. A variety of reversions and feedback loops occur in their experience, and they commented that smokers and dieters in particular often seem to go through stages one and two and then back to the start, repeatedly, in a series of 'short-circuited decision loops'. Janis and Mann seem here to have observed about the excessive appetites something akin to Hunt and Matarazzo's finding of high relapse rates for the 'addictions' after treatment, which the latter writers interpreted in terms of the extinction of new learning in the absence of firm decision-making.

Horn's (1972) view also, based on his study of cigarette smokers over a four-year period and other studies, was that the cessation of smoking was best considered not as a single event but rather as a process continuing over a period of time. Thus, if Horn's idea of the process was one of decision-making, it too was certainly not a simple one. A further element in his theory of the change process was the inclusion of the prevailing social climate as one of the major influences inhibiting or facilitating change, alongside other factors such as family, friends, co-workers, and television. His views on this subject are remarkably like Ledermann's (1956) *boule de neige* theory of the uptake and spread of drinking customs in society:

> . . . change takes place in society largely through an interactive process whereby for reasons of self-interest the individual or large numbers of individuals begin to change . . . this in itself affects institutions, and these changes then become institutionalized either through social custom or by the way of government regulation or legislation. As the change becomes institutionalized in a society it

> moves back and affects the people who are in that society so that there is a continuing process of interaction between the individualized change and the institutionalization of that change which in turn helps to create more individual change. This is how things grow and this is why changes tend to continue (p.67).

That individual change takes place in the context of a society where attitudes and customs are not static was apparent to Horn for smoking, but this fact can be easily neglected, and usually is, in discussions of changes in drinking, gambling, and other forms of drug-taking which are almost always dealt with on a purely individual level. In a sense Janis and Mann's model concerns the way individuals react to society's formal and informal attempts to control appetitive behaviour.

Of the different ways of responding to public health messages or warnings or other communications or events which forced a reappraisal, it was 'vigilance' which Janis and Mann (1977) considered mostly resulted in the best decisions. This involved searching for relevant information and objectively appraising alternatives before making a choice, and it occurred when an individual was aware of the risks involved in behaviour, was hopeful of finding a better solution, and believed there was time to search for the best solution. They recommended the full completion of a balance sheet as a pre-decisional exercise encouraging vigilance. This required that the decision-maker explored and made explicit four types of consequence: utilitarian gains and losses for self; utilitarian gains and losses for significant others; self-approval or disapproval; and approval or disapproval from significant others. They stressed that even in business decisions, ethical or non-utilitarian considerations were nearly always relevant, including questions of pride and shame, self-esteem, or whether a decision was consistent with living up to one's ideals or involved letting oneself down. Their prediction was that decision-making would be least successful, and would be most likely to lead to decisions that were later regretted, when the balance sheet was defective by containing 'gaps', unacknowledged and unpredicted consequences that were not fully taken into account when making the decision.

Janis and Mann provided the following quotation from Benjamin Franklin, writing to the scientist Joseph Priestley in 1772, in support of their balance sheet procedure:

> When those difficult cases occur, they are difficult, chiefly because while we have them under consideration, all the reasons pro and con are not present to the mind at the same time; but sometimes one set present themselves, and at other times another, the first being out of sight. Hence the various purposes or inclinations that alternatively prevail, and the uncertainty that perplexes us. To get over this, my way is to divide half a sheet of paper by a line into two columns; writing over the one Pro, and over the other Con. Then, during three or four days consideration, I put down under the different heads short hints of the different motives, that at

> different times occur to me, for or against the measure. When I have thus got them all together in one view, I endeavor to estimate their respective weights; and where I find two, one on each side, that seem equal, I strike them both out. If I find a reason pro equal to some two reasons con, I strike out the three. If I judge some two reasons con, equal to some three reasons pro, I strike out the five; and thus proceeding I find at length where the balance lies; and if, after a day or two of further consideration, nothing new that is of importance occurs on either side, I come to a determination accordingly. And, though the weight of reasons cannot be taken with the precision of algebraic quantities, yet when each is thus considered, separately and comparatively, and the whole lies before me, I think I can judge better, and am less liable to make a rash step, and in fact I have found great advantage from this kind of equation, in what may be called moral or prudential algebra (1977, p.149).

Once again we are reminded that the procedures 'invented' by modern psychology to help people control their excessive appetites are usually tapping naturally occurring remedies and types of advice which appear in disguised, or in this case undisguised, form without its help.

A limitation of the balance sheet approach is that it assumes that all sources of motive, both for and against appetitive behaviour, can be made public and cast in the form of statements which suggest understandable, even reasonable, motives. This may not always be the case, particularly in that part of the balance sheet concerned with positive motives for continuing with excessive behaviour. Habit may be based very largely upon processes that operate beyond full awareness. Indeed, in a sense the main argument of much of this book is that the disease-like quality of habitual excessive behaviour is due to circumstances which allow the flourishing of strong attachment-forming processes, which in some cases are more than a match for forces of restraint, although the latter may appear much the more reasonable and may be much more easily listed in the form of words.

Janis and Mann also described a number of methods for counteracting cognitive defences, however. One of these, the 'awareness of rationalizations' technique, involved studying lists of common rationalizations and considering carefully which applied to the self. A second, 'emotional role-playing' involved emotional rather than cognitive confrontation of defences. In experiments conducted by Janis and Mann themselves, smokers were asked to role-play a number of scenes in which they were informed that they had cancer as a result of smoking, and were prepared for surgery. Janis and Mann report that these exercises aroused considerable feeling on the part of the participants.

CHANGE AS PROBLEM-SOLVING

Another rich source of ideas about appetitive behaviour decisions is a paper by D'Zurilla and Goldfried (1971) under the title, 'Problem Solving and

Behavior Modification'. Although not directly concerned with appetitive decisions, it outlines a treatment approach which the authors advocated be used in helping people who are having difficulty solving life problems or making significant life decisions. There are clear parallels between the process they advocated and the model espoused by Janis and his colleagues. They defined problem-solving as:

> . . . a behavioral process whether overt or cognitive in nature, which (a) makes available a variety of potentially effective response alternatives for dealing with the problematic situation and (b) increases the probability of selecting the most effective response from amongst these various alternatives (p.108).

A first major assumption is that a broad social learning approach can be used to understand many kinds of 'performance deficit'. This framework supposes, they stated, that an individual must engage in trial-and-error behaviour, receive prompting or social reinforcement from others, or be influenced by behaviour models of other people in order to adopt more effective ways of acting. However:

> . . . it is at this point that most social-learning theorists fail to consider the possibility that an individual may learn an effective response to at least some problematic situations on his own without having to engage in overt trial-and-error behavior, receive guidance, or observe an effective model. We are referring to the possibility that the individual might be able to 'figure out' what he should do in these situations (p.110).

The second, and much more questionable, assumption is that people might be helped by training in general problem-solving skills. From their perusal of relevant literature, D'Zurilla and Goldfried outlined five stages in problem-solving which they considered should form the basic curriculum for such a training course. The first stage involved adopting an appropriate general orientation or 'set'. Successful problem-solving was encouraged, they stated, if there was acceptance of the fact that problematic situations constituted a normal facet of life and that it was possible to cope with them, if there was recognition of problematic situations when they occurred, and inhibition of the tendency to respond on first impulse or else to do nothing. Interestingly, these latter two tendencies correspond to two of Janis and Mann's less-than-ideal coping patterns, namely 'hypervigilance' (involving frantic searching and settling for a solution without due consideration) and 'unconflicted persistence'.

The second stage concerned clear problem definition and formulation. Amongst the ways of formulating commonly encountered problems, they listed as one kind issues involving conflict or dissonance between two or more seemingly incompatible goals, which clearly matches closely the model of appetitive behaviour problems developed here.

At the third stage—generation of alternatives—D'Zurilla and Goldfried recommended borrowing ideas from 'brainstorming', a procedure developed in the 1930s for facilitating the discovery of new ideas in groups. The rules of successful brainstorming include the suspension of criticism at the idea-generating stage, the encouragement of ideas which appear wild at first sight, the generation of a relatively large number of possible solutions, and the encouragement of combinations and improvements.

The fourth stage was the decision-making stage itself, at which the likely consequences of alternative solutions were considered, the alternatives weighed against one another, and one solution decided upon. The process outlined by D'Zurilla and Goldfried was completed by the verification stage at which the alternative decided upon at the decision-making stage was tested for its adequacy in practice.

Others who have advocated an understanding of change in terms of decision-making processes include Mausner (1973) and Broadhurst (1976), and those who have devised treatment programmes with rationales similar to that of D'Zurilla and Goldfried, but for people with excessive appetites, include Toomey (1972) for excessive drinkers and Colten and Janis (1978) for dieters.

As D'Zurilla and Goldfried admitted, we know very little about what really happens during this crucial stage of the problem-solving process. Indeed, it is an assumption in the present state of our knowledge that such a stage model best fits the human problem-solving process, where health and social behaviour decisions are concerned, and that decision-making is to be viewed as a separate stage within that process. Ideas about decision-making in psychology have relied heavily, and probably far too heavily, upon utility theory designed to describe mathematically the process of choice in economics and games. Although Edwards (1961) extended this thinking to realms in which no mathematically precise utility could be ascribed to a particular choice, but rather where utility was the product of the *subjective* estimate of the probability that an alternative would achieve a given outcome, and the *subjective* value of that outcome ($u = p \times v$ as the basis for the subjective expected utility model of human choice), it remains true that such models of decision-making focus, '. . . more on what an individual might do to improve his decision-making ability, rather than describing what he actually does in practice' (D'Zurilla and Goldfried, 1971, p.119).

Although Mausner (1973) was an advocate of a decision model of appetitive behaviour, in this case smoking change, he admitted that the process was less like the neatly shaped 'decision tree' of the theorists and more like a messy bush! It would be hard, he suggested, to describe the branches leading up to a presumed moment of decision, added to which the 'decision' might have to be remade on many occasions when the ex-smoker was faced with temptation. Nevertheless, he believed that it would be wrong to abandon decision models such as subjective expected utility (SEU) altogether:

> . . . we should not underestimate the frequency of moments of crisis in which a quantal change in subjective expected utility leads to an event in the head which we may label a 'decision to stop smoking' (p.118).

Indeed, Mausner presented evidence that a reduction in smoking (subjects were volunteers and very few stopped altogether) in a role-playing anti-smoking experiment was related to the expected utility of stopping. As in an earlier experiment (Mausner and Platt, 1971), what discriminated the reducers from the non-reducers was the reducers' markedly higher subjective expected utility for *stopping*, although the expected utility for continuing showed no difference. It appears to have been the increased expectation of benefits from stopping that aided change rather than the heightened fear of consequences. Expected improvements in health, and the expectation that there would be little difficulty in handling tension were particularly predictive. Subjects who did not predict an improvement in health and who expected difficulty in handling tension if they stopped smoking, tended not to reduce.

The failure of a quantitative SEU theory to make better predictions of smoking change need not, in this writer's view, invalidate a general decision-making model. It seems extremely unlikely that such an attempt at precision and quantification could meet with more than very limited success in practice. Even if a person has full knowledge of the benefits and losses likely to accrue from different resolutions of conflict, and even if it could be assumed that values and probabilities remain sufficiently constant to be given numbers, the task of listing and assigning numbers seems daunting. Certainly the SEU method of calculating the relative utilities of different behavioural options for a person makes a number of possibly unwarranted assumptions. For one thing it assumes a linear relationship between the perceived probability of an outcome and utility. It seems reasonable to suppose that certain outcomes (100 per cent probable) may have much more than twice the influence of outcomes with a 50 per cent probability, for example. A further assumption is that probability × value products should be added across a large number of possible outcomes in order to arrive at the best estimate of SEU for that alternative. It might however be possible, with less precision, to make predictions about *groups* of people in different circumstances.

Apart from these considerations, the Mausner and Platt model omitted a number of factors which appear to take on much importance in individual cases. For example, change decisions to do with drug use may be much influenced by the perceived likelihood of a change attempt being carried out successfully (Eiser *et al.*, 1978). This 'confidence' factor could be particularly important when an individual has previous experience of unsuccessful attempts to give up or cut down. Another factor which Eiser *et al.* suggested should be included in a more detailed model of decision-making relevant to the decision to quit smoking was the current availability of energy resources for an attempt at change. Although advice to stop smoking, and an appraisal of alternatives, may motivate an individual to want to give up smoking, consideration of a decision may be postponed until such time as there is less pressure from other activities or until such time as the person is under less stress of a personal or emotional nature. Although these additions to the model go some way towards dealing with the criticism that utility models assume rationality and the availability of perfect information (Tedeschi, 1972), it seems unlikely that such attempts at precise prediction will meet with much success.

The process of generating a range of *alternative* solutions to a problem is one that is highlighted by those who have written of the advantages of 'brainstorming', and it therefore figures large within the problem-solving approach recommended by D'Zurilla and Goldfried and others. It is interesting to consider in this light the demand for total abstinence which has been the cornerstone of self-help (Alcoholics Anonymous, Gamblers Anonymous), and clinical treatment approaches in recent times, especially when the object of behavioural excess has been alcohol or gambling activity. The requirement that a person with a drinking or gambling problem acknowledge themselves to be 'an alcoholic' or a 'compulsive gambler', and that they then submit themselves to the necessity for total abstinence, may be thought of as the very antithesis of brainstorming. The process is one of closure upon a single solution rather than the opening up of a range of possibilities for consideration. If there is validity in the view that individuals with such problems are best advised to pursue the abstinence solution, and flirt with other possibilities only to their own cost, then it has to be acknowledged that the general problem-solving approach to these kinds of problems is found wanting, at least in this most important respect.

That abstinence as a *universal* requirement for people with serious drinking problems has been challenged in the last ten or twenty years is now fairly common knowledge. This field of work has now been reviewed a number of times, for example by Heather and Robertson (1983) who found, from a survey of treatment centres in Britain, that the majority now offer help towards controlled drinking for at least some of their problem drinking clients.

In decision-making terms, the opening up of alternatives other than total abstinence makes available to an individual who is troubled by excessive appetitive behaviour a whole range of options for future behaviour. Janis and Mann's (1968) hypothetical balance sheet for a smoker (see Table 8) showed four options each representing a different behavioural choice: continuing as before, giving up altogether, switching from non-filter to filter cigarettes, and cutting down from one packet to half a packet a day. Thus, it was immediately made clear that abstinence was not the sole solution for this hypothetical smoker. Although this example was hypothetical, since that time there have been a number of suggestions as well as examples of actual clinical practice involving alternative forms of controlled smoking other than total quitting. For example, Russell (1974) has suggested that 'safer smoking' should be the goal for many people who find it impossible to abstain. Accordingly, he campaigned, successfully as it turned out, for the compulsory declaration of levels of tar in different brands of cigarette. Although it may be argued that switching to lower tar cigarettes leaves quite untouched the appetite for the activity of smoking, or for the constituent nicotine, it does make available alternative courses of action for the smoker.

More closely related to the controlled drinking development is the work of Frederiksen *et al.* (1976). They have suggested that changes can be brought about in at least three separate components of smoking behaviour. First, the substance can be modified, for example by switching to a low tar or low nicotine cigarette, or changing to a different mode of smoking such as pipe or cigar. Secondly, smoking rate can be modified, for example by reducing the number of cigarettes, pipes, or cigars consumed per day or per week. Thirdly, changes may be brought about in smoking 'topography': for example, the amount of time spent smoking a single cigarette, the number of puffs taken, or the length or depth of puffs, can all be modified. Health risks may be reduced by any one of these modifications, they argued. They reported some success in practice in achieving such 'controlled smoking' changes. Although others (e.g. Paxton, 1980) believe such successes to be no greater than those achieved by more conventional treatments, and believe on health grounds that the aim must always be abstinence from smoking, the important point here again is the one about behavioural options. Although the majority of clinicians who advise smokers may have a goal of total abstinence in mind, in practice it seems likely that most changes in smoking behaviour take place outside formal treatment, and that smokers consider the matter as one of problem-solving or decision-making and, at least early in the change process, entertain a number of options.

It was pointed out in Chapter 3 that the development of ideas about so-called 'compulsive gambing' have taken directions remarkably similar to those in the area of 'alcoholism', although they have lagged behind the latter by at least a decade or two. One crucial point of similarity has been the insistence of Gamblers Anonymous, as of Alcoholics Anonymous, and of clinicians who have treated excessive gambling, as of those who have treated 'alcoholism', that total abstinence is the only safe goal. The fact that abstinence as a goal following the development of an excessive appetite for gambling should have received less challenge than the abstinence-only view of treatment for excessive drinking (a drug as opposed to a non-drug appetite) may seem paradoxical. This is probably to be explained, however, in terms of the relative recency of interest in excessive gambling and the relative scarcity of treatment for it. As might be expected, however, reports of treatment aimed at 'controlled gambling' have begun to appear (e.g. Dickerson and Weeks, 1979).

Although temporary starvation whilst in hospital has been used as a treatment for obesity (see Chapter 5) total abstinence from food is obviously not available as more than a very short-term option for people who are concerned about the excessiveness of their eating. Attempts at modification here must be aimed at changing the kinds of food consumed, altering the pattern of eating across the hours of the day, changing the circumstances under which food is taken, and/or reducing total food intake, for example. It is no accident, therefore, that some of the earliest experiments in using behavioural 'self-control' techniques for the moderation of appetitive behaviour were employed with people who complained of excessive eating (e.g. Ferster *et al.* 1962; Stuart, 1967).

CHANGE AS SELF-CONTROL

The philosophy of self-control or self-regulation treatment is that it is possible to take control of one's *own* behaviour and by the judicious use of certain tactics and strategies to reduce excess behaviours (or indeed to increase desired behaviour such as exercising or studying which do not seem to 'come naturally'). This philosophy stands in contra-distinction to the view of treatment as an externally imposed regime which requires only a willing and co-operative subject, and it therefore provides an interesting bridge between expert treatment on the one hand and self-initiated change on the other.

Some of the procedures used by Ferster *et al.* and Stuart with obese persons illustrates the techniques which have now been used widely with a whole range of problems including most of the kinds of excessive behaviour problems discussed in Part I of this book. The procedures include *self-monitoring*: for example Stuart asked patients to keep detailed 'food data sheets' as well as 'weight range sheets' for recording weight four times every day. The main purpose of such self-monitoring is to collect data about one's own behaviour. This enables precise goals to be set on the basis of a more detailed knowledge of present behaviour, and provides a baseline against which any subsequent progress can be charted. Furthermore, Stuart made an important observation when he pointed out that weight data recorded by his patients served, '. . . as four daily reminders of the therapeutic program'. Stuart was aware that, 'Much compulsive eating is "automatic" in the sense that the patient may be unaware of the fact that he is eating', just as others have observed that smoking may become automatic. Excessive drinkers are frequently unable to report at all accurately how much they drink, and it is a common clinical observation that some kind of self-monitoring of behaviour is a signal of good intent to try to reduce an excessive behaviour.

Another major category of self-regulation techniques is that of *stimulus control*. For example, Stuart and others who have treated obesity using this kind of approach, have recommended that excessive eaters discipline themselves to eat only at mealtimes, sitting down at a place at a table laid properly for a meal, and that they school themselves not to pair eating with other activities such as watching television, reading, talking on the telephone, or cooking. Patients are asked to make eating a 'pure experience', thus breaking important associations with other activities, and in the process increasing further their awareness of eating. Similarly, excessive drinkers have been advised, on the basis of close analysis of their drinking, to confine drinking to certain times of day, to drinking with certain people, or in certain places associated with moderate rather than excessive drinking (e.g. Miller and Munoz, 1976).

There is a further large category of self-control tactics which might be termed *response control*. Setting targets such as eating low calorie foods more often and high calorie foods less often, or sipping alcoholic drinks rather than gulping them, or drinking only low alcohol content beverages (e.g. beer rather than spirits), would be examples. Also included in this category would be suggestions for engaging in alternative behaviours at times of particular temptation. For example, Stuart recommended that a neighbour be called or a paper read at 10 a.m. if that was a time when eating was particularly likely to occur. Arranging to be at home and to engage in some group project on Saturday afternoons was such a technique claimed to be particularly beneficial by a group of men living together in a hostel and attempting to overcome their excessive gambling (Orford, 1975).

This self-control movement in psychology stems from the behavioural tradition and has been largely concerned with the kinds of tactics outlined above, plus others such as 'self-reward' and 'self-punishment' (Thoresen and Mahoney, 1974). It has been less concerned with the strategic decisions which the model being developed here assumes underlie attempts at self-control, and which may be the basis of the 'resolve' which William James (1891) considered necessary in order to, '. . . launch ourselves with as strong and decided an initiative as possible' (p.123), when acquiring a new habit or leaving off an old one. A number of writers, however, have considered self-control in this wider sense. In their important contribution Kanfer and Karoly (1972) defined self-control as that special case of change in which a person wishes to bring about a reduction in the occurrence of a 'high-probability' behaviour. Necessary for this process is a degree of self-monitoring of behaviour, not necessarily in the technical sense of keeping a record of behaviour, but in the general sense of being aware of behaviour, thinking about it, and evaluating it. Kanfer and Karoly suggested that chains or sequences of actions involving such behaviours might be run off smoothly, automatically, and without self-monitoring until such time as, '. . . a choice point is reached, when an external event interrupts and refocusses one's attention, when one's activation level changes or when the expected consequences of behaviour are not forthcoming . . .' (p.429). Once such a point was reached behaviour became subject to attempts at self-control, and behaviour was then monitored or 'edited' by comparison with stated intentions, plans, predictions, promises, or resolutions. These were often embodied in a kind of 'performance promise' or 'contract'. Viewing self-control as a process that involves the negotiation of a contract with oneself or with others is potentially very fruitful because it helps to tie together the otherwise separate strands of 'spontaneous' self-control, therapy-induced control, and control by important others. The knot that ties them together is the contract:

> Basically, a contract is an agreement that describes particular behaviours that must be engaged in by the contractors, under specific conditions. Typically, some mode of enforcement is provided. Non-fulfilment of the terms of the contract is clearly identifiable and the imposition of sanctions (consequences) is agreed upon in advance. A contract provides one means of social monitoring that clearly incorporates the elements of discriminative and contingency control. Our lives are fraught with situations of a contractual nature, varying in specificity and controlling power for enforcement (for example,

employer–employee, buyer–seller, teacher–pupil, parent–child, and, most relevant for the current argument, therapist–client) (pp.430–1).

Kanfer and Karoly proceeded to list a number of circumstances which they hypothesized promoted the making of intention statements. Again this list serves to remind us of the very general nature of the processes being discussed. Furthermore, there are a number of points of similarity with the models of Janis and colleagues and others discussed above. The first circumstance on their list, for example, occurred when an individual received cues that signalled the conflictual nature of current behaviour (being reminded of the link between smoking and cancer, for example, or being told of a friend who died of a drug overdose). This circumstance, they believed to be, '. . . an invariant early component of the self-control sequence' (p.432). The second circumstance occurred when a person suffered aversive effects of behaviour (a coughing fit for a smoker or a hangover for a drinker, for example). Other circumstances in their list are helpful because they serve, as does the concept of 'dissonance' discussed in Chapter 11, to make sense of the sometimes apparently devious behaviour of a person in conflict over excessive appetitive behaviour. For example, they hypothesized that intention statements would be particularly likely when a person was satiated with respect to the behaviour in question or when the probability of performing the behaviour was low (e.g. someone who thinks their sexual behaviour to be excessive following several exhausting sexual encounters, or someone who declares an intention to give up gambling when their money has run out), when the probability of social approval for making intention statements was high, when the intention statement was made to a person who was not in a position to monitor future behaviour, when the behaviour in question was infrequent or in the distant future, or when making such a statement enabled the person to get out of trouble. Like Eiser *et al.* (1978), Kanfer and Karoly suggested that intention statements were unlikely to be made if the probability of execution of the new behaviour was generally known to be low, or if the person had a history of previously unsuccessful attempts at control. Interestingly, they had rather less to say about the conditions that make for successful carrying out of intentions. They did, however, acknowledge that 'sticking to the bargain' was a major problem, and they speculated that overt, publicly made, commitments—as for example in Weight Watchers or Alcoholics Anonymous—might be more effective than covert promises.

Logan (1973) is another who has considered self-control in wider perspective. Specifically he was concerned with those, '. . . important decisions . . . involving a conflict between immediate gratification and the long-range best interests of the individual and/or society' (p.127). Amongst such intrinsically rewarding activities, eating, drinking, and sexual activity ranked high, he argued, and were particularly likely to be the subjects of self-control attempts. His particular contribution was the positing of a general self-control drive, based upon experiences in life in which the inability to control behaviour has been associated with discomfort, fear, or frustration.

Premack (1970) is yet another who has discussed self-control in its broader meaning. His discussion of the mechanisms of self-control took as its starting point the contrast between the failure of behaviour therapists to modify smoking behaviour in the laboratory, and on the other hand the survey reports that millions of people had given up smoking voluntarily. He concluded that current behaviour theory was radically incomplete, and that people in the real world exercised control over their behaviour by mechanisms other than those which had been put into practice in the laboratory and the behaviour therapy clinic. His particular contention was that the circumstances for self-control of smoking in the real world consisted of some combination of knowledge of the smoking–cancer link, which served merely as a catalyst for change, coupled with some sort of humiliating experience (realizing that one was putting money into the pockets of cigarette manufacturers, or that one was encouraging one's children to smoke, for example). Central to Premack's formulation, as to the one being developed here, were the concepts of conflict and decision. According to Premack, whatever the nature of a decision, 'Its prime operational consequence is self-instruction' (p.116). Internal anti-smoking statements occurred, and the individual might be likened to two people, one the behavioural agent, the other the critic who offers the agent advice, 'Don't do that', or 'Do, do that'. Like others who have written about the self-control process, Premack considered that self-instruction could serve to restore thought to behaviour sequences which, as a result of frequent occurrence had become automatic or thoughtless.

Premack was concerned to clarify the relationship between cognitive mechanisms, such as decision-making, and conditioning or learning processes. He cautioned that decisions, although they could play a major role in modifying established behaviour patterns, should not be thought of as magical events that could abolish at one sweep all the control that months or years of learning had established. He rejected both the view that either cognitive processes or conditioning represents the true process, the other being false or trivial, and the view that they are essentially the same processes described in different language.

In view of the danger that a problem-solving or decision-making approach to self-control may be seen as overly cognitive and lacking in reference to emotional elements, Premack's emphasis upon the importance of emotion is also most welcome. Although his specific theory may be criticized for overemphasis upon 'humiliation' as the key emotion involved, his general remarks on the subject are highly relevant. He suggested that the emotion associated with the discovery of being a member of 'an ethically repugnant class' (or, it might be added, of being in a very high risk group for major illness, or of being close to financial ruin) would be strongest on the first occasion and might weaken progressively thereafter. However, if self-instruction were successful, and if the decisional processes were instigated early on and successfully, this emotion would have little chance of being habituated. Thus, it was important, if the emotional component was to be preserved, that early success occurred. Although not well worked out, these ideas may go some way towards helping explain the high rate of relapse which is usually found to follow treatment for excessive behaviour problems.

From a decision-making viewpoint it seems that the majority of new behavioural decisions are especially vulnerable within the first few weeks or months and fail to be consolidated on a permanent basis. In the natural course of events such resolutions succumb to pressures created by stressful events, moods of depression and anxiety, and social pressures of one kind or another. Hence the typical group relapse curve.

Research on the circumstances surrounding relapse has been carried out by Sjoberg and his colleagues in Sweden. Sjoberg and Johnson (1978), for example, described in detail the 'breakdown of the will' or volitional breakdown, that occurred for most of ten people whom they studied who had made the 'decision' to give up smoking. Like Janis and Mann they assumed that the initial act of giving up smoking was based on a process of 'balanced information processing', a 'decision', requiring 'high quality information processing'. The process of volitional breakdown which nine of their ten subjects subsequently described to them was not of such a kind, however. Indeed, Sjoberg and Johnson depicted it as one characterized by 'low quality information processing' and 'twisted reasoning' mostly brought about under 'mood pressure':

> Strength of the will is experienced as an important determinant in accounting for success in the achievement of goals. To have a strong will means being able to stick to an initial well-balanced decision under various forms of pressure that tend to give rise to twisted short-sighted reasoning, to be able to maintain values and moral convictions in the face of threat and temptation (p.150).

Some, but by no means all, relapsed under external pressure such as a family row or hearing bad news, but nearly all produced evidence of cognitive distortions. Most of these fell into one of two categories: telling themselves that they could get away with smoking just a little (e.g. 'a pipe now and then is OK', 'OK to accept an offered cigarette, but not to buy cigarettes myself'); and delaying the attempt to quit.

Sjoberg and Johnson subscribed to the view of Astin (1962), and Heilizer (1964) and others on the importance of conflict, but viewed its importance in terms of mental energy and cognitive distortion:

> The stronger the conflict the stronger is the mood pressure, and the more likely is a twisted cognitive functioning which may ultimately lead to a breakdown of the will. . . . The wish which forms the basis of decision is invested with more energy the stronger the motivation is. Energy leads to more efficient attention, effort, etc, and also to greater resources available to the cognitive system (pp.151–2).

What was needed was not improved knowledge about the effects of appetitive behaviour, nor improved cognitive processing or aids to decision. The need was to find the mental energy to sustain a difficult decision in the face of emotional stress.

Under mood pressure, mental energy was diverted, there might be, '. . . a narrowing of the perspectives in time and in values and commitments . . .' (p. 151), and the kind of twisted reasoning which most of their subjects described might take place, Sjoberg and Johnson also described, as one of the results of such volitional breakdowns, what they called a 'domino effect'. After the initial breakdown, the second, third, and subsequent breakdowns occur more easily. Indeed, after one or two breakdowns the initial 'high quality' decision may easily be abandoned altogether. They attributed this effect to the threat to a person's self-concept which occurs as a result of this experience of failure. Whatever its causes, they appear to be describing exactly the same phenomenon which Cummings *et al.* (1980) have referred to as the 'abstinence violation effect' for people attempting to abstain from alcohol.

Research with excessive eaters has also shown the importance of emotional stress in precipitating relapse. Loro and Orleans (1981) found that the stresses of school or work pressure or problems in personal relationships were the circumstances most often reported as precipitants of eating 'binges'. Stuart (1967) had earlier counselled that those attempting to self-control over-eating should learn to identify 'danger periods' between meals when arousal was high as these would be the times when the probability of the most habitual or well-practised response was increased. This idea, that heightened arousal increases the likelihood of occurrence of the most over-learned act, often the very act that is excessive in frequency and is to-be-controlled, is one that crosses the various excesses we have considered in this book and recurs in clinical accounts of 'alcoholics', 'compulsive gamblers', and drug 'addicts', for example. The 'typology of dangerous situations' for excessive drinkers developed by Litman *et al.* (1977), for example, included, (1) unpleasant mood states such as anxiety and depression, (2) external situations and euphoric feelings, (3) social anxiety, and (4) lessened cognitive vigilance and rationalizations.

In a further report on a study of ten excessive drinkers who were relatively socially stable, Samsonowitz and Sjoberg (1981) confirmed their own previous findings as well as that of Loro and Orleans (1981) with excessive eaters, Litman *et al.* (1977, 1979a) with excessive drinkers, and that of Marlatt and Gordon (1979) with excessive drinkers, smokers, and heroin addicts, that relapse is most likely under conditions of adverse emotional arousal. In this study Samsonowitz and Sjoberg also examined the techniques used to resist relapse. The most commonly reported technique among this group was 'bringing values to mind'. As the authors of this report stated, this kind of decision can be regarded as a 'negative choice', i.e. a choice between the action of drinking and non-action of abstaining. This creates volitional problems, and bringing to mind the positive consequences that would result from maintaining the decision, or negative consequences of going back on the decision, seemed to be helpful. Other strategies used by the majority of this group were engaging in conscious planning and preparation prior to the decision to give up, avoiding difficult and tempting situations, and performing a particular activity, including both physical and mental activities, in order to divert attention from temptation. The number of relapses reported correlated inversely and significantly with the number of techniques reported. Furthermore, the degree of a person's social stability correlated positively with the number of techniques employed, and the number of techniques used by this group of relatively socially stable people was significantly greater than the number reported in a previous study of socially unstable or 'skid row' drinkers. The latter group had been particularly unlikely, by comparison, to use the bringing to mind of values.

In a paper summarizing his work with different excessive appetites, Sjoberg (1980) neatly summed up the conflict of a person whose appetitive behaviour is excessive. He referred to *wishes* or *wants* that have an, '. . . inherent tendency to attract (or repel) . . .' (p.124), and *values* or *shoulds* that refer to, '. . . acts that are strived for (or avoided) due to a sense of obligation . . .' (p.124).

With his emphasis upon humiliation, Premack's (1970) understanding of the self-control process was also highly dependent upon the potentially behaviour-controlling functions of a set of beliefs about right and wrong conduct, or conscience. He concluded his chapter by considering three limitations of conscience. The first was 'ignorance of the law': for example, although a person might be strongly opposed to setting young people a bad example, he or she might not be aware that smoking in the presence of children sets an example. Secondly, a person might, through lapse in attention, discover him or herself in the middle of the to-be-controlled act. Thirdly, and of most interest here, a person might still 'succumb to temptation' despite full knowledge and complete attention. The self-control process is simply insufficient to suppress the behaviour. Although the adverse emotion may shortly return, for the moment it is, 'supplanted by different emotion'. Although this amounts to little more than a restatement of the conflict view of strongly appetitive behaviour, it leads to a postulate about 'spontaneous' change which is in keeping with Winick's (1962) theory of the 'maturing out' of drug addiction:

> Thus, at 45 an individual may suddenly become a model husband for no reason other than that the emotional voltage is now able to cope with the weakened challenges. Similarly, people who have been unable to quit smoking at one age may suddenly prove able at a later age (Premack, 1970).

This discussion leads on to a consideration of the role of higher-order attitudes and values, and hence of 'spiritual' factors in behaviour change. In Chapter 14 the proposition will be considered that the moral aspects of the appetitive behaviour change process have been insufficiently acknowledged in the past.

CHAPTER FOURTEEN

Giving up Excess as Moral Reform

I should rely both upon medical and moral influences. Certain medical treatment may be used, which will make the brain stronger after a time, and then moral and regular habits will come in after abstinence; but . . . I think that nothing is more pernicious than the practice of sending dipsomaniacs to country retreats, where they are allowed to fish and shoot, and pass their time in a listless and inactive way; as a rule, I believe that this mode of life paralyses the will and relaxes all energy of character. Therefore I think that it could only be in a public institution where hard work could be enforced, and where certain additional burdens and extra interests might be brought to bear upon them that benefits could be expected. (Dr Browne replying to a question put by the Select Committee on Habitual Drunkards, 1872).

. . . society and its agencies have always had a consistent response, in that in the same breath they are able to say the homeless alcoholic is 'sad, mad *and* bad'. Each agency seems to carry within it the seeds of these three elements. Courts punish but also remand for medical reports; hostels take in but also turn out a man when he is drunk; doctors heal but then lecture a man as to what will happen if he continues to drink; clergymen pray for him and then give him the price of a cup of tea. Missions and psychiatry coexist painlessly and effortlessly. (Cook, 1975, p.172).

CONDUCT AND ATTITUDE REORGANIZATION

Particularly stimulating amongst those who have written about the spiritual elements of the change process are the ideas of Sarbin and Nucci on what they call the self-reconstitution processes (1973). Their argument was that a change in status from that of 'confirmed' smoker to that of 'confirmed' ex- or former smoker involved more than a mechanistic habit change or simple isolated decision, but rather involved the taking on of a new self-identity. This was because, '. . . the degree to which the person incorporates the label "smoker" . . . into his overall self-concept determines whether he can or cannot easily dispense with smoking behaviour' (p.182). Such a view is in line with consistency theories of attitude organization and change. Because attitudes are not isolated, conduct change will be more likely, and more likely to stick in the long term, if related attitudes (particularly attitudes about the self and/or superordinate attitudes or values) bolster rather than oppose the reordered set of beliefs about the appetitive object and its consumption. If A believes he is an X kind of person, and also that X kinds of people are usually heavy gamblers, then it would be inconsistent and hence difficult for him to hold strongly to the view of himself as a non- or light gambler. A similar view, linking maintenance of behaviour with the self-concept, has been put forward by Fransella (1972) for eating.

Sarbin and Nucci described a number of major themes which they claimed existed in descriptions of most successful programmes of conduct reorganization whether these be religiously, politically, or therapeutically motivated. Essentially they saw three central processes in successful reconstitution: (a) symbolic death; (b) surrender; and (c) re-education (re-birth). What they described was a kind of conversion process that began when the previous social identity was acknowledged to be bankrupt. 'Hitting rock bottom', a state believed by Alcoholics Anonymous to be necessary before change can occur, is perhaps one kind of symbolic death, whilst Premack's 'humiliation' is another. The individual 'surrendered' to the conduct reorganization programme, and in particular to a group or individual who provided a role model for the new self. The role model might be a group of other individuals, an '. . . abstract referent in a transcendental or theological system' (p.186), or an individual 'teacher' or 'guide' (sponsor, priest, therapist, shaman, doctor, etc.). The teacher had, '. . . the legitimate or coercive power to administer reinforcements and also the expert power to guide the participant into proper role behaviour' (p.186). Public testimony was a widely used method.

Sarbin and Nucci illustrated the process by reference to a description of the Spiritual Exercises of Ignatius Loyola. The exercises took 4 weeks, the first being devoted to thoughts of sin and its consequences, with due attention being paid to surroundings—a darkened cell, solitary confinement, prostration. The second week concentrated on the Saviour as a means to salvation and at the end of this week, the climax of the exercises, an election for Christ or the devil was made. Meditations during the third week confirmed the election to Christ, and the fourth concentrated on the positive values of life eternal. Sarbin and Nucci considered that similar components were to be found in such conduct reorganization systems for drug 'addicts' as Synanon, and in Alcoholics Anonymous, and they proceeded to outline a suitable 14-day retreat programme of conduct reorganization for confirmed smokers. Unfortunately, there is no evidence that Sarbin and Nucci put their proposals into practice, and we can only speculate that had they done so, and had their programme been credible to a reasonable proportion of their pupils (they admit that, 'The current period in history may indeed be an inappropriate time to resurrect religious metaphors', p.195), then their methods would have met with at least the same success rate as more conventional procedures.

The importance of Sarbin and Nucci's original ideas for our present discussion lies in their view that decision-making of a more or less rationalistic kind goes little way towards accounting for changes in excessive behaviours.

As beliefs associated with major world religions constitute some of the most all-embracing sets of beliefs about social conduct and the self, amounting to comprehensive moral or ethical systems or 'attitudes to life', it should come as no surprise to find strong moral reform or spiritual change elements in those programmes or organizations that appear to have had the greatest impact in the control of excessive appetites, nor to find that giving up excess is not infrequently accompanied by a reversal or change in religious sentiment or observance. In terms of consistency theory, spiritual change may be seen as a widespread logical change in a whole set of attitudes about right and wrong conduct. Such a sweeping change may be necessary to support a radical reversal of conduct in one particular area, such as sexual behaviour or the consumption of drugs. Conformity to the Christian religion has been shown in numerous surveys in predominantly Christian countries to be related to a lower level of indulgence in alcohol, drugs and other forms of appetitive consumption (Gorsuch and Butler, 1976; Jolly and Orford, 1983). Belief in the importance of self-control and restraint, and a belief in the rightness of a relatively ascetic way of life, probably provide the intervening logic between religious belief and appetitive moderation (Thorner, 1953). According to Thorner,

> The essence of the ascetic pattern . . . is hostility toward spontaneous, impulsive enjoyment of life and what it has to offer; active and purposive control over the emotions, with consideration for the ethical consequences of one's actions; and a life-long, systematic, rational ordering of the moral life, oriented toward and subordinated to a supernatural goal . . . It is because of the profound importance of emotional control that ascetic Protestants manifest moral and emotional intensity in their roles as prohibitionists. They experience misgivings over breaches in discipline, and interpret submission to the 'appetites' as a sign of moral weakness. Tobacco and liquor are felt to be chinks in the armor of impulse control, faults that open the gate to delinquency and hinder social and moral improvement . . . (p.167, 169).

It was Anna Freud's (1936) view too that asceticism was a defence which functioned to protect a person against the internal threat of forbidden impulses (Janis and Mann, 1977).

In line with Sarbin and Nucci's (1973) thesis that change attempts must employ a theme acceptable to their times, it seems likely from historical accounts that the mid-nineteenth century, both in Britain and the United States, saw many dramatic changes in drinking behaviour at least, brought about by evangelical religious means. In particular, the taking of abstinence pledges appears to have played a major part. Although it is impossible to know whether old-fashioned pledge-taking met with equal or higher success rates in comparison with modern 'treatments', it does seem that the former was sometimes on a rather larger scale. McPeek (1972), for example, described the effects of the early American temperance movement in the 1820s and 1830s. The annual report of the American Temperance Society in 1833 claimed, he tells us, that in its five years of existence the Society had sobered up 5,000 known drunkards. Within three years of becoming the American Temperance Union in 1836, claims were being made that as many as 350,000 people had signed their abstinence pledge. Perhaps the best known of all religious temperance movements of that time was the Washington Temperance Society which originated in 1840 and which, before its demise not many years later, was claiming between 150,000 and 250,000 pledged members. The Washingtonians held meetings which sound to have been not dissimilar to those of Alcoholics Anonymous 100 years later, but by comparison with AA they adopted a much more actively proselytizing stance: each new recruit was to go out and obtain new pledges (McPeek, 1972; Sagarin, 1969).

It was at about the same time that one of the most famous temperance reformers, Father Mathew of Cork, was active in Ireland (see Chapter 2). Both McPeek and Sagarin mentioned his claimed achievements, as did Longmate (1968). That representatives of 'the trade' tried to break up his later meetings in England testifies to his effectiveness. In comparison with the influence of Father Mathew, the present-day effect of individual practitioners who painstakingly 'treat' the 'disease' of 'alcoholism' seems ludicrously insignificant.

Despite the seemingly very different style of temperance-wrought changes of the 1830s and 1840s in comparison with those brought about with the help of professional treatment in the 1970s and 1980s, there are intriguing hints that the basic change processes have not altered. Exaggerated claims of treatment effectiveness were being made then as now. McPeek quoted from a report of the Washington Temperance Society in 1841:

> The question is often asked, and with a great deal of propriety, too, Do they hold out who sign the pledge? We answer, No. Some—and be assured, the number is very small—go back to drinking again; but as soon as it is known to any of the society that this is the case, the backslider is waited upon by some friend, who seldom fails to induce him to sign the pledge again and commence anew, and then the fact of his having violated the pledge fills him with shame and repentance and is the means of his adhering more rigidly to it (McPeek, 1972, p.409).

On the other hand, McPeek was able to cite a prohibitionist senator who, fifty years later, could view the Washingtonians' success with greater objectivity:

> In a few years 600,000 drunkards have been reformed, of whom, however, all but 150,000 returned to their cups. The moral of this movement is that we must save the boy if we would be sure of the man . . . To be sure, 150,000 reformed men had adhered to their pledges and were saved; but what are 150,000 among so many? (McPeek, p.411).

The senator put the follow-up success rate at around 25 per cent. One history of the temperance movement, entitled *Battling with the Demon*, which McPeek cited, estimated that around seven out of ten of those who received temperance medals from Father Mathew in his campaigns relapsed into their old habits. The similarity between these estimates of around 25–30 per cent who managed sustained change in drinking habits following exhortation and pledge-taking within a religious context, and the percentages of success estimated by Hunt and his colleagues (e.g. Hunt and Matarazzo, 1973) and other observers of the modern treatment scene, is striking.

In this context it may be remarked that there has been a strange neglect in the modern literature on excessive appetites, of pledge-taking and its effects. This is presumably because the belief that excessive drinkers 'need treatment' is inconsistent with the expectation that anything as apparently simple and unclinical as taking a pledge could be instrumental in 'curing' a 'disease'. Yet pledge-taking involves at least a decision to take the pledge (and presumably to a greater or lesser degree an intention to stand by it) as well as a verbal commitment to behaviour, two factors important for attitude change (e.g. Bennett, 1955). An article in the *Journal of Social Psychology* (Hallaq, 1976) suggests, however, the possibility of a renewed interest in pledge-taking as an instrument of appetitive behaviour change. Hallaq obtained written pledges from 148 smokers that they would abstain from smoking during one hour of their choosing every day during one month. The interviewers who obtained the pledges explained that their work, '. . . was motivated by their concern for community welfare' (p.147). Whether such a modern rationale carries the same force as did nineteenth-century temperance campaigning seems doubtful, and unfortunately insufficient details are presented in Hallaq's report to enable its effectiveness to be judged.

In an even more recent paper entitled, 'The Great American Smoke-out', Dawley and Finkel (1981) described some of the effects of the American Cancer Society's day on which the whole nation (United States) was urged to sign a non-smoking pledge for one day. A 'phoned follow-up one year later (1978) had suggested that approximately a third of the nation's smokers had participated, with a third of them succeeding for that day. In 1979, a follow-up was made of 125 people who had taken the pledge at one particular medical centre in New Orleans. Eighty-two had tried not to smoke on the day itself and

60 of these said that they had succeeded for that day. Twenty-six of these 60 reported returning to smoking the following day and at 2 months follow-up 11 had not returned to smoking.

Although there has otherwise been a neglect of pledge-taking as such in recent times, modern behaviourally oriented therapists do speak of establishing behaviour 'contracts' between client and therapist, husband and wife, or patient and hospital staff. Where excessive appetitive behaviour is the focus, these frequently contain items stating the requirement of reduced or eliminated appetitive behaviour, and they are often carefully written out, and signed by the different parties to the contract.

There is also a large body of research in social psychology devoted to the effectiveness of 'persuasive communications' in changing attitudes (McGuire, 1980) and this has had some application to excessive smoking and to excessive eating. Much of the original work on the value of 'fear arousal' in attitude change was carried out with smoking cessation or reduction as the object (Leventhal, 1970) and there has been more recent interest in doctors as 'credible' sources of advice about smoking (Russell *et al.*, 1979). With weight reduction as the aim, Ley *et al.* (1974) carried out a programme of research to test such variables as degree of comprehensibility of the attitude change message, the degree of fear arousal intended and achieved, the position of the fear-arousing element in the overall communication, the number of times the message is repeated, and the mode of presentation (personal, tape, or written). Clear conclusions are few, but the interesting point for present purposes is the way excessive smokers and eaters have been considered suitable cases for this kind of persuasive object-focused attitude change whilst excessive gamblers, heterosexuals, alcohol users, and drug users have on the whole been seen as more suitable for intensive institutional management, psychological treatment, or self-help groups.

It is the present argument that modern forms of 'treatment' for excessive behaviour are not as dissimilar in their essentials to the nineteenth-century ways of changing people's behaviour as modern practitioners would like to suppose. There are numerous instances to be found of treatments which, when described, are seen to incorporate powerful consciousness-raising and attitude-changing elements which seem much more likely to be the active treatment ingredients than the components or processes supposedly active according to the treatment's theoretical rationale. If the effective functions of most treatments are to focus attention on the excessive behaviour, to instil the belief and to provide many repetitions of the message that the behaviour needs to be controlled, and to engender the expectation that it can be controlled, this would explain the rather similar outcomes following the whole range of apparently very varied treatments.

That some very technical-sounding procedures are really just varieties of attitude-changing or enhancing is best illustrated by descriptions of some of the more elaborate behavioural techniques such as Stuart's (1967) self-control treatment for over-eating, and Barker and Miller's (1968) aversion therapy for compulsive gambling. Amongst a number of attitude change elements in Stuart's method were the 'food data sheets' and 'weight range sheets' filled in by his patients which provided both data and 'daily reminders of the program'. This was important particularly as Stuart had observed, as Hunt and Matarazzo (1970) and others have noted about some smokers, that, 'Much compulsive eating is "automatic", in the sense that the patient may be unaware of the fact that he is eating' (p.358). This and a number of other parts of the procedure, for example making eating 'a pure experience' unconnected with other activities such as TV-watching or reading, must have had the effect, whatever their intended purpose, of re-establishing awareness or thought about a previously habitual and 'un-thoughtful' behaviour. Two further examples of apparently technical 'procedures', which in all probability are really examples of attitude control which people use in modified form to control their unwanted urges in the natural course of events without formal treatment, are verbal 'self-instruction' and 'coverant sensitization' (Cautela, 1971). As an example of the former, Stuart instructed his patients, when tempted to repeat, 'I can control my eating by engaging in other activities which I enjoy'. His paper contains a splendid example of the latter technique involving a woman who had difficulty giving up a favourite type of 'cookie' at a certain time each day. She was instructed to imagine vividly taking the forbidden item from its package, putting it to her lips, crunching it, tasting it, and then to switch to imagining, equally vividly, her husband seducing another woman, a great fear admitted at the initial interview!

Imagery can in fact be a powerful means of influencing aspects of behaviour and experience which are normally thought of as being beyond voluntary control. For example, instructions to imagine that water placed on the tongue is sour or that citric acid is tasteless can produce an elevation or reduction in salivary response, respectively, and instructions to dream about specific topics can produce the desired effect (Cautela, 1971). This is part of the rationale behind Cautela's 'covert conditioning' treatment for excessive appetites in which once again the symbolic or attitude-changing elements are starkly apparent. A dissonant smoker, for example, might be instructed to imagine the following scene:

> As soon as you start reaching for the cigarette, you get a nauseous feeling in your stomach. You begin to feel sick to your stomach, as if you are about to vomit. You touch the pack of cigarettes and bitter spit comes into your mouth. When you take the cigarette out of the pack some pieces of food come into your throat. Now you feel sick and have stomach cramps. As you are about to put the cigarette in your mouth, you puke all over the pack of cigarettes. The cigarette in your hand is very soggy and full of green vomit. There is a stink coming from the vomit. Snots are coming from your nose. Your hands feel all slimy and full of vomit. The whole desk is a mess. Your clothes are all full of puke. You get up from your desk and turn away from the vomit and cigarettes. You immediately

> begin to feel better being away from the vomit and the cigarettes. You go to the bathroom and wash up and feel great being away from the vomit and the cigarettes (Cautela, p.113).

The commitment to carrying out such a 'treatment' and the process of going through this routine repetitively (Cautela recommended ten 'trials' a session for a number of sessions with practice between times) could scarcely have been better arranged for enhancing a new-found attitude towards the at-one-time attractive appetitive object. Whatever the effectiveness of this procedure in conditioning an aversive response (as Cautela supposed), it contains, like Boswell's discourse against fornication (Chapter 6), all the ingredients of experiments for inducing dissonance (see Kelman and Baron, 1974), and its major impact was almost certainly the bolstering of a negative set towards smoking which must already have been developing in order for the 'patient' to be willing to enter treatment in the first place.

Alternating with each aversive scene would be an 'escape' or 'self-control' scene. For the typical smoker, for example:

> You are at your desk working and you decide to smoke, and as soon as you decide to smoke you get this funny sick feeling in the pit of your stomach. You say to yourself, 'The hell with it, I'm not going to smoke!' As soon as you decide not to smoke, you feel fine and proud that you resisted temptation (p.114).

These aversion therapy 'treatments', because of their technical appearance (which probably added to their 'magic'), scientific rationale, and flamboyant methods, illustrate the attitude-enhancing elements of treatment very nicely, but it is the present argument that most if not all 'treatments' for excessive appetites, whatever their form, work in the same way, principally by virtue of the commitment which the patient makes to entering and undergoing some form of 'therapeutic' procedure the purpose of which is to help control the excessive behaviour.

Perhaps because he was an ordained minister, John Gardner (see Chapter 2) could appreciate the symbolic elements in the aversion therapy he received:

> The great boon, for me anyway, was the feeling of freshness which accompanied the treatment: the body was livelier, eyes clearer, and a new alertness took the place of the former mental lethargy. Even more than this were the spiritual benefits. To one who had lived and thought for much of his life in terms of sacramental symbolism, it was easy to see how the sudden, sharp expulsion of alcohol, and its attendant poisons, from the body, could be allied with the exorcism of that devil-desire to drink: and on each fresh appointment with the trolley of drinks there was a decisive sense of waking to a new life.

> I have heard people moan about the horrors of the aversion treatment; even read novels which describe it in much more graphic terms than those I have used here. But, on looking back, I recall those hours of sickness, sweat and churning bowels with some pleasure. Uncomfortable? Yes, of course. But the removal of a malignant tissue is uncomfortable; the cutting away of a diseased organ is not pleasant; and, if it offers you the chance of living a full and useful life, the discomfort is as a tiny grain of sand (Gardner, 1964, p.215).

Very few studies of formal treatment have involved asking people for their own views on how change occurs. One which is particularly interesting, however, because it involved both people who were attempting to give up smoking alone and those who had enrolled in one or other of two treatment programmes (aversion and behavioural management) is that by Di Clemente and Prochaska (1982). There were some differences consistent with treatment rationale. For example, those in the behavioural-management group rated 'social management' (getting other people involved in efforts to stop) as relatively more important than those in other groups, with the self-quitting group rating it least highly. On the other hand, most of the results support the view that the essential elements of change are not peculiar to 'treatment', let alone to any one particular form of treatment. Rated as most important, on average, by all three groups, were 'self-liberation' (e.g. 'it was really a day-to-day commitment not to smoke and to stay away from cigarettes that helped me to quit smoking'), 'counter-conditioning' (finding other ways to relax and deal with tension), and 'feedback' (becoming aware of the reasons for smoking). Thus, feedback was rated highly by those enrolled in the two forms of treatment, although neither was designed particularly to produce insight. Similarly, finding alternatives to smoking was rated highly by the self-quitting group, although they were given no help in finding alternatives.

In particular, the commitment process of 'self-liberation' was given the highest ratings overall and Di Clemente and Prochaska expressed surprise that this process has received such little attention in writings on therapeutic change. They were particularly puzzled as to why aversion clients should rate self-liberation so highly. They were along the right lines, I believe, when they suggested that, '. . . the ordeal of undergoing unpleasant procedures either reflected or increased the personal commitment of the subjects' (p.141). A number of years ago, as a probationer clinical psychologist, I was involved in administering aversion therapy (Orford, 1971b), and became convinced that any effectiveness of the procedure was due to the personal commitment to change held by the client, which was then strongly reinforced by undergoing a procedure which appeared very scientific, very elaborate, apparently very convincing, probably rather frightening at first, and certainly designed as a direct attack upon the client's attraction to the appetitive object. It therefore comes as no surprise at all to me that anti-smoking aversion clients should rate the factor of commitment so highly.

A further point of interest in Di Clemente and Prochaska's study arose from asking their subjects to rate the importance of different change processes for each of three different stages: the 'decision to quit' period, the 'active change' period, and the 'maintenance' period. Verbal processes such as 'feedback' and 'education' (information from Health Education campaigns for example) were rated as highly important during the initial decision period, but were thought relatively unimportant after that, whilst behavioural processes such as 'counter-conditioning', 'social-managament', and 'stimulus control' were rated as more important during the later two periods, particularly during the 'active change' period. Once again, 'self-liberation' emerged as generally the most important process of all, particularly during the 'active change' period and the 'decision' period.

SELF-HELP

The argument that the change process is not to be understood most readily by accepting the supposed rationales or taking too seriously the techniques of modern physical or psychological treatments, but rather by an appreciation of the factors that are common to a variety of forms, whether religious, medical, or 'spontaneous', is supported by the prominence of self-help in the spectrum of modern forms of help for excessive appetites. Those who have analysed the self-help movement, such as Sagarin (1969) in his intriguing book, *Odd Man In: Society's Deviants in America*, have described the way in which Alcoholics Anonymous, the best known self-help organization in the field of appetitive behaviour change, has been used as a model for many similar organizations for gamblers, over-eaters, ex-prisoners, psychiatric patients, and numerous other special groups. AA itself is a quite remarkable phenomenon. Although it is impossible to know the true success rate of the organization, it must be counted uniquely successful in organizational terms. It has already survived for over four decades, and has spread to all parts of the United States and to over 50 other countries. In Britain, membership has continued to rise in recent years (Robinson, 1979).

The importance of a religious, or at least spiritual, element in the AA programme is apparent in two ways. First, this element is made quite explicit in the 12 steps which are to be followed by members and which constitute the core of the process. God, or 'a Higher Power', are mentioned in no less than 6 of the 12 steps, and although new members are instructed to interpret the expression 'Higher Power' in any way they like, religious or otherwise, the religious connotation is clear.

Secondly, it is possible to trace the lineage of many modern self-help organizations, via AA, back to the Oxford Group Movement, a worldwide and still functioning organization, originally known as the First Century Christian Fellowship and later as Moral Re-Armament (Sagarin, 1969; Glaser, 1973; Kaufman and de Leon, 1978). The founder and guiding light of the Oxford Group Movement was Dr Frank Buchman, who patterned his operation upon his idea of what Christianity was like before the advent of the organized Church, and it was from this source that AA received its ideas of self-examination, acknowledgement of character defects, restitution for harm done to others, and working with others. Amongst the key practices of the Oxford Group Movement was 'sharing', by which was meant the open confession of sins at large public meetings or smaller 'house parties'. Recounting one's life story, but in a particular stylized form which confirmed the organization's view of the central and damaging role of the appetitive activity, formed a major part of the group activities of both Alcoholics Anonymous (Robinson, 1979) and Gamblers Anonymous (Scodel, 1964). A key practice, 'guidance', meant the acceptance of divine inspiration as the sole indication of action. People who accepted such guidance were said to be under 'God control', although Glaser remarks that Dr Buchman and the hierarchy of the organization appeared to be the filters through which God made his wishes known to the movement's members.

'Changing', or conversion to the beliefs of the movement, was generally held to be a sudden, dramatic, emotional, or public experience, and as Sarbin and Nucci (1973) found to be true of many organizations for conduct change, persons who had been converted were spoken of as 're-born' or 'second-born'. The movement also attempted to inculcate in its members four absolute values: absolute honesty, absolute purity, absolute unselfishness, and absolute love. The introduction to the second edition of *Alcoholics Anonymous*, the fellowship's 'Big Book' (1955), contains The Doctor's Opinion, the testimony of Dr Silkworth who influenced one of the founder members of AA. Particularly interesting is the sentence:

> We doctors have realised for a long time that some form of moral psychology was of urgent importance to alcoholics but . . . with our ultra-modern standards, our scientific approach, we are perhaps not well equipped to apply the powers of good that lie outside our synthetic knowledge (p.xxv).

That successful passage through the programme involves a wide-ranging moral reform (Gusfield, 1962) is made clear in many subsequent passages in the book. For example, 'Selfishness—self-centeredness! That, we think, is the root of our troubles . . . the alcoholic is an extreme example of self-will run riot . . .' (p.62). 'Admitting' to another human being was, 'a humbling experience', and very necessary. This might take the form of a religious confession or it might be done with a doctor, a psychologist, or maybe a family member or friend (but not to someone who would be hurt by it), but it must be entirely honest.

Even in Al-Anon, for family members of 'alcoholics', members are encouraged to make a, 'searching and fearless moral inventory' of themselves, and to correct, 'years of entrenched patterns of negative thinking and doing', although it may be the passing of information about alternative ways of reacting to common problems, plus the support which members can give each other, which is most effective (Ablon, 1974). Robinson (1979) concluded from his study of AA that a vital function of membership was belonging to a group for whom to be an 'alcoholic' was not purely to be a member of Premack's (1970) 'morally repugnant class' but was to be a member of a valued fellowship that was turning something to be ashamed of into something to be proud of—destigmatization or reconstructing the problem, as Robinson called it.

Whatever the essence of the change process that is occurring, it must be acknowledged that, at least in the case of self-help groups, it takes place within a group or social context, and this is an aspect which has usually been considered by those who have studied self-help groups to be of vital significance (e.g. Bales, 1945; Robinson, 1979). It may be that what is important here is the support which other group members can provide. Consistent with the foregoing discussion, however, is a slightly different view, namely that the group provides a new set of attitudes and values, and it is to the group's ideology or 'will' that the novice must submit if he or she is to become a successful member. These two views of the social role of the self-help organization are not as incompatible as they may at first seem. Janis and Rodin (1979) have described 'social support' as a resource which combines friendship with demands for conformity. 'Support' does not come without strings, but imposes certain obligations upon those who are in receipt of it.

Otto and Orford (1978) and Volkman and Cressey (1968) have interpreted the impact upon their residents of small hostels or halfway houses for drug addicts, compulsive gamblers, and alcoholics, in terms of the re-socializing influence of living with a group of people who are subscribing to an ideology of change. They draw attention to the similarity between their ideas and those who have supported the *differential association theory* of the development and remission of delinquent behaviour. This theory (Sutherland and Cressey, 1970) gives maximum weight, in explaining how delinquency is taken up and given up, to the social influence of the peer group at different stages in a person's life and delinquent career.

As already mentioned (see Chapter 9), the theory of differential association has been applied directly by Akers *et al.* (1979) to the taking up of drug use. Thus, the account of excessive appetitive behaviour comes full circle. The same factors which have been shown to be the most important in accounting for the differential uptake of appetitive behaviours turn out to have a good claim to be amongst the most important in accounting for the giving up of excessive forms of appetitive behaviour later on. Arguably at least, it is the behaviours a person sees modelled by his or her closest associates, and the attitudes and values to which he or she is most intimately exposed, that have most influence at times of change.

Glaser's purpose in his paper (1973) was to trace the lineage of modern drug-free therapeutic communities, of which Synanon in California appears to have been the first, and other communities such as Daytop Village in New York and Phoenix Houses in New York and Britain were later examples. The link with AA is via the founder of Synanon, Charles Dederich, who was himself a graduate of AA. According to Glaser, '. . . it is clear that Synanon evolved out of

Alcoholics Anonymous' (p.6). It was Glaser's view that Synanon introduced some important innovations in translating the AA type of self-help approach into a form that might work with drug addicts:

> Alcoholics Anonymous espouses a God-centred theology, whilst Synanon espouses a secular ideology. In terms of the increasing secularization of civilized life, this change may eventually do more to involve people in self-help movements than any other single step. However the change is one of content. The form is the same. Whether secular or sacred, a form common to all of these organizations is an intensely-held, highly cherished belief system. In an age in which science has made serious (if unwarranted) inroads upon all sorts of mythological systems, the offering of just such a system may partly explain the growing popularity of these programs. Before Dederich, the programs had Religion; now they have religion. The change is one from theology to sociology, which is less of a change than one might suppose. Incidentally, the essentially religious nature of these programs . . . may partly explain the opposition to them by the mental health professions, which are famously and fashionably irreligious (pp.9–10).

Sagarin contrasted self-help organizations which were intent on promoting the reduction of deviance in their members with those, like the homophile organizations, which were dedicated to protecting the interests of deviants who were mainly intent upon continuing their preferred behaviour unhampered. The former type:

> . . . condemns sternly, both moralistically and scientifically, painting the road of eternal damnation that awaits anyone who slips backward . . . deviance-reducing groups exert extreme pressure through inner-group loyalty; they thus develop a pattern of over-conformity in suppressing the controversial behaviour itself . . . [this] results in harsher condemnation of deviance than is found in the general population . . . (pp.22–3).

Whilst Robinson (1979), for example, defended AA's lack of statistics regarding successful outcomes on the grounds that to collect the kind of data necessary for an evaluation would infringe the principle of anonymity central to this particularly resilient and popular form of self-help, Sagarin was generally critical of the way self-help organizations had been allowed to make claims which were clearly 'self-serving' and exaggerated. He found it unusual that they had had, '. . . a sort of immunity from serious scientific study . . .', which would not be surprising were it not for, '. . . the complicity of the social scientists in these patently false presentations' (pp.234–5). He thought it possible that this 'uncritical whitewash' of the tenets of such self-help programmes for appetitive conduct reorganization might actually have hindered progress by helping to maintain such views as that excessive appetitive behaviour constitutes disease or that the only person who can help someone with an excessive appetite is someone who has suffered from that condition themselves.

Sagarin also pointed to the irony that an organization born in part of the Oxford Group Movement which believed that all men were sinners and responsible for their sins, should have reversed that belief and should now ask, '. . . the individual to define as disease exactly that aspect of his life . . . for which he himself is primarily responsible' (p.46).

In his description of what he called the 'inspirational' group therapy of Gamblers Anonymous, Scodel (1964) also noted the spiritual nature of the programme and the way frequent mention was made of newly acquired religiosity incorporated into the person's pronouncement of a reformation of character. The, '. . . renunciation of hedonism and the (avowed) internalization of new, austere values' (p.117), is also a major theme which he noted in group meetings. Frequent mention of adulterous sexual behaviour is also made, as it was with great regularity at Oxford Group confessionals (Glaser, 1973). Of particular interest is the way in which the question of disease, and hence of responsibility for behaviour, is handled in an organization of people who have been 'addicted' to a non-drug activity. Here, the view of excessive appetitive behaviour as a special condition appears to be underpinned by a belief in the theory that the person so afflicted is a 'compulsive loser'. This serves as a denial that the compulsive gambler is motivated in the same way as the casual punter or gambler and affirms his status as a person with a special abnormality. In this case the idea of being motivated to lose as a form of self-punishment, has been borrowed from a poorly supported psychoanalytic hypothesis of Bergler's (1957; see Chapter 8 above), in the same way as the allergy view of alcoholism was borrowed by Alcoholics Anonymous from an unsubstantiated medical hypothesis (Alcoholics Anonymous, 1955).

A close reading of the teachings of Alcoholics Anonymous also serves to link the spiritual approach to appetitive behaviour change with the tactical self-control approach of modern behavioural psychologists. In the AA Big Book (1955) it is stated that before becoming members the, '. . . needed power was not there. Our human resources, as marshalled by the will, were not sufficient . . .' (p.45). By admitting personal powerlessness over the problem (step 1) and putting trust in a higher power however that be defined (step 2),

> . . . we have ceased fighting anything or anyone—even alcohol . . . we will find that this has happened automatically . . . our new attitude . . . has been given us without any thought or effort on our part. It just comes! That is the miracle of it . . . (pp.84–5).

On the other hand, will-power may be exercised in the direction of improving the spiritual condition. Indeed this is the, '. . . proper use of the will' (p.85). In other words 'will-power' may be employed to do things *incompatible* with continued appetitive behaviour, and hence, as is advocated in the behavioural self-control approach, the need for a concept of volition, and the possibility that man operates upon his environment rather than being totally determined by it, is not removed, but the employment of will is pushed back to a new arena where it can more easily be exercised. The appetitive compulsion is too great to exercise an effort of will in order to restrain it directly at the point of maximum temptation, but tactics may be adopted away from the heat of the action which make temptation less likely or which make alternative behaviour more probable. How does this analysis fit with a decisional view of the change process? It almost suggests a completely contrary view. It is as if the subjugation of one's will to a 'higher power' frees the self from an agonizing decision. Perhaps decision-making is actually *avoided* in this way? Difficult decisions of this kind may perhaps be taken by default, or by acting so that the need for decision is circumvented?

That the AA approach does not preclude the use of tactics, some of which bear a remarkable resemblance to behavioural self-control tactics, and including others which are clearly designed to bolster a totally contrary view of alcohol to the one once espoused, is illustrated by much of AA literature. For example, a pamphlet entitled, *15 Points for an Alcoholic to Consider when Confronted with the Urge to Take a Drink* (Alcoholics Anonymous, undated), includes the following items:

> Don't for a split second allow yourself to think: 'Isn't it a pity or a mean injustice that I can't take a drink like so-called normal people'.
>
> Don't allow yourself to either think or talk about any real or imagined pleasure you once did get from drinking.
>
> Don't permit yourself to think a drink or two would make some bad situation better, or at least easier to live with. Substitute the thought: 'one drink will make it worse—one drink will mean a drunk' . . .
>
> Catalogue and re-catalogue the positive enjoyments of sobriety . . .
>
> Cultivate a helpful association of ideas: Associate a drink as being the single cause of all the misery, shame and mortification you have ever known. . . .

The value of thought control for habit development or change was recognized by Emile Coué, William James, and others, before the advent of either AA or modern behavioural self-regulation methods. A succinct statement of Coué's view—'Our actions spring not from our Will but from our Imagination'—appears on the title page of the 1960 reprinting of Coué's, *Self-Mastery Through Conscious Auto-Suggestion*, and Brooks', *The Practice of Auto-Suggestion by the Method of Emile Coué*, both originally published in 1922. Coué's central suggestion was that when people 'will' to do things, being conscious of applying *effort*, they are likely to fail: but when they are convinced that they will do something—what Coué calls 'imagination', although Brooks thinks this is a misleading word and prefers to call it 'thought' ('expectation' might do as well)—then the action is performed *without effort* (recall Bruch's, 1974, woman over-eater whose 'body became stiff' with the effort of resisting eating—Chapter 5). Coué's first two laws of action were, first, that when the will and the imagination are antagonistic, it is always the imagination which wins, without exception; and, secondly, that in the conflict between the will and the imagination, the force of the imagination is in, '. . . direct ratio to the square of the will', a proposal which he emphasized was, '. . . not rigorously exact . . .'! His advocacy of what might now be termed 'self-talk' or 'self-instruction' is well known, especially his use of the statement: 'Every day, in every respect, I am getting better and better' (Coué and Brooks, 1960, p.23).

Even earlier, William James' observations on the subject of habit should ring many bells for latter-day students of excessive appetitive behaviour, once due allowance is made for the style and language of the times in which he was writing. He made much of the fact that the development of habitual behaviour caused a diminution of conscious attention over action, and that habitual acts consisted of chains of behaviour, each event 'calling up' the next, '. . . without any alternative offering itself, and without any reference to the conscious will . . .' (James, 1891, p.114). In considering how habits might be changed, James was much impressed by a chapter on, 'The Moral Habits', by Professor Bain. He took from this chapter two maxims. The first was quoted at the beginning of Chapter 13. The second was:

> *Never suffer an exception to occur till the new habit is securely rooted in your life.* Each lapse is like the letting fall of a ball of string which one is carefully winding up; a single slip undoes more than a great many turns will wind again . . . (pp.122–3, his emphasis).

He cited Professor Bain as believing that moral habits could be distinguished from others by the, '. . . presence of two hostile powers . . .'. The task in habit change was to regulate these so that one had, '. . . a series of uninterrupted successes, until repetition [had] fortified it to such a degree as to enable it to cope with the opposition, under any circumstances' (cited by James, p.123). That James was concerned with the general question of moral improvement is illustrated by his final suggestion, concerning habits of the will, that we should:

> *Keep the faculty of effort alive in you by a little gratuitous exercise every day.* That is, be systematically ascetic or heroic in little unnecessary points, do every day or two something for no other reason than that you would rather not do it, so that when the hour of dire need draws nigh, it may find you not unnerved and untrained to stand the test. Asceticism of this sort is like the insurance which a man pays on his house and goods (p.126, his emphasis).

Rosen and Orenstein (1976) reported finding from a similar period an equivalent of the modern behavioural procedure of 'thought-stopping' used in a case of excessive sexuality. The example comes from Lewis who in 1875 reported treating a man preoccupied with thoughts of nude women and sexual intercourse. He told his patient to:

> Fix it in your mind that a sensual idea is dangerous, harmful; then the instant one comes it will startle you. By an effort you change the subject immediately . . . If there is a moment's doubt, spring up and engage in some active exercise of the body. Each effort will be easier, until after a week or two you will have . . . complete control of your thoughts.

THE COEXISTENCE OF TREATMENT AND MORAL REFORM

Even in 1985 agencies of relatively recent origin, rooted in a modern professional mental health perspective, and others of longer standing with origins in religious and moral reform, coexist side by side. This is nowhere more obvious than in the agencies that serve vagrant excessive drinkers. Wiseman (1970) has given a vivid description of the range of facilities used by skid row 'alcoholics' in a U.S. Western Coast City. Amongst these were the county jail, the state mental hospital, a welfare home for homeless men, and, amongst a variety of others, a Christian missionaries' work and residence centre for handicapped men. Despite the very different perspectives on excessive drinking held by these various institutions, men passed rapidly from one to another, and despite the contrasting beliefs and ideologies of those who worked in them, to those that used them they were interchangeable to a large degree. This state of affairs reflects our continuing confusion about the very nature of excessive appetite itself. As Cook has put it in his book, *Vagrant Alcoholics*, 'Missions and psychiatry coexist painlessly and effortlessly' (1975, p.172).

The Salvation Army, at its height at around the time William James was writing, is an organization that has been active in the field of controlling appetitive behaviour. As outlined in General Booth's book, *In Darkest England, and the Way Out* (1890), its purpose was to rescue large numbers of the 'sinking classes' from a sea of misery and temptation to excess in which drunkenness, gambling, adultery, and fornication figured large. Over eighty years later, a self re-appraisal, *In Darkest England Now* (Salvation Army, 1974), appeared largely in the form of questions posed by an unidentified interviewer with answers mostly by Salvation Army workers, officers, and clients. The questioner seemed preoccupied with the question whether change towards 'social work' or 'community work' in the intervening years was inconsistent with Booth's exhortation to, 'go for souls and go for the worst'. With monotonous uniformity, all respondents replied that the spiritual, mental, physical, economic, and other aspects of man are interdependent, and that the Salvation Army is continuing to save souls by doing social work. The 'penitent form' at which people kneel, confess, and are 'saved' is mentioned a number of times, and of it a Salvation Army Captain says:

> [It] is a good place at which to make public decisions . . . But these life-changing decisions can take place in personal conversation, perhaps over coffee, or kneeling in a sitting room . . . We should not be too rigid about this, or legislate as to where conversion has to take place. It can be in a home. But of course, this decision can be confirmed in front of all the congregation at the hall (p.127).

It is no accident that Gusfield (1962) wrote of the need for a 'repentent role' as part of the process of 'moral passage' out of deviance, and that Sagarin (1969) referred to users of those self-help organizations which seek for their members to conform to the norms of society, as 'penitents'.

Hemming (1969), in his discussion of conflicts over sexual and other kinds of behaviour, has pointed out how hygienic and moral values are still mixed together to this day in official orientations towards many areas of conduct, and has described the clash which occurs when those who adopt what is essentially a short-term utilitarian value approach to matters of sexual conduct, such as abortion, are opposed by others (Mrs Whitehouse and the Television Viewers' Association for example) who adopt attitudes based on moral values.

It may be the ability of self-help organizations to fuse the disease and the moral perspectives that has been a major source of their organizational success, for as the argument of earlier chapters suggests, each perspective on its own has serious shortcomings in accounting for excessive appetitive behaviour. Together they come nearer to an adequate formulation. The combined philosophy is sufficiently seductive to have attracted very large numbers of excessive drinkers, gamblers, drug-users, over-eaters, and people troubled by excessive sexual behaviour. Hence, such organizations are able to provide a multitude of face-to-face groups, as well as a widespread reference group with its own considerable literature, sharing a consensus about the right decision to take with regard to appetitive behaviour, sharing an approach to life which bolsters that decision, and providing a forum within which a pledge or commitment is made. The circumstances are therefore right for a profound attitude and behaviour change, likened by one observer of Alcoholics Anonymous (Tiebout, 1944) to a conversion phenomenon.

Tiebout's analyses of the process of change occurring at Alcoholics Anonymous (Tiebout, 1944, 1961) were reprinted by the National Council on Alcoholism (U.S.A.) and his ideas appear in AA literature (e.g. 1955). He defined conversion as a psychological event in which there was, '. . . a major shift in personality manifestation' (1944, p.2). Previously the person's attitudes were predominantly hostile and negative, but after the conversion process they were largely positive and affirmative. The shift might come about rapidly and dramatically, as in old-style religious conversion, but more typically took place over a longish period of time. Before conversion, 'alcoholics' had a tendency,

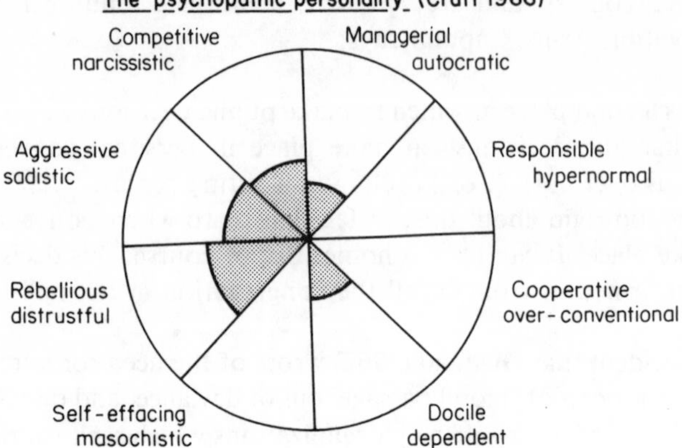

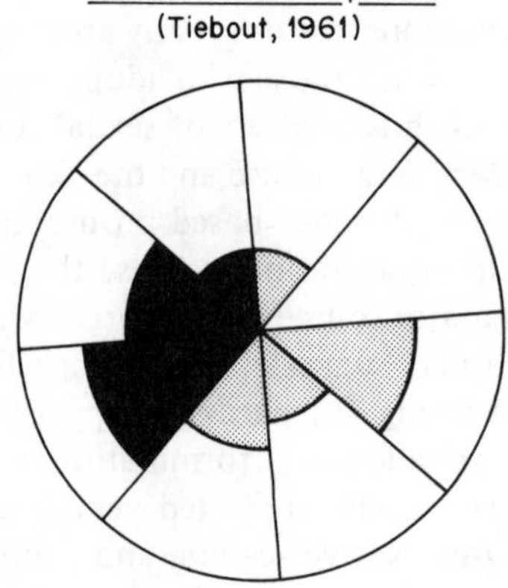

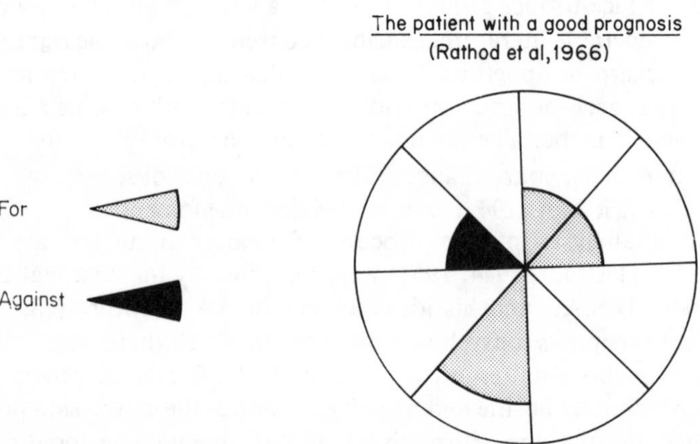

Figure 12 *(caption opposite)*

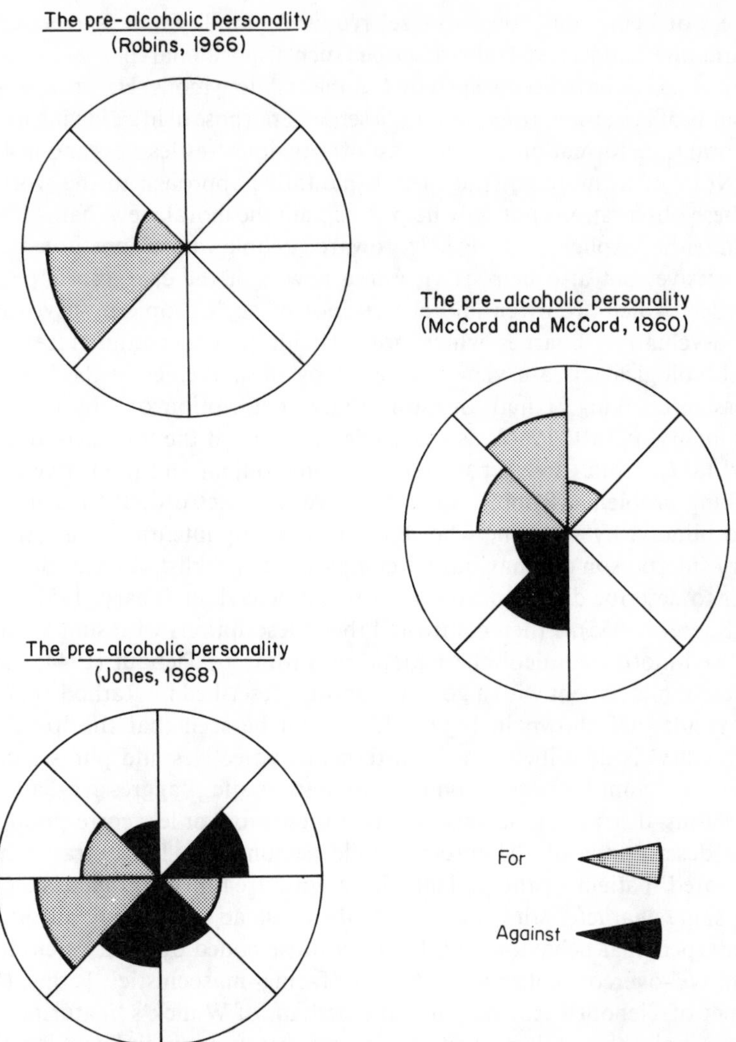

Figure 12 Leary Interpersonal Behaviour Circle depictions of the 'well-motivated alcoholic patient', the 'alcoholic patient with a good prognosis', the 'pre-alcoholic personality', and the 'psychopathic personality' (based on data and descriptions in Tiebout, 1961; Rathod *et al.*, 1966; Robins, 1966; McCord and McCord, 1960; Jones, 1968; and Craft, 1966).

he observed, to be tense and depressed, aggressive, oppressed with a sense of inferiority, whilst at the same time harbouring feelings of superiority, lonely and isolated, egocentric and self-centred, defiant, and walled-off from others. Defiance and '. . . the projections which produce and maintain it . . .' (p.7), he considered to be particularly typical and important. In Freudian terms, the individual had a 'big ego' typical of infantile narcissism. Successful passage through the AA programme involved a process of 'ego reduction', and this process of being 'cut down to size' required humility and 'surrender' to the programme. Scodel (1964) also described such dispositional changes in individuals who claimed to have been helped by Gamblers Anonymous. He wrote of people's accounts of acquiring 'tranquillity', 'a sense of purpose in life', having undergone 'a moral transformation', having cast off previous 'restlessness and instability', in favour of a 'more trusting, less exploitative approach to the world'.

These observations not only help to explain the moral view that is frequently taken, either explicitly or covertly, towards people whose appetitive behaviour is excessive, but also help us view in a new light the charges of 'personality disorder' which are often laid at the door of such people by psychoanalysis and psychiatry—charges which are difficult to understand if seen from a quasi-biological disease view. Intrigued by these themes in the literature on excessive drinking, I had an authoritative description of 'the psychopathic personality' (Craft, 1966), as well as descriptions of the 'pre-alcoholic personality' taken from three separate major longitudinal and predictive studies of drinking problems (Robins, 1966; McCord and McCord, 1960; Jones, 1968), rated blindly, by someone who did not know my intentions, in terms of the Leary Interpersonal Behaviour Circumplex—a checklist of terms developed in order to describe different aspects of social behaviour (Leary, 1957; La Forge and Suczek, 1955). I then contrasted these descriptions with similar ratings of the 'well-motivated alcoholic patient' according to Tiebout (1944, 1961) and the 'alcoholic patient with a good prognosis' described by Rathod *et al.* (1966). The results are shown in Figure 12. It can be seen that the 'psychopathic personality' is described largely in terms of adjectives and phrases coded on Leary's Circumplex in the 'competitive–narcissistic', 'aggressive–sadistic' and 'rebellious–distrustful' octants, and that these more or less correspond with the three descriptions of the 'pre-alcoholic personality'. In contrast, the 'well-motivated' patient or the patient with a good treatment prognosis lacks these very same characteristics, but is described instead as showing all other types of interpersonal behaviour, particularly those coded on Leary's circle as 'co-operative–overconventional' and 'self-effacing–masochistic'. Is this, then, the essence of Tiebout's 'conversion', and perhaps of Winick's 'maturing' as well?

The main theme here is the contrast between discipline, control, and conformity on the one hand, and uncontrolled non-conformity on the other. This dominant theme is to be seen at work whenever attempts are being made to help or coerce people to moderate excessive appetitive behaviour. In our study of therapeutic hostels (Otto and Orford, 1978), for example, we were struck by the way in which staff descriptions of the progress of individual residents seemed to reflect an idea of far-reaching changes in values and conduct. Stopping drinking and staying stopped was only a part of it, and a part to which relatively little reference was made. More frequently mentioned were categories of behaviour which we termed 'responsible involvement' (e.g. 'putting in a lot', 'playing his part', 'part of the house'), 'sense, insight and openness' (e.g. 'realistic', 'thoughtful', 'an appropriate attitude', 'forthcoming'), and 'sociability' (*not*, for example, 'aggressive, bitter', 'cunning, manipulative, exploiting', 'attention-seeking, cock-of-the-walk').

That a moral perspective coexists with a disease view even when excessive drinking, longest accepted as a disease amongst the group of excessive appetites, is treated within a psychiatric setting in the present day, is well illustrated by Davies' (1979) analysis of doctor–patient encounters. In particular he suggested, on the basis of his findings, that the notion of 'motivation' provides the cover under which the moral view operates. Analyses of tape-recorded encounters in two outpatient 'alcoholism' clinics suggested that psychiatrists operate with a kind of counselling style during which they invite a patient to provide information and opinions about the nature of the problem, its aetiology, its management, and the nature of the patient's role and the doctor's role and responsibility in its management. This is consistent with a view of treatment as a process that involves the patient in taking as much responsibility as the doctor, and is consistent with the problem-solving approach to psychological problems taken by D'Zurilla and Goldfried (1971) amongst others.

There was evidence too that the therapists employed the concept of motivation, and did so in the 'static' way of which Sterne and Pittman were critical some years ago (1965). Although attributions of motivation were seldom made explicitly during the consultations themselves, they were made clear in comments made to the research worker afterwards. From the excerpts which Davies provided, it is quite clear that many of these attributions were strongly evaluative and moralistic. For example:

> . . . he's willing to do something about it . . .
>
> . . . appears to be accepting his drink problem and is sincerely determined to do something about it.
>
> . . . she seems to realise that she must stop drinking . . . she means well . . .
>
> I found [his] attitude to his drink problem a very sensible and constructive one.

In contrast to:

> . . . the wife's point about him being selfish. She is so right . . . He's trying to make a good impression to the court.
>
> . . . making all of the usual noises . . . He's really an irresponsible psychopathic citizen.
>
> What a dreadful person . . . I can't decide whether he is an inadequate personality or an inadequate psychopath. He's certainly terribly immature. He's no motivation whatsoever.

> . . . appears to have no insight at all into the severity of his drink problem . . .

Davies concluded:

> . . . The data presented in this paper suggests that patients' will-power, strength or weakness of character, and self-responsibility are the basic constituent features of the psychiatric treatment of alcoholism. In this respect the health and alcoholism literature's suggestion that alcoholism is 'like any other illness' appears to be rather inexact (p.457).

Treatment appears to consist largely of 'non-specific' elements: helping patients gain new insight into their lives and emotional needs. To patients, Davies comments, this may, '. . . seem like moral work' (p.456).

Davies points out that the nature of these encounters between doctors and patients does not conform to the Parsonian model of the sick role in which the professional applies skill and knowledge and remains objective and affectively neutral, in return for which the patient is obliged to show motivation to get well, to seek technically competent help, and to put trust in the professional (Parsons, 1951). What was going on in these exchanges corresponded more closely, he suggested, to the 'mutual participation' model of doctor–patient interaction put forward by Szasz and Hollender (1956) to describe a type of exchange in which it is the doctor's role to help the patient to help himself and the patient's role to participate in this partnership.

It is consistent with the model of excessive appetitive behaviour developed here that the maintenance of affective neutrality will be difficult in the face of such behaviour, provided the behaviour is confronted at all. Some psychoanalysts (Adams, 1978) refuse, perhaps wisely, to give advice on such matters as drug or alcohol use and avoid making such issues the focus of discussion in treatment. They may, thereby, retain the kind of non-judgemental relationship considered by them to be essential for progress. Few others, who come into contact with excessive appetitive behaviour, retain this composure, however.

At the opposite extreme from the non-interventionist psychotherapist are those, notably close family, who bear the fullest brunt of excessive behaviour and must make some reaction to it. The varied reactions of family members to a person within their midst whom they identify as having a drinking problem (Orford *et al.*, 1975; Wilson C., 1982) testify both to the virtual impossibility of remaining neutral under such circumstances, and to the availability of a number of different positions or roles which can be adopted. Family members usually try out a variety of such 'coping' responses but rarely remain neutral. Many such responses may be seen as falling into one of two general classes; those that represent attempts at coercion or control of the excessive behaviour or the person displaying it, and those that represent a kind of defeatist withdrawal from or avoidance of the person whose behaviour is identified as being excessive.

Although many treatment personnel attempt to maintain a non-judgemental acceptance of the person whilst at the same time confronting the issue of the excessive behaviour, this is not always easy and sometimes therapists are placed in a position that makes this balance almost impossible to maintain. For example, on the basis of his research at London 'drug dependency' clinics (DDCs), Stimson (1978) has pointed to the dilemma for staff working there. The question of control, which is an underlying issue whenever excessive appetitive behaviour is confronted, is brought out in stark relief in such settings. In such clinics in Britain, the staff are required to report users of certain drugs such as heroin to the Home Office. Besides which, one of the avowed aims of DDCs, set up under the 1967 Dangerous Drugs Act, was the control of the availability of dangerous drugs and the prevention of the development of a black market. That staff in this case are in the business of social control for the benefit of society as a whole is inescapable.

Stimson described a clash of perspectives between staff and patients, the central conflict being the users' need for drugs, and the staff's desire to control prescribing and to wean individuals away from drugs if possible:

> In the experience of the staff most addicts are liars . . . the situation is one that will generate lying on both sides. The upshot is that clinic staff distrust patients and are ever on the lookout against being conned by them (p.60).

Stimson saw this situation as arising because staff had a monopoly over the resource wanted by the clients, namely drugs. Although this situation must undoubtedly make the conflict greater, the breakdown in trust and communication is very similar to that found in many families where one member has a problem of excessive drug-taking, drinking, or gambling, and the real source of conflict is the confrontation between one person with an excessive appetite and another who wants him or her to give up this behaviour, or at least moderate it. If the latter is also a person in a position to supply the former's appetitive needs, then this scenario may be intensified, but it is in essence the same.

Saxon *et al.* (1978) have described a similar kind of dilemma for staff of methadone maintenance treatment programmes in the United States. They described how a counsellor is torn between the requirement to establish an alliance with a client whilst at the same time having to monitor the latter's drug use. An early task, according to Saxon *et al.*, was to establish that the client did have the two-year history of opiate addiction that needed to be proved before methadone could be prescribed. Apart from this interrogating, and potentially alienating role, counsellors were usually also required to observe the client while giving a urine specimen at periodic intervals, and also to obtain proof of employment by examining, for example, a stub from a current pay cheque.

Although such a programme, with its strict rules and procedures, points it up in obvious form, this potential confusion between roles in relation to someone whose appetitive behaviour is excessive is inherent in the behaviour itself. Indeed, it is a part of the argument of this book that excessive appetitive behaviours simultaneously invite a number of responses, including some that are punitive and others that are non-judgemental. These roles can be split and played by different parties, or they can be combined in the one person, as in the case of the methadone programme counsellor or 'drug dependency' clinic staff member. The different possible modes of responding to excess are often displayed in clear contrast by different family members or different agents in society. One member of a family may take a more controlling role, another that of sympathetic ally; the bookmaker supplies the means, the magistrate the punishment, the psychologist the mitigating plea in court.

Edwards (1977) and also Kurland (1978) have discussed the issue of compulsion in the treatment of excessive drug users. In the United States there has been vigorous debate and legal battles over the efficacy and ethics of compulsory treatment (Kurland, 1978). In Britain, according to Edwards (1977), the question has often been posed but has not obtained wide support and in recent years has slipped out of sight. Dr Branthwaite was one member of the Rolleston Committee (1926b) who championed the cause of compulsion but received little support. Edwards tells us that at an early meeting of the committee he expressed the view:

> My general opinion is that drug cases are so difficult to control that they cannot be treated satisfactorily on any voluntary basis. They are so unreliable and untrustworthy that their word cannot possibly be taken, and under these circumstances I feel that cases of addiction should be dealt with in very much the same manner as persons of unsound mind.

Although this view has not carried the day, then or now, Edwards has encouraged us to question whether 'treatment' for drug 'addiction', and much the same question could be asked of 'treatment' for excessive drinkers and gamblers, is conducted purely on a voluntary basis or whether it is not the case that an involuntary, but poorly acknowledged, system of 'treatment' is in existence concurrently. How many 'addicts', he asked, are given custodial sentences for drug offences or for offences such as petty theft, closely connected with their addiction? How often are probation orders conferred with a 'condition' of treatment attached? How often are 'addicts' detained in a mental hospital under any provision of the Mental Health Act? And, lastly, how frequently is the 'addict's' compliance in a 'voluntary' treatment forced by threat or manipulation?

With our understanding of excess as behaviour which repeatedly violates norms of control and moderation, it is predictable that there should always be the possibility of coercion by family, friends, or the law. Excessive appetitive behaviour is out-of-control behaviour and thus it constantly invites attempts at control. These efforts at restraint are not confined to other people or institutions, however. Indeed, much of the argument of the later chapters of this book has been that the person who experiences an excessive appetite is often the one who is most critical of her own behaviour and the one who exercises the firmest self-control. If it is the case that excessive appetitive behaviour is in itself paradoxical, a further paradox is contained in the fact that the conflict it creates has within it the seeds of change. Drug 'addiction', 'compulsive gambling', 'alcoholism', unwanted smoking, over-eating, and 'hypersexuality', can all be very troublesome, often to the point of threatening life and relationships. But each carries with it the possibility of positive change, often sudden and dramatic but more often slow and uncertain, sometimes with expert help but usually without it.

CHAPTER FIFTEEN

Summary

> Hippocrates: . . . In [Mark Twain's] days, Americans were level-headed people. They knew the difference between a habit, like drinking or drug-taking, and a disease, like cancer or rheumatism. Now they prattle about 'alcoholism' and 'drug abuse' as diseases. What nonsense!
>
> Socrates: It's worse than nonsense. It's an outright lie. . . . Don't despair. Perhaps they'll reject this folly and reaffirm their dedication to individual dignity. Perhaps. (From a fictional modern dialogue on drug education conceived by Thomas Szasz, 1978, p.14).
>
> . . . if we are to be as prudent as may be, might not wisdom indicate an experimental procedure in which we commit ourselves to the disease view [of alcoholism] on a trial basis and judge finally the soundness of our definition by its consequences? (Seeley, 1962, p.593).

How do we stand more than 20 years after Seeley suggested we give a disease view a trial period? Does the review conducted in these pages suggest that we have a coherent alternative to offer to the many people and practitioners who have become disaffected with a disease model, or must we agree with Shaffer and Burglass (1981) who concluded in the epilogue to their collection of, *Classic Contributions in the Addictions*, that the field of addiction studies was in a pre-paradigm state where almost any information was relevant and where there was an absence of leading theory? Have modern behavioural and social sciences produced insights which would have aided Walter in an understanding of his sexual excess, Dostoevsky his gambling mania, Lilian Roth her 'alcoholism', the worried parents their son or daughter's drug 'addiction', or members of weight groups their over-eating? Or must we reluctantly admit that the conclusion of all this endeavour has been a re-statement of what was intuitively obvious to these individuals, with some additional but disparate facts and theories thrown in to add to their confusion?

The argument of the preceding chapters may be summarized as follows.

1. There exists *a range of appetitive activities* which can become excessive. These include eating, heterosexual activity, and gambling. Although these activities appear very different, the experiences of those who are excessive are similar in many respects. Even in the case of drugs, a simple division into those that are 'addictive' and those that are not is no longer tenable, and any consideration of the nature of excessive appetitive behaviour must embrace drugs such as alcohol, tobacco, and the 'minor' tranquillizing drugs, each of which has at sometime or another been excluded from consideration by those who would have us confine our attention to a more limited class of phenomena.

2. The degree of a person's involvement in each of these appetitive activities has *multiple interacting determinants*. These include features of character or personality, but some of the strongest determinants are social or ecological, including the availability of opportunities for activity and the normative influence of friends. This wide range of determinants includes those that operate to restrain activity, or which offer disincentives, as well as those which operate to promote activity, or which offer incentives. Fear of the effects of drugs or religious views about the use of alcohol may act as restraints, for example. Friends' views and availability may promote behaviour for one person but restrain activity for another. This way of looking at things is clearly identifiable as a form of social learning theory (Akers *et al.*, 1979). In contrast to this social view, the clinical or disease model has tended to focus more narrowly upon those aspects of individual personality which were thought to promote appetitive behaviour, and has tended to neglect social and ecological variables and factors which act to restrain.

3. Each of the major appetitive activities considered can serve *numerous personal functions* for different individuals, and even within the same person. These include forms of mood modification as well as the enabling of many different forms of self expression and the enhancing of many different kinds of self-identity. Cross-cultural and historical perspectives are invaluable in pointing to the different meanings which can be attached to the same activity, and to the different routes which may be taken towards excess. Even within one culture at one time, however, the personal uses to which appetitive activities may be put varies greatly depending among other things upon age, gender, and social class. Seen in this light, it is little wonder that single factor theories of the origins of excessive appetitive behaviour have met with such little success. Tension reduction, as an example, turns out to be a highly complex and controversial matter. A strong case can be made for eating and gambling as potentially anxiolytic activities.

4. *A longitudinal perspective is vital* for understanding appetitive behaviour and excess. Changes in behaviour are the rule rather than the exception, and frequently occur as part of a developmentally normal change in a whole

constellation of attitudes, experiences, values, and activities. Leaving home, going to college, joining the armed forces, getting married, are amongst the landmarks in this developmental process. Normative changes in behaviour may be upward or downward depending upon age and stage (Jessor and Jessor, 1977). Different personal functions may be served by the same activity at different stages for the same individual, and different personal and social factors may be predictive of different transitions from one life stage to another. This relatively new emphasis upon appetitive behaviour as a dynamic, changing process through time provides further grounds for mistrusting simple predispositional theories of excessive behaviour.

5. *Population distribution curves* for extent of involvement in a number of appetitive activities take a similar, and markedly skewed, form with a mode representing abstinence or very moderate indulgence. There are two, not mutually exclusive, explanations for the shape of these curves which support the present model of appetitive behaviour. One is that these are reversed J-shaped conformity curves demonstrating the effect of restraint, control, and impediment, deterring the manifestation of behaviour promoted by a variety of biological and social influences. This supports the relevance of a balance-of-forces type of social learning theory.

6. An alternative explanation is that appetitive behaviour is subject to *the law of proportionate effect* whereby the influence of a new behaviour-promoting event is proportional to the cumulative effect of previous influences. Operant learning theory, with its various schedules of positive and negative reinforcement, provides ample grounds for expecting that a developmental process of increasing attachment to appetitive behaviour might occur. This is particularly persuasive when account is taken of the many opportunities which appetitive behaviour settings provide for the operation of discriminative stimuli, and the abundant opportunities that exist for the development of behaviour-enhancing expectations, attributions, and fantasies. Such a learning process, which would satisfy the law of proportionate effect, would be expected to develop under circumstances of relatively strong inclination and relatively weak restraint.

7. This developmental *process of increasing attachment* is manifest in the form of increasingly generalized activity and the erosion of the discriminations which maintain normally moderate activity. Activity becomes more widely cue-linked, serves a wider range of personal functions, is more likely to serve intrinsic, personal, non-social purposes, and may become automatic and functionally autonomous. Although there is this possibility of a progressive increase in attachment to activity, this process is much more varied in length and effect than was suggested by some earlier progression theories. Furthermore, whilst the habit component may become an important one, original social and personal motives for appetitive behaviour continue to operate to a greater or lesser extent.

8. The development of an *altered biological response* as a result of exposure is clearly established in the case of some drugs, and is less clearly established in the case of others. However, the role of altered biological response in understanding the development of strong affective–behavioural–cognitive

attachment to a drug is controversial. Biological and psychological systems are inseparable, and there is good reason to suppose that increasing attachment to a non-drug appetitive activity will affect physiological responses, and vice versa. The integration of biological change and learning is relevant to all excessive appetites. Lessened control over behaviour, felt desire, or craving for the object of the activity, and increasingly stereotyped behavioural patterns, are major features of all excesses, and in their modern more complex forms notions of loss of control, craving, and narrowed behavioural repertoire are applicable to drug and non-drug appetites alike.

9. Strong and relatively indiscriminate attachment to appetitive behaviour runs increased *risk of incurring costs* which may be physical or social, immediate or longer term, affecting the self or others. Costs are personally and socially relative, however, depending upon numerous factors including age, sex, values, social roles, and circumstances. Excess is not an absolute, but is personally and socially defined. Reaction against, or criticism of, appetitive activity is necessary in order for it to be labelled 'addiction' or 'dependence'. Excessive appetitive behaviour is an example of deviance, but deviancy theory alone is insufficient without the inclusion of the possibility of the development of increased attachment. The incurring of costs or harm from behaviour may amplify the process of increasing attachment, for example by encouraging alterations of role and social group, and by weakening relationships with sources of social control and restraint. Costs may, on the other hand, reduce attachment by shifting the balance of incentives and disincentives in a direction that encourages increased moderation.

10. The balance-of-forces social learning model suggests that ambivalence is likely to characterize appetitive behaviour at all levels. The development of increased attachment, plus the incurring of costs, may result in a more obvious, and personally disturbing, *conflict of motives*. This may be depicted as an avoidance–approach conflict with the approach gradient rising more steeply towards the point of consumption or activity. This may help to explain the feeling of being restrained, of decisional conflict, and moral dilemma, and the apparently impulsive nature of loss of control and relapse. Many of the behaviours which give rise to charges of bad character or 'personality disorder' amongst those with excessive appetites can be attributed to the cognitive dissonance created by unresolved conflict.

11. Change in appetitive behaviour in the direction of greater moderation or abstinence is a naturally occurring response to the ambivalence, conflict, or dilemma which attends the appetites. Such changes may occur at all stages, and at all levels of attachment to the activity. The changes are best construed as *personal decisions*, and are influenced by factors in the everyday social setting, changes in roles and circumstances, humiliating and other change-promoting events, social coercion, changes in motives with age, and communications from a variety of sources.

12. There is agreement that making such decisions is a *multi-stage process* involving at least making the initial decision or finding the initial solution to

a problem, and later maintenance or commitment. The initial decision may be reached suddenly or slowly, but it is likely to involve vigilant information processing and monitoring of or attention to behaviour, as opposed to defensive avoidance (Janis and Mann, 1977). Particularly when attachment has been strong, decisions are likely to be vulnerable and many breakdowns and reversions to earlier stages of the decision-making process are to be expected, particularly under conditions of mood arousal and low vigilance. Similar relapse curves showing high rates of breakdown shortly after treatment for different excessive appetitive behaviours bear out these expectations. Chronic excessive appetitive behaviour may be viewed as the result of a series of failed opportunities for committed decision-making.

13. Particularly with very difficult decisions, when attachment is strong and costs high, conflict is extreme and change involves not only high quality information processing but also *self-reconstitution*, the adoption of a new identity, a shift of attitudes and values across a wide range of issues. Change-supporting agencies have often taken a religious form. In addition, self-help, therapeutic community, and other helping agencies combine moral–religious and medical–disease ideas and have historical links with religiously based organizations. They frequently involve tactics of public testimony, thought control, and submission to the will of an external agent such as a group or a 'higher power'. The emphasis upon movement from a personal stance of egocentrism and hedonism to one of humility and asceticism further illustrates the view that change in appetitive behaviour constitutes a kind of moral passage.

14. Besides these naturally occurring processes, modern forms of *expert treatment* play a modest part in excessive appetitive behaviour change. There exists a very wide range of treatment rationales and procedures but they produce a rather similar and modest result in the short term, although careful research suggests they have some effectiveness. Evidence suggests that factors common to different treatments, such as the client's engagement in attending to behaviour, positive engagement in a treatment programme, the feeling of being listened to and understood, involvement of family, and the expectation of change, are the more effective ingredients. Modern professional and traditional religious–moral agencies and ideas co-exist. That professional treatment for excessive appetitive behaviour is partly moral work is not officially acknowledged.

The reader will judge whether this model, or way-of-looking-at excessive drinking, gambling, drug-taking, eating, and sexuality enhances our understanding or confuses further. Disease models have produced undoubted benefits. How else could the medical profession be convinced that an excessive drinker was a suitable case for special and sympathetic consideration, or the wife of an excessive gambler be persuaded that her husband's beastliness was attributable to his modifiable gambling rather than to his unmodifiable character, without recourse to some notion of sickness? But it seems that well-established disease models, such as that of 'alcoholism', have not reduced stigma, and in the end have not convinced the doctors and the lawmakers (as witnessed by the exclusion of excessive drinking from the category mental disorder in the recent U.K. Mental Health Act; Bluglass, 1983).

Of even greater importance, disease models are now retarding our understanding. They put too great a weight upon the experience of clinical cases and insufficient upon the far more numerous instances of troublesome appetitive behaviour in the general population. They have elevated the role of expert, particularly medical, help out of all proportion to its real significance, and they have over-emphasized the one factor of altered biological response, or 'physical addiction', and have hence neglected the psychological mechanisms involved in the development of strong attachment to appetitive activity. As a result they have narrowed our sights upon excessive drug use, and particularly upon a few categories of drugs thought to have major 'addiction' potential, and have prevented us from developing a satisfactory science of addiction in the more generally understood lay sense of that word. In particular they have hindered a useful cross-fertilization of ideas between alcohol, drug, gambling, eating, and sexual behaviour studies. It is towards this much overdue rapprochement that this book has aimed to make a contribution.

References

Abel, E. (1980). Fetal Alcohol Syndrome, Behavioral Teratology, *Psychological Bulletin*, **87**, 29–50.

Abelson, R. (1963). Computer Simulation of 'Hot' Cognition, in *Computer Simulation of Personality* (Eds. S. Tomkins and S. Messick), Wiley, New York (cited by Janis and Mann, 1977).

Ablon, J. (1974). Al-Anon Family Groups: Impetus for Learning and Change through the Presentation of Alternatives, *American Journal of Psychotherapy*, **28**, 30–45.

Adams, J. (1978). *Psychoanalysis of Drug Dependence: Understanding and Treatment of a Particular Form of Pathological Narcissism*, Grune & Stratton, New York.

Adler, N. and Goleman, D. (1969). Gambling and Alcoholism: Symptom Substitution and Functional Equivalency, *Quarterly Journal of Studies on Alcohol*, **30**, 733–736.

Advisory Committee to the Surgeon General (1964). *Smoking and Health*, Department of Health, Education and Welfare, U.S. Public Health Service Publication 1103, Washington D.C., U.S. Government Printing Office.

Aitchison, J. and Brown, J. (1966). *The Lognormal Distribution*, Cambridge University Press, Cambridge.

Akers, R., Krohn, M., Lanza-Kaduch, L., and Radosevich, M. (1979). Social Learning and Deviant Behavior: a Specific Test of a General Theory, *American Sociological Review*, **44**, 636–655.

Alcoholics Anonymous (1955). *AA: the Story of how Many Men and Women have Recovered from Alcoholism*, AA Stirling Area Services (second edition).

Alcoholics Anonymous (Undated). 15 Points for an Alcoholic to Consider when Confronted with the Urge to Take a Drink.

Alcott, W. (1853). *The Physical and Moral Effects of Using Tobacco as Luxury*, Harned, New York (cited by Jaffe, 1977).

Alexander, B., Beyerstein, B., Hadaway, P., and Coambs, R. (1981). The Effect of Early and Later Colony Housing on Oral Ingestion of Morphine in Rats, *Pharmacology, Biochemistry, and Behavior*, **15**, 571–576 (cited by Alexander and Hadaway, 1982).

Alexander, B. and Hadaway, P. (1982). Opiate Addiction: the Case for an Adaptive Orientation, *Psychological Bulletin*, **92**, 367–381.

Allbutt, T. (1870). On the Abuse of Hypodermic Injections of Morphia, *The Practitioner*, **5**, 327–331.

Allport, F. (1934). The J-Curve Hypothesis of Conforming Behaviour, *Journal of Social Psychology*, **5**, 141–181.

Allport, G. (1961). *Pattern and Growth in Personality*, Holt, New York.
American Medical Association Committee on Alcoholism and Addiction and Council on Mental Health (1965). Dependence on Barbituates and other Sedative Drugs, *Journal of the American Medical Association*, **193**, 673–677 (cited by Wesson and Smith, 1977, p.56).
American Medicine (1915). Editorial, November, 799–800 (cited by Brecher, 1972, p.50).
Anonymous (1966). *My Secret Life*. Grove Press, New York.
Archard, P. (1979). *Vagrancy, Alcoholism and Social Control*, Macmillan, London.
Armor, D., Polich, J., and Stambul, H. (1978). *Alcoholism and Treatment*, Wiley, New York (originally 1976, Santa Monica, Rand Corporation).
Aronfreed, J. (1968). *Conduct and Conscience: the Socialisation of Internalised Control over Behaviour*, Academic Press, New York.
Ashton, J. (1898, orig. 1619). *The Nicker Nicked, or the Cheats of Gaming Discovered*. Cited by Ashton, History of Gambling in England (cited by France, C., The Gambling Impulse, *American Journal of Psychology*, **13**, 1902, 364–407).
Ashwell, M. (1978). Commercial Weight Loss Groups, in *Recent Advances in Obesity Research, II*, Proceedings of the Second International Congress on Obesity, October 1977, Washington D.C. (Ed. G. Bray), Newman, London.
Ashwell, M. and Etchell, L. (1974). Attitude of the Individual to his own Body Weight, *British Journal of Preventive and Social Medicine*, **28**, 127–132.
Astin, A. (1962). 'Bad Habits' and Social Deviation: a Proposed Revision in Conflict Theory, *Journal of Clinical Psychology*, **18**, 227–231.
Athey, G. and Coyne, L. (1979). Toward a Rapprochement of Empirical and Clinical Enquiry in Evaluation of Psychologically Oriented Alcoholism Treatment, *Alcoholism: Clinical and Experimental Research*, **3**, 341–350.
Auerback, A. (1968). Satyriasis and Nymphomania, *Medical Aspects of Human Sexuality*, **September 1968**, 39–45.
Baasher, T. (1981). The Use of Drugs in the Islamic World, *British Journal of Addiction*, **76**, 233–243.
Bacon, S. (1973). The Process of Addiction to Alcohol: Social Aspects, *Quarterly Journal of Studies on Alcohol*, **34**, 1–27.
Bales, R. (1945). Social Therapy for a Social Disorder — Compulsive Drinking, *Journal of Social Issues*, **1**, 14.
Balint, M. *et al.* (1970). *Treatment or Diagnosis: a Study of Repeat Prescriptions in General Practice*, Tavistock, London.
Bandura, A. (1977). *Social Learning Theory*, Prentice-Hall, Englewood Cliffs, New Jersey.
Bannister, D. (1975). Preface, in *Issues and Approaches in the Psychological Therapies* (Ed. D. Bannister), Wiley, London.
Banting, W. (1863). *Letter on Corpulence Addressed to the Public*, Harrison, London (cited by Bray, G., 1978, To Treat or Not to Treat — That is the Question, in *Recent Advances in Obesity Research, II*, Proceedings of the Second International Congress on Obesity, Washington D.C., October 1977, Ed. G. Bray, Newman, London).
Barbeyrac, J. (1737). *Traite du jeu*, 3 vols, Amsterdam. Cited by France, C., The Gambling Impulse, *American Journal of Psychology*, **13**, 1902, 364–407.
Barker, J. and Miller, M. (1968). Aversion Therapy for Compulsive Gambling, *Journal of Nervous and Mental Disease*, **146**, 285–302.
Baron, R. (1968). Attitude Change through Discrepant Action: a Functional Analysis, in *The Psychological Foundations of Attitudes* (Eds. A. Greenwald, T. Brock, and T. Ostrom), Academic Press, New York.
Barry, H. (1976). Cross-Cultural Evidence that Dependency Conflict Motivates Drunkenness, in *Cross-Cultural Approaches to the Study of Alcohol: an Interdisciplinary Perspective* (Eds. M. Everett, J. Waddell, and D. Heath), Mouton, The Hague.

Becker, H. (1963). Becoming a Marihuana User, in *Outsiders* (Ed. H. Becker), Free Press, New York.

Behar, D. and Winokur, G. (1979). Research in Alcoholism and Depression: a Two-way Street under Construction, in *Psychiatric Factors in Drug Abuse* (Eds. R. Pickens and L. Heston), Grune and Stratton, New York.

Bennett, E. (1955). Discussion, Decision, Commitment, and Consensus in 'Group Decision', *Human Relations*, **8**, 251–274.

Bennett, J. (1981). The Experience of the Campaign on the Use and Restriction of Barbiturates, in *The Misuse of Psychotropic Drugs* (Eds. R. Murray, H. Ghodse, C. Harris, D. Williams, and P. Williams), Gaskell, The Royal College of Psychiatrists, London.

Bem, D. (1967). Self-perception: an Alternative Interpretation of Cognitive Dissonance phenomena, *Psychological Review*, **74**, 183–200.

Bergin, A. (1971). The Evaluation of Therapeutic Outcomes, in *Handbook of Psychotherapy and Behavior Change* (Eds. A. Bergin and S. Garfield), Wiley, New York.

Bergin, A. and Lambert, M. (1978). The Evaluation of Therapeutic Outcomes, in *Handbook of Psychotherapy and Behavior Change: an Empirical Analysis* (Eds. S. Garfield and A. Bergin), Wiley, New York.

Bergler, E. (1958). *The Psychology of Gambling*, Harrison, London.

Bernstein, D. (1970). The Modification of Smoking Behavior: an Evaluative Review, in *Learning Mechanisms in Smoking* (Ed. W. Hunt), Aldine, Chicago.

Bernstein, D. and McAllister, A. (1976). The Modification of Smoking Behavior: Progress and Problems, *Addictive Behaviors*, **1**, 89–102.

Berridge, V. (1977a). Opium and the Historical Perspective, *The Lancet*, **9 July 1977**, 78–80.

Berridge, V. (1977b). Fenland Opium Eating in the Nineteenth Century, *British Journal of Addiction*, **72**, 275–284.

Berridge, V. (1977c). Our Own Opium: Cultivation of the Opium Poppy in Britain, 1740–1823, *British Journal of Addiction*, **72**, 90–94.

Berridge, V. (1978). Opium Eating and the Working Class in the Nineteenth Century: The Public and Official Reaction, *British Journal of Addiction*, **73**, 107–112.

Berridge, V. (1979). Morality and Medical Science: Concepts of Narcotic Addiction in Britain, 1820–1926, *Annals of Science*, **36**, 67–85.

Berridge, V. and Rawson, N. (1979). Opiate Use and Legislative Control: a Nineteenth Century Case Study, *Social Science and Medicine*, **13A**, 351–363.

Bigelow, G. and Liebson, I. (1972). Cost Factors Controlling Alcoholics' Drinking, *Psychological Record*, **22**, 305–310.

Björk, S. (1950). Alcoholism from the Psychological Viewpoint, *Svenska Lakartidn*, **47**, 1018–1026 (cited by Jellinek, 1960, p.58).

Blaxter, M. (1978). Diagnosis as Category and Process: the Case of Alcoholism, *Social Science and Medicine*, **12**, 9–17.

Bluglass, R. (1983). *A Guide to the Mental Health Act 1983*, Churchill Livingstone, London.

Bolen, D. and Boyd, W. (1968). Gambling and the Gambler: a Review and Preliminary Findings, *Archives of General Psychiatry*, **18**, 617–630.

Booth, W. (1970, orig. 1890). *In Darkest England, and the Way Out*, Knight, London.

Bowers, W. (1968). Normative Constraints on Deviant Behavior in the College Context, *Sociometry*, **31**, 370–385.

Boyd, W. and Bolen, D. (1970). The Compulsive Gambler and Spouse in Group Psychotherapy, *International Journal of Group Psychotherapy*, **20**, 77–90.

Bray, G. (Ed.) (1978). *Recent Advances in Obesity Research, II*, Proceedings of the Second International Congress on Obesity, October 1977, Washington D.C., Newman, London.

Brecher, E. and the Editors of Consumer Reports (1972). *Licit and Illicit Drugs: the Consumers Union Report on Narcotics, Stimulants, Depressants, Inhalants, Hallucinogens, and Marijuana—including Caffeine, Nicotine and Alcohol*, Little, Brown and Co., Toronto.

Briddell, D., Rimm, D., Caddy, G., Krawitz, G., Sholis, D., and Wunderlin, R. (1978). Effects of Alcohol and Cognitive Set on Sexual Arousal to Deviant Stimuli, *Journal of Abnormal Psychology*, **87**, 418–430.

Brill, L., Nash, G., and Langrod, J. (1972). The Dynamics of De-addiction—a Pilot Study, in *Major Modalities in the Treatment of Drug Abuse* (Eds. L. Brill and L. Lieberman), Behavioral Publications, New York (cited by Kurland, 1978).

British Medical Journal (1968). Compulsive Gambler, Leading Article, **13 April 1968**, 69.

Broadhurst, A. (1976). Applications of the Psychology of Decisions, in *Theoretical and Experimental Bases of the Behaviour Therapies* (Eds. M. Feldman and A. Broadhurst), Wiley, Chichester.

Bromet, E. and Moos, R. (1977). Environmental Resources and the Post-treatment Functioning of Alcoholic Patients, *Journal of Health and Social Behaviour*, **18**, 326–338.

Brotman, R., Meyer, A., and Freedman, A. (1965). An Approach to Treating Narcotic Addicts based on Community Mental Health Diagnosis, *Comprehensive Psychiatry*, **6**, 104 (cited by Kurland, 1978).

Bruch, H. (1974). *Eating Disorders: Obesity, Anorexia Nervosa, and the Person Within*, Routledge & Kegan Paul, London.

Bullough, V. (1977). Sex Education in Medieval Christianity, *Journal of Sex Research*, **13**, 185–196.

Bunzel, R. (1940). The Role of Alcoholism in Two Central American Cultures, *Psychiatry*, **3**, 361–387.

Bynner, J. (1969). *The Young Smoker*, HMSO, London.

Cahalan, D. (1970). *Problem Drinkers*, Jossey-Bass, San Francisco.

Cahalan, D. and Room, R. (1974). *Problem Drinking Among American Men*, College and University Press, New Haven.

Campbell, D. and Watson, J. (1978). A Comparative Study of 18 Glue Sniffers, *Community Health*, **9**, 207–210.

Cappell, H. and Herman, C. (1972). Alcohol and Tension Reduction: a Review, *Quarterly Journal of Studies on Alcohol*, **33**, 33–64.

Carlin, A. and Armstrong, H. (1968). Aversive Conditioning: Learning or Dissonance Reduction?, *Journal of Consulting and Clinical Psychology*, **32**, 674–678.

Carstairs, G. (1968). Compulsive Gambler, Letter, *British Medical Journal*, **April 1968**, 239.

Carstairs, S. (1954). Daru and Bhang: Cultural Factors in the Choice of Intoxicant, *Quarterly Journal of Studies on Alcohol*, **15**, 220–237.

Cartwright, A. (1980). The Attitudes of Helping Agents towards the Alcoholic Client, *British Journal of Addiction*, **75**, 413–431.

Cartwright, A. (1981). Are Different Therapeutic Perspectives important in the Treatment of Alcoholism?, *British Journal of Addiction*, **76**, 347–362.

Cartwright, A., Shaw, S., and Spratley, T. (1975). Designing a Comprehensive Community Response to Problems of Alcohol Abuse, Report to the Department of Health and Social Security by the Maudsley Alcohol Pilot Project, London.

Cautela, J. (1971). Covert Conditioning, in *The Psychology of Private Events* (Eds. A. Jacobs and L. Sachs), Academic Press, London.

Chafetz, M., Blane, H., and Hill, M. (Eds.) (1970). *Frontiers of Alcoholism*, Science House, New York.

Chein, I., Gerard, D., Lee, R., and Rosenfeld, E. (1964). *Narcotics, Delinquency and Social Policy: The Road to H*, Basic Books, New York.

Cherrington, E. (1920). *The Evolution of Prohibition in the USA*, American Issue Press, Westville, Ohio (cited by Levine, 1978, pp.153–154).

Chesser, E. (1974). The Nymphomaniac: Always Willing—Why?, *Sexology*, **40**, 10–14.

Chick, J. (1980). Is there a Unidimensional Alcohol Dependence Syndrome?, *British Journal of Addiction*, **75**, 265–280.

Churches' Council on Gambling (1960–1968). Annual Reports of the Churches' Council on Gambling, CCG, London (cited by Cornish, 1978).

Coates, T. (1977). Theory, Research, and Practice in Treating Obesity: Are they Really All the Same?, *Addictive Behaviors*, **2**, 95–103.

Coffey, T. (1966). Beer Street: Gin Lane: Some Views of Eighteenth Century Drinking, *Quarterly Journal of Studies on Alcohol*, **27**, 669–692.

Cohen, M., Liebson, I., Faillace, L., and Speers, W. (1971). Alcoholism: Controlled Drinking and Incentives for Abstinence, *Psychological Reports*, **28**, 575–580.

Cohen, S. (Ed.) (1971). *Images of Deviance*, Penguin, Harmondsworth, Middlesex.

Cohen, S. (1979). Inhalents and Solvents, in *Youth Drug Abuse: Problems, Issues and Treatment* (Eds. G. Beschner and A. Friedman), Lexington Books, Lexington, Mass.

Cole, C. and Spanier, G. (1973). Induction into Mate-swapping: a Review, *Family Process*, **12**, 279–289.

Colten, M. and Janis, I. (1978). Effects of Self Disclosure and the Decisional Balance Sheet Procedure in a Weight Reduction Clinic, in *Counselling on Personal Decisions: Theory and Field Research on Helping Relationships* (Ed. I. Janis), Yale University Press, New Haven, Connecticut.

Conger, J. (1951). The Effect of Alcohol on Conflict Behavior in the Albino Rat, *Quarterly Journal of Studies on Alcohol*, **12**, 1–29.

Connell, P. (1958). *Amphetamine Psychosis*, Oxford University Press, Oxford.

Cook, T. (1975). *Vagrant Alcoholics*, Routledge & Kegan Paul, London.

Cooper, A., Ismail, A., Phanjoo, A., and Love, D. (1972). Antiandrogen Therapy in Deviant Hypersexuality, *British Journal of Psychiatry*, **120**, 59–63.

Cooperstock, R. and Lennard, H. (1979). Some Social Meanings of Tranquiliser Use, *Sociology of Health and Illness*, **1**, 331–347.

Cornish, D. (1978). *Gambling: a Review of the Literature and its Implications for Policy and Research* (Home Office research study, 42), HMSO, London.

Costello, R. (1980). Alcoholism Treatment Effectiveness: Slicing the Outcome Variance Pie, in *Alcoholism Treatment in Transition* (Eds. G. Edwards and M. Grant), Croom Helm, London.

Cotton (1674). *Compleat Gamester*. Cited by Ashton, History of Gambling in England (cited by France, C., The Gambling Impulse, *American Journal of Psychology*, **13**, 1902, 364–407).

Coué, E. and Brooks, C. (1960, orig. 1922). Self-Mastery through Conscious Auto-Suggestion, in *Self-Mastery through Conscious Auto-suggestion by Emile Coué, and The Practice of Auto-suggestion by the Method of Emile Coué* (Ed. C. Brooks), Unwin, London.

Craft, M. (Ed.) (1966). *Psychopathic Disorders and their Assessment*, Pergamon, Oxford.

Crawford, G., Hughes, P., and Kohler, M. (1978). The Dynamics of Heroin Spread in Endemic Neighbourhoods, in *Drug Abuse: Modern Trends, Issues and Perspectives* (Eds. A. Schecter, H. Alksne, and E. Kaufman), Marcel Dekker, New York.

Crisp, A. (1978). Some Psychiatric Aspects of Obesity, in *Recent Advances in Obesity Research, II*, Proceedings of the Second International Congress on Obesity, October, 1977, Washington D.C. (Ed. G. Bray), Newman, London.

Crisp, A. and McGuiness, B. (1976). Jolly Fat: Relation between Obesity and Psychoneurosis in a General Population, *British Medical Journal*, **i**, 7–10.

Crisp, A. and Stonehill, E. (1970). Treatment of Obesity with Special reference to Seven Severely Obese Patients, *Journal of Psychosomatic Research*, **14**, 327–345.

Cronkite, R. and Moos, R. (1978). Evaluating Alcoholism Treatment Programs: an Integrated Approach, *Journal of Consulting and Clinical Psychology*, **46**, 1005–1019.

Crothers, T. (1911). A Review of the History and Literature of Inebriety: the First Journal and its Work up to the Present Time, *Journal of Inebriety*, **33**, 139–151 (cited by Jellinek, 1960, p.3).

Cummings, C., Gordon, J., and Marlatt, G. (1980). Relapse: Prevention and Prediction, in *The Addictive Behaviors: Treatment of Alcoholism, Drug Abuse, Smoking and Obesity* (Ed. W. Miller), Pergamon Press, Oxford.

Curlee, J. (1969). Alcoholism and the 'Empty Nest', *Bulletin of the Menninger Clinic*, **33**, 165–171.

Daily Mirror (1981). Is Sex Driving You Mad: They've Thought of a New Way to take the Lust out of Life, **Saturday, 12 September 1981**.

Davidson, H. (1964). Rationalizations for Continued Smoking, *New York State Journal of Medicine*, **15 December 1964**, 2993–3001.

Davies, J. (1982). The Transmission of Alcohol Problems in the Family, in *Alcohol and the Family* (Eds. J. Orford and J. Harwin), Croom Helm, London.

Davies, P. (1979). Motivation, Responsibility and Sickness in the Psychiatric Treatment of Alcoholism, *British Journal of Psychiatry*, **134**, 449–458.

Dawley, H. and Finkel, C. (1981). The Great American Smokeout: a Follow-up Report, *Addictive Behaviors*, **6**, 153–154.

de Alarcon, R. (1969). The Spread of Heroin Use in a Community, *Bulletin on Narcotics*, **21**, 17–22.

de Jong, W. (1980). The Stigma of Obesity: the Consequences of Naive Assumptions Concerning the Causes of Physical Deviance, *Journal of Health and Social Behavior*, **21**, 75–87.

de Lint, J. (1977). The Frequency Distribution of Alcohol Consumption: an Overview, in *The Ledermann Curve*, Report of a Symposium held in London, January, Alcohol Education Centre, London.

de Lint, J. and Schmidt, W. (1971). Consumption Averages and Alcoholism Prevalence: a Brief Review of Epidemiological Investigations, *British Journal of Addictions*, **66**, 97–107.

Department of the Environment (1976). *Drinking and Driving: Report of the Departmental Committee* (The Blennerhassett Report), HMSO, London.

Department of Health, Education, and Welfare, Public Health Service (U.S.) (1977). Definitions and Methods: Definitions of Obesity and Methods of Assessment, in *Behavioral Treatments of Obesity* (Ed. J. Foreyt), Pergamon, Oxford.

Department of Health and Social Security (1981). *Prevention and Health: Drinking Sensibly*, HMSO, London.

de Quincey, T. (1897, orig. 1822). The Confessions of an English Opium Eater, in *The Collected Writings of Thomas De Quincey, Vol. III* (Ed. D. Masson), Black, London.

Dews, P. (1973). The Behavioral Context of Addiction, in *Psychic Dependence: Definition, Assessment, in Animals and Man, Theoretical and Clinical Implications* (Eds. L. Goldberg and F. Hoffmeister), Springer-Verlag, Heidelberg.

Dickerson, M. (1974). The Effect of Betting Shop Experience on Gambling Behaviour, Unpublished Ph.D. thesis, University of Birmingham.

Dickerson, M. and Weeks, D. (1979). Controlled Gambling as a Therapeutic Technique for Compulsive Gamblers, *Behavior Therapy and Experimental Psychiatry*, **10**, 139–141.

Dicks, H. (1967). *Marital Tensions: Clinical Studies towards a Psychological Theory of Interaction*, Routledge & Kegan Paul, London.

Di Clemente, C. and Prochaska, J. (1982). Self-change and Therapy Change of Smoking Behavior: a Comparison of Processes of Change in Cessation and Maintenance, *Addictive Behaviors*, **7**, 133–142.

Dole, V. and Nyswander, M. (1965). A Medical Treatment for Diacetylmorphine (heroin) Addiction, *Journal of the American Medical Association*, **193**, 646 (cited by Kurland, 1978).

Downes, D., Davies, B., David, M., and Stone, P. (1976). *Gambling, Work and Leisure: a Study across Three Areas*, Routledge & Kegan Paul, London.

Drew, L. (1968). Alcoholism as a Self-Limiting Disease, *Quarterly Journal of Studies on Alcohol*, **29**, 956–966.

Duffy, J. (1977). Estimating the Proportion of Heavy Drinkers, in *The Ledermann Curve*, Report of a Symposium held in London, January, Alcohol Education Centre, London.

Duval, S. and Wicklund, R. (1972). *A Theory of Objective Self-Awareness*, Academic Press, New York.

Dwyer, J., Feldman, J., and Mayer, J. (1970). The Social Psychology of Dieting, *Journal of Health and Social Behaviour*, **11**, 269–287.

Dwyer, J., Feldman, J., Seltzer, C., and Mayer, J. (1969). Body Image in Adolescents: Attitudes toward Weight and Perception of Appearance, *Journal of Nutrition Education*, **1**, 14–19 (cited by Dwyer *et al.*, 1970).

Dwyer, J. and Mayer, J. (1970). Potential Dieters: Who Are They?, *Journal of the American Dietetic Association*, **56**, 510–514.

D'Zurilla, T. and Goldfried, M. (1971). Problem Solving and Behavior Modification, *Journal of Abnormal Psychology*, **78**, 107–126.

Eckholm, E. (1977). The Unnatural History of Tobacco, *Natural History*, **86**, 22–32.

Edwards, G. (1968). The Problem of Cannabis Dependence, *The Practitioner*, **200**, 226–233.

Edwards, G. (1971). Social Background to the Use and Abuse of Alcohol and Drugs: Professional Aspects, in *Alcoholism and Drug Dependence*, Proceedings of the 29th International Congress, Sydney, Australia, February 1970 (Eds. L. Kiloh and D. Bell), Butterworth, Australia.

Edwards, G. (1974a). Drugs, Drug Dependence and the Concept of Plasticity, *Quarterly Journal of Studies on Alcohol*, **35**, 176–195.

Edwards, G. (1974b). The Handling of the Delinquent Alcoholic: the Play of Expectations, Paper read at the International Symposium on the Integrated Treatment of Alcoholics, Brussels, May.

Edwards, G. (1976). Cannabis and the Psychiatric Position, in *Cannabis and Health* (Ed. J. Graham), Academic Press, London.

Edwards, G., Chandler, J., and Hensman, C. (1972a). Drinking in a London Suburb I: Correlates of Normal Drinking, *Quarterly Journal of Studies on Alcohol*, **Suppl No. 6**, 59–93.

Edwards, G., Chandler, J., Hensman, C., and Peto, J. (1972b). Drinking in a London Suburb II: Correlates of Trouble with Drinking Among Men, *Quarterly Journal of Studies on Alcohol*, **Suppl No. 6**, 94–119.

Edwards, G., Chandler, J., and Peto, J. (1972c). Motivation for Drinking Among Men in a London Suburb, *Psychological Medicine*, **2**, 260–271.

Edwards, G. and Gross, M. (1976). Alcohol Dependence: Provisional Description of a Clinical Syndrome, *British Medical Journal*, **i**, 1058–1061.

Edwards, G., Gross, M., Keller, M., Moser, J., and Room, R. (Eds.) (1977). *Alcohol-Related Disabilities*, World Health Organization Offset Publication No. 32, World Health Organization, Geneva.

Edwards, G. and Guthrie, S. (1967). A Controlled Trial of In-patient and Out-patient Treatment of Alcohol Dependence, *Lancet*, **i**, 555–559.

Edwards, G., Hawker, A., Hensman, C., Peto, J., and Williamson, V. (1973). Alcoholics Known or Unknown to Agencies: Epidemiological Studies in a London Suburb, *British Journal of Psychiatry*, **123**, 169–183.

Edwards, G., Orford, J., Egert, S., Guthrie, S., Hawker, A., Hensman, C., Mitcheson, M., Oppenheimer, E., and Taylor, C. (1977). Alcoholism: a Controlled Trial of 'Treatment' and 'Advice', *Journal of Studies on Alcohol*, **38**, 1004–1031.

Edwards, G., Williamson, V., Hawker, A., Hensman, C., and Postoyan, S. (1968). Census of a Reception Centre, *British Journal of Psychiatry*, **114**, 1031.

Edwards, J. and Holgate, S. (1979). Dependency upon Salbutamol Inhalers, *British Journal of Psychiatry*, **134**, 624–626.

Edwards, W. (1961). Behavioral Decision Theory, *Annual Review of Psychology*, **12**, 473–498.

Einstein, S. and Geritano, W. (1972). Treating the Drug Abuser: Problems, factors and alternatives, *International Journal of the Addictions*, **7**, 321–331 (cited by Wesson and Smith, p.56)

Eisenstein, V. (1956). Sexual Problems in Marriage, in *Neurotic Interaction in Marriage* (Ed. V. Eisenstein), Tavistock, London.

Eiser, J., Sutton, S., and Wober, M. (1978). 'Consonant' and 'Dissonant' Smokers and the Self-Attribution of Addiction, *Addictive Behaviors*, **3**, 99–106.

Elliott, S. (1977). The Implications of Follow-up Data for Current Conceptions of Obesity and its Treatment, Paper presented at the Annual Conference of the British Psychological Society, Exeter, April.

Ellis, A. (1951). *The Folklore of Sex*, Charles Boni, New York.

Ellis, A. (1975, orig. 1962). *Reason and Emotion in Psychotherapy*, Lyle Stuart, Secaucus, New Jersey.

Ellis, A. and Sagarin, E. (1965). *Nymphomania: A Study of the Oversexed Woman*, Ortolan, London.

Emrick, C. (1975). A Review of Psychologically Oriented Treatment of Alcoholism. II: The Relative Effectiveness of Different Treatment Approaches and the Effectiveness of Treatment versus No Treatment, *Journal of Studies on Alcohol*, **36**, 88–109.

Endler, N. (1975). The Case for Person-Situation Interaction, *Canadian Psychological Review*, **16**, 12–21.

Erikson, M. (1960). The Utilization of Patient Behavior in the Hypnotherapy of Obesity: Three Case Reports, *American Journal of Clinical Hypnosis*, **3**, 112–116.

Eysenck, H. (1952). The Effects of Psychotherapy: an Evaluation, *Journal of Consulting Psychology*, **16**, 319–324.

Eysenck, H. (1970). Personality and Attitudes to Sex: a Factorial Study, *Personality*, **1**, 355–376.

Eysenck, H. (1971a). Personality and Sexual Adjustment, *British Journal of Psychiatry*, **118**, 593–608.

Eysenck, H. (1971b). Masculinity–Femininity, Personality and Sexual Attitudes, *The Journal of Sex Research*, **7**, 83–88.

Eysenck, H. and Beech, R. (1971). Counterconditioning and Related Methods, in *Handbook of Psychotherapy and Behavior Change* (Eds. A. Bergin and S. Garfield), Wiley, New York.

Eysenck, H. and Eysenck, S. (1969). *Personality Structure and Measurement*, Routledge & Kegan Paul, London.

Feldman, M. and MacCulloch, M. (1971). *Homosexual Behaviour: Therapy and Assessment*, Pergamon, Oxford.

Fenichel, O. (1945). *The Psychoanalytic Theory of Neuroses*, Norton, New York.

Ferster, C., Nurnberger, J., and Levitt, E. (1962). The Control of Eating, *Journal of Mathetics*, **1**, 87–109. Reprinted in: Goldfried, M. and Merbaum, H. (Eds.) (1973). *Behaviour Change through Self-control*, Holt, Rinehart & Winston, New York.

Fingarette, H. (1981). Legal Aspects of Alcoholism and Other Addictions: Some Basic Conceptual Issues, *British Journal of Addiction*, **76**, 125–132.

Finney, J., Moos, R., and Mewborn, C. (1980). Posttreatment Experiences and treatment Outcome of Alcoholic Patients six months and two years after Hospitalisation, *Journal of Consulting and Clinical Psychology*, **48**, 17–29.

Fleck, L. (1970). The 12-year struggle against alcoholism in France, in *World Dialogue on Alcohol and Drug Dependence* (Ed. E. Whitney), Beacon Press, Boston.

Ford, C. and Beach, S. (1952). *Patterns of Sexual Behaviour*, Eyre and Spottiswoode, London.

Foreyt, J. (Ed.) (1977). *Behavioral Treatments of Obesity*, Pergamon, Oxford.
Foreyt, J. and Frohwirth, R. (1977). Introduction, in *Behavioral Treatments of Obesity* (Ed. J. Foreyt), Pergamon, Oxford.
France, C. (1902). The Gambling Impulse, *American Journal of Psychology*, **13**, 364–407.
Fransella, F. (1972). *Personal Change and Reconstruction: Research on a Treatment of Stuttering*, Academic Press, London.
Frederiksen, L., Miller, P., and Peterson, G. (1977). Topographical Components of Smoking Behaviour, *Addictive Behaviors*, **2**, 55–61.
Frederiksen, L., Peterson, G., and Murphy, W. (1976). Controlled Smoking: Development and Maintenance, *Addictive Behaviors*, **1**, 193–196.
Freud, A. (1946, orig. 1936). *The Ego and Mechanisms of Defense*, International University Press, New York (cited by Janis and Mann, 1977).
Gallup (1976). *Gambling in Britain*, Social Surveys (Gallup Poll) Ltd, London (cited by Cornish, 1978).
Gardner, J. (1964). *Spin the Bottle: the Autobiography of an Alcoholic*, Muller, London.
Garrow, J. (1978). The Regulations of Energy Expenditure in Man, in *Recent Advances in Obesity Research, II*, Proceedings of the Second International Congress on Obesity, Washington D.C., October 1977 (Ed. G. Bray), Newman, London.
Gath, D. (1969). The Male Drunk in Court, in *The Drunkenness Offence*, (Eds. D. Gath, T. Cook, and C. Hensman), Pergamon, Oxford.
Gayford, J. (1975). Wife Battering: a Preliminary Study of 100 Cases, *British Medical Journal*, **i**, 194–197.
Ghinger, C. and Grant, M. (1982). Alcohol and the Family in Literature, in *Alcohol and the Family* (Eds. J. Orford and J. Harwin), Croom Helm, London.
Ghodse, H. (1977). Drug Dependent Individuals Dealt with by London Casualty Departments, *British Journal of Psychiatry*, **131**, 273–280.
Gibbens, T. and Silberman, M. (1970). Alcoholism Among Prisoners, *Psychological Medicine*, **1**, 73.
Glaser, F. (1973). Some Historical Aspects of the Drug-Free Therapeutic Community, Unpublished paper presented at a Conference on Intervening in Drug Misuse: the Therapeutic Community and other Self-Help Efforts, at Saddlebrook, New Jersey, May.
Glaser, F. (1980). The Core Shell Model and the Matching Hypothesis, in *Alcoholism Treatment in Transition* (Eds. G. Edwards and M. Grant), Croom Helm, London.
Glatt, M. (1958). The English Drink Problem: Its Rise and Decline through the Ages, *British Journal of Addiction*, **55**, 51–65.
Glatt, M. (1975). *Alcoholism: a Social Disease*, Teach Yourself Books, London.
Golden, J. (1968). What is Sexual Promiscuity?, *Medical Aspects of Human Sexuality*, **October 1968**, 37–53.
Golüke, U., Landeen, R., and Meadows, D. (1981). A Simulation Model of Drinking Behaviour, *British Journal of Addiction*, **76**, 289–298.
Gomberg, E. (1979). Problems with Alcohol and Other Drugs, in *Gender and Disordered Behavior: Sex Differences in Psychopathology* (Eds. E. Gomberg and V. Franks), Bruner/Mazel, New York.
Goodwin, D. (1970). The Alcoholism of F. Scott Fitzgerald, *Journal of the American Medical Association*, **212**, 86–90.
Goodwin, D. (1971). The Alcoholism of Eugene O'Neill, *Journal of the American Medical Association*, **216**, 99–104.
Goodwin, D. (1976). *Is Alcoholism Hereditary?*, Oxford University Press, New York.
Goodwin, D. (1979). The Cause of Alcoholism and Why It Runs in Families, *British Journal of Addiction*, **74**, 161–164.
Goorney, A. (1968). Treatment of a Compulsive Horse Race Gambler by Aversion Therapy, *British Journal of Psychiatry*, **114**, 329–333.

Gorsuch, R. and Butler, M. (1976). Initial Drug Abuse: a Review of Predisposing Social Psychological Factors, *Psychological Bulletin*, **83**, 120–137.

Grant, M. (1979). Prevention, in *Alcoholism in Perspective* (Eds. M. Grant and P. Gwinner), Croom Helm, London.

Grant, M., Plant, M., and Williams, A. (Eds.) (1983). *Economics and Alcohol: Consumption and Controls*, Croom Helm, London.

Gray, J. (1975). *Elements of a Two-Process Theory of Learning*, Academic Press, London.

Gross, A. (1978). The Male Role and Heterosexual Behaviour, *Journal of Social Issues*, **34**, 87–107.

Gunn, J. (1968). Compulsive Gambler, Letter, *British Medical Journal*, **April, 1968**, 240.

Gusfield, J. (1962). Status Conflicts and the Changing Ideologies of the American Temperance Movement, in *Society, Culture and Drinking Patterns* (Eds. D. Pittman and C. Snyder), Wiley, New York.

Haberman, P. (1969). Drinking and other Self-indulgences: Complements or Counter-attractions, *International Journal of the Addictions*, **4**, 157–167.

Habitual Drunkards, Report of a Select Committee (1968, orig. 1872), in: *British Parliamentary Papers*, Irish University Press.

Hallaq, J. (1976). The Pledge as an Instrument of Behavioral Change, *Journal of Social Psychology*, **98**, 147–148.

Hamburger, W. (1951). Emotional Aspects of Obesity, *Medical Clinics of North America*, **35**, 483–499.

Hardy, K. (1964). An Appetitional Theory of Sexual Motivation, *Psychological Review*, **71**, 1–18.

Hardy, Thomas (1866). *The Life and the Death of the Mayor of Casterbridge*, Macmillan, London.

Harris, E. (1853). *Tobacco: the Effects of its Use as a Luxury on the Physical and Moral Nature of Man*, Harned, New York (cited by Jaffe, 1977).

Harris, M. and Hallbauer, E. (1973). Self directed Weight Control through Eating and Exercise, *Behaviour Research and Therapy*, **11**, 523–529.

Harrison, B. (1971). *Drink and the Victorians*, Faber & Faber, London.

Hawks, D., Mitcheson, M., Ogborne, A., and Edwards, G. (1969). Abuse of Methylamphetamine, *British Medical Journal*, **ii**, 715–721.

Heath, D. (1976). Anthropological Perspectives on Alcohol: an Historical Review, in *Cross-Cultural Approaches to the Study of Alcohol: an Interdisciplinary Perspective* (Eds. M. Everett, J. Waddell, and D. Heath), Mouton, The Hague.

Heather, N. and Robertson, I. (1981). *Controlled Drinking*, Methuen, London (Revised Edition, 1983).

Heilizer, F. (1964). Conflict Models, Alcohol, and Drinking Patterns, *Journal of Psychology*, **57**, 457–473.

Hemming, J. (1969). *Individual Morality*, Nelson, London.

Henry, J. and Henry, Z. (1953). Doll Play of Pilaga Indian Children, in *Personality in Nature, Society, and Culture* (2nd edn) (Eds. C. Kluckholn, H. Murray, and D. Schneider), Knopf, New York (cited by Hardy, 1964).

Hensman, C. (1969). Problems of Drunkenness Amongst Male Recidivists, in *The Drunkenness Offender* (Eds. D. Gath, T. Cook, and C. Hensman), Pergamon, Oxford.

Herman, C. and Polivy, J. (1975). Anxiety, Restraint, and Eating Behavior, *Journal of Abnormal Psychology*, **84**, 666–672.

Herman, R. (1976). *Gamblers and Gambling: Motives, Institutions and Controls*, Lexington Books, Lexington, Mass.

Hershon, H. (1977). Alcohol Withdrawal Symptoms in Drinking Behaviour, *Journal of Studies on Alcohol*, **38**, 953–971.

Higgins, R. and Marlatt, G. (1975). Fear of Interpersonal Evaluation as a Determinant of Alcohol Consumption in Male Social Drinkers, *Journal of Abnormal Psychology*, **84**, 644–651.

Hingson, R. and Day, N. (1977). Comment on 'Alcoholism: a Controlled Trial of Treatment and Advice', *Journal of Studies on Alcohol*, **38**, 2206–2211.

Hirschi, T. (1969). *Causes of Delinquency*, University of California Press, Berkeley, California.

Hobson, J. (1905). The Ethics of Gambling, in *Betting and Gambling: a National Evil* (Ed. B. Rowntree), Macmillan, London.

Hochbaum, G. (1965). Psychosocial Aspects of Smoking with Special Reference to Cessation, *American Journal of Public Health*, **55**, 692–697 (cited by Reinert, 1968).

Hodgson, R. and Rachman, S. (1976). The Modification of Compulsive Behaviour, in *Case Studies in Behaviour Therapy* (Ed. H. Eysenck), Routledge & Kegan Paul, London.

Hodgson, R., Rankin, H., and Stockwell, T. (1979b). Alcohol Dependence and the Priming Effect, *Behaviour Research and Therapy*, **17**, 379–387.

Hodgson, R., Rankin, H., and Stockwell, T. (1979c). Craving and Loss of Control, in *Alcoholism: New Directions in Behavioral Research and Treatment* (Eds. P. Nathan, G. Marlatt, and T. Loberg), Plenum, New York.

Hodgson, R., Stockwell, T., and Rankin, H. (1979a). Can Alcohol Reduce Tension?, *Behaviour Research and Therapy*, **17**, 459–466.

Hollister, L., Motzenbacker, F., and Degan, R. (1961). Withdrawal Reactions from Chlordiazepoxide ('Librium'), *Psychopharmacologia*, **2**, 63–68.

Hore, B. and Plant, M. (Eds.) (1981). *Alcohol Problems in Employment*, Croom Helm, London.

Horn, D. (1972). Determinants of Change, in *The Second World Conference on Smoking and Health* (Ed. G. Richardson), Pitman Medical, London.

Horn, J. and Wanberg, K. (1969). Symptom Patterns Related to Excessive Use of Alcohol, *Quarterly Journal of Studies on Alcohol*, **30**, 35–58.

Huba, B., Wingard, J., and Bentler, P. (1979). Beginning Adolescent Drug Use and Peer and Adult Interaction Patterns, *Journal of Consulting and Clinical Psychology*, **47**, 265–276.

Huenemann, R., Shapiro, L., Hampton, M., Mitchell, B., and Behnke, A. (1966). A Longitudinal Study of Gross Body Composition and Body Conformation and their Association with Food and Activity in a Teenage Population, *American Journal of Clinical Nutrition*, **18**, 325–338 (cited by Dwyer *et al.*, 1970).

Hull, J. (1981). A Self-Awareness Model of the Causes and Effects of Alcohol Consumption, *Journal of Abnormal Psychology*, **90**, 586–600.

Hull, J. and Levy, A. (1979). The Organization Functions of the Self: an Alternative to the Duval and Wicklund Model of Self-Awareness, *Journal of Personality and Social Psychology*, **37**, 756–768.

Hunt, H. (1968). Prospects and Possibilities in the development of Behavior Therapy, in *Ciba Foundation Symposium on the Role of Learning in Psychotherapy* (Ed. R. Poster), Churchill, London (cited by Hunt and Matarazzo, 1973).

Hunt, L., Farley, E., and Hunt, R. (1979). Spread of Drug Use in Populations of Youths, in *Youth Drug Abuse: Problems, Issues and Treatment* (Eds. G. Beschner and A. Friedman), Lexington Books, Lexington, Mass.

Hunt, W. and Bespalec, D. (1974). Relapse Rates after Treatment for Heroin Addiction, *Journal of Community Psychology*, **2**, 85–87.

Hunt, W. and General, W. (1973). Relapse Rates after Treatment for Alcoholism, *Journal of Community Psychology*, **1**, 66–68.

Hunt, W. and Matarazzo, J. (1970). Habit Mechanisms in Smoking, in *Learning Mechanisms in Smoking* (Ed. W. Hunt), Aldine, Chicago.

Hunt, W. and Matarazzo, J. (1973). Three Years Later: Recent Developments in the Experimental Modification of Smoking Behavior, *Journal of Abnormal Psychology*, **81**, 107–114.

Huxley, A. (1954). *The Doors of Perception*, Harper, New York.

Hyman, M. (1979). The Ledermann Curve: Comments on a Symposium, *Journal of Studies on Alcohol*, **40**, 339–347.

Ikard, F. and Tomkins, S. (1973). The Experience of Affect as a Determinant of Smoking Behavior: a Series of Validity Studies, *Journal of Abnormal Psychology*, **81**, 172–181.

Inglis, B. (1976). *The Opium War*, Hodder & Stoughton, London.

Inquiry Into Drunkenness, Report from the Select Committee (1968, orig. 1834), in *British Parliamentary Papers*, Irish University Press.

International Narcotic Education Association (1936). Los Angeles (cited by Edwards, 1968).

Iwawaki, S. and Eysenck, H. (1978). Sexual Attitudes among British and Japanese Students, *Journal of Psychology*, **98**, 289–298.

Jacobs, P. (1978). Epidemiology Abuse: Epidemiological and Psychosocial Models of Drug Abuse, in *Drug Abuse: Modern Trends, Issues and Perspectives* (Eds. A. Schecter, H. Alksne, and E. Kaufman), Marcel Dekker, New York.

Jaffe, J. (1977). Tobacco Use as a Mental Disorder: the Rediscovery of a Medical Problem, in *Research on Smoking Behavior* (Eds. M. Jarvik, J. Cullen, E. Gritz, T. Vogt, and L. West), National Institute on Drug Abuse Research Monograph 17, U.S. Dept of Health, Education and Welfare, NIDA, Rockville, Maryland.

Jahoda, G. and Cramond, J. (1972). *Children and Alcohol: a Developmental Study in Glasgow*, HMSO, London.

James, King, The First (1604). *A Counterblaste to Tobacco* (cited by Jaffe, J., 1977).

James, W. (1891). The *Principles of Psychology, Vol. 1*, Macmillan, London.

James, W. (1976). *Research on Obesity: a Report of the Department of Health and Social Security/Medical Research Council Group*, HMSO, London.

Janis, I. and Mann, L. (1968). A Conflict Theory Approach to Attitude Change and Decision Making, in *Psychological Foundations of Attitudes* (Eds. A. Greenwald, T. Brock, and T. Ostrom), Academic Press, New York.

Janis, I. and Mann, L. (1977). *Decision-making: a Psychological Analysis of Conflict, Choice, and Commitment*, Free Press, New York.

Janis, I. and Rodin, J. (1979). Attribution, Control, and Decision-making: Social Psychology and Health Care, in *Health Psychology: a Handbook: Theories, Applications and Challenges of a Psychological Approach to the Health Care System* (Eds. G. Stone, F. Cohen, and N. Adler), Jossey-Bass, San Francisco.

Jarvik, M. (1970). The Role of Nicotine in the Smoking Habit, in *Learning Mechanisms in Smoking* (Ed. W. Hunt), Aldine, Chicago.

Jasinski, D., Haertzen, C., and Isbell, H. (1971). *Annals of the New York Academy of Sciences*, **191**, 196–205.

Jauhar, P. (1981). Non-opiate Abuse among Opiate Addicts, in *The Misuse of Psychotropic Drugs* (Eds. R. Murray, H. Ghodse, C. Harris, D. Williams, and P. Williams), Gaskell, The Royal College of Psychiatrists, London.

Jellinek, E. (1952). The Phases of Alcohol Addiction, in Expert Committee on Mental Health, Alcoholism Sub-Committee, World Health Organisation Technical Report Services, No. 48, Geneva.

Jellinek, E. (1960). *The Disease Concept of Alcoholism*, Hillhouse, New Jersey.

Jessor, R., Collins, M., and Jessor, S. (1972). On Becoming a Drinker: Social-Psychological Aspects of an Adolescent Transition, in *Nature and Nurture in Alcoholism* (Ed. F. Seixas), New York Academy of Sciences, New York.

Jessor, R. and Jessor, S. (1977). *Problem Behaviour and Psycho-Social Development: a Longitudinal Study of Youth*, Academic Press, New York.

Jessor, R., Jessor, S., and Finney, J. (1973). A Social Psychology of Marijuana Use: Longitudinal Studies of High School and College Youth, *Journal of Personality and Social Psychology*, **26**, 1–15.

Jolly, S. and Orford, J. (1983). Religious Observance, Attitudes towards Drinking, and Knowledge about Drinking, amongst University Students, *Alcohol and Alcoholism,*, **18**, 271–278.

Jones, E. and Davis, K. (1965). From Acts to Dispositions: the Attribution Process in Person Perception, in *Experimental Social Psychology, Vol. 2* (Ed. L. Berkowitz), Academic Press, New York.

Jones, J. *The Mysteries of Opium Revealed*, cited by Sonnedecker, G. (1958). Emergence and Concept of Opiate Addiction, in *Narcotics and Drug Addiction Problems* (Ed. R. Livingstone), Public Health Service Publication No. 1050, U.S. Department of Health, Education and Welfare Washington, D.C. (cited by Kurland, 1978, pp.1–2).

Jones, M. (1968). Personality Correlates and Antecedents of Drinking Patterns in Adult Males, *Journal of Consulting and Clinical Psychology*, **32**, 2–12.

Jurek, K. (1974). Some Causes of Moral Disorder in Youth, *Psychologia a Patopsychologia Dietata*, **9**, 171–176 (Language: Czechoslovakian, English Abstract).

Kalin, R., McClelland, D., and Kahn, M. (1965). The Effect of Male Social Drinking on Fantasy, *Journal of Personality and Social Psychology*, **1**, 441–452.

Kallick, M., Suits, D., Dielman, T., and Hybels, J. (1979). *A Survey of American Gambling Attitudes and Behavior*, University of Michigan, Survey Research Centre, Institute for Social Research.

Kammeier, M., Hoffmann, H., and Loper, R. (1973). Personality Characteristics of Alcoholics as College Freshmen and at Time of Treatment, *Quarterly Journal of Studies on Alcohol*, **34**, 390–399.

Kandel, D. (Ed.) (1978). *Longitudinal Research on Drug Use: Empirical Findings and Methodological Issues*, Hemisphere, Washington.

Kanfer, F. and Karoly, P. (1972). Self-control: a Behavioristic Excursion into the Lion's Den, *Behavior Therapy*, **3**, 389–433.

Kaplan, H. (1974). *The New Sex Therapy*, Brunner/Mazel, New York.

Kaplan, H. I. and Kaplan, H. S. (1957). The Psychosomatic Concept of Obesity, *Journal of Nervous and Mental Disorder*, **125**, 181–201.

Kaufman, E. and de Leon, G. (1978). The Therapeutic Community: a Treatment Approach for Drug Abusers, in *Treatment Aspects of Drug Dependence* (Ed. A. Schecter), CRC Press, West Palm Beach, Florida.

Keller, M. (1972). On the Loss-of-Control Phenomenon in Alcoholism, *British Journal of Addiction*, **67**, 153–166.

Kelly, G. (1955). *The Psychology of Personal Constructs, Vol. 1, A Theory of Personality*, Norton, New York.

Kelman, H. and Baron, R. (1974). Moral and Hedonic Dissonance: a Functional Analysis of the Relationship between Discrepant Action and Attitude Change, in *Readings in Attitude Change* (Eds. S. Himmelfarb and A. Eagly), Wiley, New York.

Kendell, R. (1979). Alcohclism: a Medical or a Political Problem?, *British Medical Journal*, **10 February, 1979**, 367–371.

Kerr, N. (1889). *Inebriety, its Etiology, Pathology, Treatment and Jurisprudence*, 2nd edn, London (cited by Berridge, 1979, p.76).

Kessel, N. (1965). Self Poisoning, *British Medical Journal*, **ii**, 1629.

Keutzer, C. (1968). Behaviour Modification of Smoking: the Experimental Investigation of Diverse Techniques, *Behaviour Research and Therapy*, **6**, 137–157.

Khan, A. and Gupta, B. (1979). A Study of Malnourished Children in Children's Hospital Lusaka (Zambia), *Journal of Tropical Pediatrics and Environmental Child Health*, **25**, 42–45.

Kielholz, P. (1973). Addictive Behaviour in Man, in *Psychic Dependence: Definition, Assessment in Animals and Man, Theoretical and Clinical Implications* (Eds. L. Goldberg and F. Hoffmeister), Springer-Verlag, Heidelberg.

Kiloh, L. and Brandon, S. (1962). Habituation and Addiction to Amphetamines, *British Medical Journal*, **ii**, 40.

Kingsley, R. and Wilson, G. (1977). Behavior Therapy for Obesity: a Comparative Investigation of Long-term Efficacy, *Journal of Consulting and Clinical Psychology*, **45**, 288–298.

Kinsey, A., Pomeroy, W., and Martin, C. (1948). *Sexual Behaviour in the Human Male*, Saunders, Philadelphia.

Kinsey, A., Pomeroy, W., Martin, C., and Gebhard, P. (1953). *Sexual Behaviour in the Human Female*, Saunders, Philadelphia.

Klass, E. (1978). Psychological Effects of Immoral Actions: the Experimental Evidence, *Psychological Bulletin*, **85**, 756–771.

Kosviner, A. and Hawks, D. (1977). Cannabis Use amongst British University Students. II: Patterns of Use and Attitudes to Use, *British Journal of Addiction*, **72**, 41–57.

Kosviner, A., Hawks, D., and Webb, M. (1973). Cannabis Use Amongst British University Students. I: Prevalence Rates and Differences Between Students Who Have Tried Cannabis and Those Who Have Never Tried It, *British Journal of Addiction*, **69**, 35–60.

Krafft-Ebbing, R. von (1965). *Psychopathia Sexualis* (English Translation by F. Klaf), Stein and Day, New York.

Kronhausen, E. and Kronhausen, P. (1967). *Walter, The English Casanova: A Presentation of his Unique Memoirs 'My Secret Life'*, Polybooks, London.

Kumar, R. and Stolerman, I. (1977). Experimental and Clinical Aspects of Drug Dependence, in *Handbook of Psychopharmacology, Vol. 7* (Eds. I. Iversen, S. Iversen, and S. Snyder), Plenum, New York.

Kurland, A. (1978). *Psychiatric Aspects of Opiate Dependence*, CRC Press, West Palm Beach, Florida.

Lader, M. (1981). Benzodiazepine Dependence, in *The Misuse of Psychotropic Drugs* (Eds. R. Murray, H. Ghodse, C. Harris, D. Williams, and P. Williams), Gaskell, The Royal College of Psychiatrists, London.

La Forge, R. and Suczek, R. (1955). The Interpersonal Dimensions of Personality: an Interpersonal Check-List, *Journal of Personality*, **24**, 94.

Laschet, U. (1973). Antiandrogen in the Treatment of Sex Offenders: Mode of Action and Therapeutic Outcome, in *Contemporary Sexual Behaviour: Critical Issues in the 1970s* (Eds. J. Zubin and J. Money), Johns Hopkins University Press.

Laurie, P. (1967). *Drugs: Medical, Psychological and Social Facts*, Penguin, Harmondsworth, Middlesex.

Leary, T. (1957). *Interpersonal Diagnosis of Personality: A Functional Theory and Methodology for Personality Evaluation*, Ronald Press, New York.

Le Dain Commission (1972). *Cannabis: a Report of the Commission of Inquiry into the Non-medical Use of Drugs*, Information Canada, Ottawa.

Ledermann, S. (1956). *Alcool, Alcoolisme, Alcoolisation*, Presses Universitaires de France, Paris (cited by de Lint, 1977, and by Schmidt, 1977).

Leland, J. (1982). Sex Roles, Family Organisation and Alcohol Abuse, in *Alcohol and the Family* (Eds. J. Orford and J. Harwin), Croom Helm, London.

Lemert, E. (1951). *Social Pathology*, McGraw-Hill, New York.

Leon, G. (1976). Current Directions in the Treatment of Obesity, *Psychological Bulletin*, **83**, 557–578.

Leon, G. and Roth, L. (1977). Obesity: Psychological Causes, Correlations, and Speculations, *Psychological Bulletin*, **84**, 117–139.

Leventhal, H. (1970). Findings and Theory in the Study of Fear Communications, in *Advances in Experimental Social Psychology, Vol. 5* (Ed. L. Berkowitz), Academic Press, New York.

Leventhal, H. and Cleary, P. (1980). The Smoking Problem: a Review of the Research and Theory in Behavioral Risk Modification, *Psychological Bulletin*, **88**, 370–405.

Levine, H. (1978). The Discovery of Addiction: Changing Conceptions of Habitual Drunkenness in America, *Journal of Studies on Alcohol*, **39**, 143–176.

Levinstein, E. (1878). *Morbid Craving for Morphia*, London (cited by Berridge, 1979, p.73).

Levitt, E. (1973). Nymphomania, *Sexual Behaviour*, **March 1973**, 13–17.

Lewin, K. (1935). *Dynamic Theory of Personality*, McGraw-Hill, New York.

Lewin, K. (1947). Frontiers in Group Dynamics: Concept, Method, and Reality in Social Science; Social Equilibria and Social Change, *Human Relations*, **1**, 5–42.

Lewin, L. (1964, orig. 1924). *Phantastica: Narcotic and Stimulating Drugs*, Dutton, New York (cited by Jaffe, 1977).

Lewis, A. (1936). Problems of Obsessional Illness, *Proceedings of the Royal Society of Medicine*, **29**, 325.

Lewis, D. and Duncan, C. (1958). Expectation and Resistance to Extinction of a Lever-pulling Response as a Function of Percentage Reinforcement and Number of Acquisition Trials, *Journal of Experimental Psychology*, **55**, 121–128 (cited by Cornish, 1978).

Lewis, J. (1971). Promiscuous Women, *Sexual Behaviour*, **November 1971**, 75–80.

Lewis, J. (1972). Commentary on J. L. McCary, Nymphomania: a Case History, *Medical Aspects of Human Sexuality*, **6**, 202–203.

Ley, P. (1978). Psychological and Behavioural Factors in Weight Loss, in *Recent Advances in Obesity Research, II*, Proceedings of the Second International Congress on Obesity, Washington D. C., October 1977 (Ed. G. Bray), Newman, London.

Ley, P. (1980). The Psychology of Obesity: Its Causes, Consequences and Control, in *Contributions to Medical Psychology, Vol. 2* (Ed. S. Rachman), Pergamon, Oxford.

Ley, P., Bradshaw, P., Kincey, J., Couper-Smartt, H., and Wilson, M. (1974). Psychological Variables in the Control of Obesity, in *Obesity* (Eds. W. Burland, P. Samuel, and J. Yudkin), Churchill Livingstone, London.

Ley, P., Whitworth, M., Skilbeck, C., Woodward, R., Pinsent, R., Pike, L., Clarkson, M., and Clark, P. (1976). Improving Doctor Patient Communications in General Practice, *Journal of the Royal College of General Practitioners*, **26**, 720–724.

Lichtenstein, E. and Rodrigues, M. (1977). Long-term Effects of Rapid Smoking Treatment for Dependent Cigarette Smokers, *Addictive Behaviors*, **2**, 109–112.

Lindesmith, A. (1947). *Opiate Addiction*, Principa, Broomington, Indiana (cited by Kurland, 1978).

Lindner, R. (1950). The Psychodynamics of Gambling, *Annals of the American Academy of Political and Social Science*, **269**, 93.

Lisansky, E. (1960). The Etiology of Alcoholism: the Role of Psychological Predisposition, *Quarterly Journal of Studies on Alcohol*, **21**, 314–343.

Litman, G. (1976). Behavior Modification Techniques in the Treatment of Alcoholism: a Review and Critique, in *Research Advances in Alcohol and Drug Problems* (Eds. R. Gibbins, Y. Israel, H. Kalant, R. Popham, W. Schmidt, and R. Smart), Wiley, New York.

Litman, G., Eiser, J., Rawson, N., and Oppenheim, A. (1977). Towards a Typology of Relapse: a Preliminary Report, *Drug and Alcohol Dependence*, **2**, 157–162.

Litman, G., Eiser, J., Rawson, N., and Oppenheim, A. (1979a). Differences in Relapse Precipitants and Coping Behaviour between Alcohol Relapsers and Survivors, *Behaviour Research and Therapy*, **17**, 89–94.

Litman, G., Eiser, J., and Taylor, C. (1979b). Dependence, Relapse and Extinction: a Theoretical Critique and a Behavioral Examination, *Journal of Clinical Psychology*, **35**, 192–199.

Logan, F. (1973). Self-Control as Habit, Drive and Incentive, *Journal of Abnormal Psychology*, **81**, 127–136.

Longmate, N. (1968). *The Water Drinkers: a History of Temperance*, Hamish Hamilton, London.

Loro, A. and Orleans, C. (1981). Binge Eating in Obesity: Preliminary Findings and Guidelines for Behavioral Analysis and Treatment, *Addictive Behaviors*, **6**, 155–166.

Luce, B. and Schweitzer, S. (1977). The Economic Costs of Smoking-Induced Illness, in *Research on Smoking Behaviour* (Eds. M. Jarvik, J. Cullen, E. Gritz, T. Vogt, and L. West), National Institute on Drug Abuse Research Monograph 17, U.S. Dept. of Health, Education and Welfare, NIDA, Rockville, Maryland.

Ludwig, A. and Wikler, A. (1974). Craving and Relapse to Drink, *Quarterly Journal of Studies on Alcohol*, **35**, 108–130.

MacAndrew, C. and Edgerton, R. (1970). *Drunken Comportment: a Social Explanation*, Nelson, London.

MacMaster (1883). *History of the People of the United States, Vol. I* (cited by France, 1902).

Maddox, G. and Liederman, V. (1969). Overweight as a Social Disability with Medical Implications, *Journal of Medical Education*, **44**, 214–220 (cited by Dwyer *et al.*, 1970).

Maletzky, B. and Klotter, J. (1976). Addiction to Diazepam, *International Journal of the Addictions*, **11**, 95–115.

Marcus, S. (1966). *The Other Victorians: A Study of Sexuality and Pornography in Mid-Nineteenth-Century England*, Weidenfeld and Nicolson, London.

Marks, J. (1978). *The Benzodiazepines: Use, Overuse, Misuse and Abuse*, Medical and Technical Publishers, Lancaster.

Marlatt, G., Demming, B., and Reid, J. (1973). Loss of Control Drinking in Alcoholics: An Experimental Analogue, *Journal of Abnormal Psychology*, **81**, 233–241.

Marlatt, G. and Gordon, J. (1979). Determinants of Relapse: Implications for the Maintenance of Behavior Change, in *Behavioral Medicine: Changing Health Lifestyles* (Ed. P. Davidson), Brunner/Mazel, New York.

Marshall, D. (1971). Sexual Behaviour in Mangaia, in *Human Sexual Behaviour: the Range and Diversity of Human Sexual Experience Throughout the World as Seen in Six Representative Cultures* (Eds. D. Marshall and R. Suggs), Basic Books, New York.

Marshall, D. and Suggs, R. (Eds.) (1971). *Human Sexual Behaviour: The Range and Diversity of Human Sexual Experience Throughout the World—As Seen in Six Representative Cultures*, Basic Books, New York.

Marshall, M. (1976). A Review and Appraisal of Alcohol and Kava Studies in Oceania, in *Cross-Cultural Approaches to the Study of Alcohol: an Interdisciplinary Perspective* (Eds. M. Everett, J. Waddell, and D. Heath), Mouton, The Hague.

Masserman, J. and Yum, K. (1946). An Analysis of the Influence of Alcohol in Experimental Neurosis in Cats, *Psychosomatic Medicine*, **8**, 36–52.

Masters, W. and Johnson, V. (1970). *Human Sexual Inadequacy*, Little, Brown, Boston.

Matarazzo, J. (1973). Some Commonalities among the Preceding Reports of Studies on the Psychology of Smoking, in *Smoking Behavior: Motives and Incentives* (Ed. W. Dunn), Wiley, New York.

Mausner, B. (1973). An Ecological View of Cigarette Smoking, *Journal of Abnormal Psychology*, **81**, 115–126.

Mausner, B. and Platt, E. (1971). *Smoking: a Behavioral Analysis*, Pergamon, New York.

Mayer, J. (1968). *Overweight: Causes, Cost and Control*, Prentice-Hall, New Jersey.

Mayfield, D. and Coleman, L. (1968). Alcohol Use and Affective Disorder, *Diseases of the Nervous System*, **29**, 467–474.

McCary, J. (1972). Nymphomania: a Case History, *Medical Aspects of Human Sexuality*, **6**, 192–210.

McClelland, D., Davis, W., Kalin, R., and Wanner, E. (1972). *The Drinking Man*, Free Press, New York.

McCord, W. and McCord, J. (1960). *Origins of Alcoholism*, Stanford University Press, Stanford, California.

McFall, R. and Hammen, C. (1971). Motivation, Structure and Self-monitoring: Role of Non-specific Factors in Smoking Reduction, *Journal of Consulting and Clinical Psychology*, **37**, 80–86.

McGoldrick, E. (1954). *Management of the Mind*, Houghton, Mifflin, Boston (cited by Jellinek, 1960, p.59).

McGuire, M., Mendelson, J., and Stein, S. (1966). Comparative Psychosocial Studies of Alcoholic and Non-alcoholic Subjects Undergoing Experimentally Induced Ethanol Intoxication, *Psychosomatic Medicine*, **28**, 13–26.

McGuire, W. (1980). Communication and Social Influence Processes, in *Psychological Problems: The Social Context* (Eds. M. Feldman and J. Orford), Wiley, Chichester.

McKennell, A. and Thomas, R. (1967). *Adults' and Adolescents' Smoking Habits and Attitudes*, Government Social Survey, HMSO, London.

McKirnan, D. (1977). A Community Approach to the Recognition of Alcohol Abuse: the Drinking Norms of Three Montreal Communities, *Canadian Journal of Behavioral Science*, **9**, 108–122.

McKirnan, D. (1978). Community Perspectives on Deviance: Some Factors in the Definition of Alcohol Abuse, *American Journal of Community Psychology*, **6**, 219–238.

McPeek, F. (1972). The Role of Religious Bodies in the Treatment of Inebriety in the United States, in *Alcohol, Science and Society: 29 Lectures with Discussions as Given at the Yale Summer School of Alcohol Studies*, Greenword Press, Westport, Conn.

Meichenbaum, D. (1977). *Cognitive-Behaviour Modification: an Integrative Approach*, Plenum, New York.

Mendelson, J. and Mello, N. (1966). Experimental Analysis of Drinking Behaviour of Chronic Alcoholics, *Annals of the New York Academy of Sciences*, **133**, 828–845.

Messenger, J. (1971). Sex and Repression in an Irish Folk Community, in *Human Sexual Behaviour: the Range and Diversity of Human Sexual Experience Throughout the World as Seen in Six Representative Cultures* (Eds. D. Marshall and R. Suggs), Basic Books, New York.

Meyer, A., Friedman, L., and Lazarsfeld, P. (1973). Motivational Conflicts Engendered by the On-Going Discussion of Cigarette Smoking, in *Smoking Behavior: Motives and Incentives* (Ed. W. Dunn), Winston, Washington.

Meyer, V. and Crisp, A. (1977). Aversion Therapy in Two Cases of Obesity, in *Behavioral Treatments of Obesity* (Ed. J. Foreyt), Pergamon, Oxford.

Miller, G. and Agnew, N. (1974). The Ledermann Model of Alcohol Consumption: Description, Implications and Assessment, *Quarterly Journal of Studies on Alcohol*, **35**, 877–898.

Miller, I. (1969). The Don Juan Character, *Medical Aspects of Human Sexuality*, **April 1969**, 43–46.

Miller, N. (1944). Experimental Studies of Conflict, in *Personality and the Behavior Disorders* (Ed. J. Hunt), Ronald, New York.

Miller, P. (1979). Interactions Among Addictive Behaviors, *British Journal of Addiction*, **74**, 211–212.

Miller, P. (1980). Theoretical and Practical Issues in Substance Abuse Assessment and Treatment, in *The Addictive Behaviors: Treatment of Alcoholism, Drug Abuse, Smoking and Obesity* (Ed. W. Miller), Pergamon, New York.

Miller, W. (1980). The Addictive Behaviors, in *The Addictive Behaviors: Treatment of Alcoholism, Drug Abuse, Smoking and Obesity* (Ed. W. Miller), Pergamon, New York.

Miller, W. and Munoz, R. (1976). *How to Control Your Drinking*, Prentice-Hall, Englewood Cliffs, New Jersey.

Miller, W. and Taylor, C. (1980). Relative Effectiveness of Bibliotherapy, Individual and Group Self-Control Training in the Treatment of Problem Drinkers, *Addictive Behaviors*, **5**, 13–24.

Minihan, M. (1967). *Dostoevsky: His Life and Work by Konstantin Mochulsky*, Princeton University Press, Princeton, New Jersey.

Minkowich, A., Weingarten, L., and Blum, G. (1966). Empirical Contributions to a Theory of Ambivalence, *Journal of Abnormal Psychology*, **71**, 30–41.

Mitcheson, M., Hawks, D., Davison, J., Hitchens, L., and Malone, S. (1970). Sedative Abuse by Heroin Addicts, *Lancet*, **i**, 606.

Money, J. (1970). Use of an Androgen-depleting Hormone in the Treatment of Male Sex Offenders, *Journal of Sex Research*, **6**, 165–172.

Moody, G. (1972). *The Facts about the 'Money Factories'*, Churches' Council on Gambling, London.

Moody, G. (1974). *Social Control of Gambling*, Churches' Council on Gambling, London.

Moran, E. (1970). Gambling as a Form of Dependence, *British Journal of Addiction*, **64**, 419–428.

Moran, E. (1975). Pathological Gambling, in *Contemporary Psychiatry*, *British Journal of Psychiatry*, **Special Publication No. 9**, Royal College of Psychiatrists, London.

Morganstern, K. (1977). Cigarette Smoke as a Noxious Stimulus in Self-managed Aversion Therapy for Compulsive Eating: Technique and Case Illustration, in *Behavioral Treatments of Obesity* (Ed. J. Foreyt), Pergamon, Oxford.

Morrison, D. and Tracey, M. (1980). Beyond Ecstasy: Sex and Moral Protest, in *Changing Patterns of Sexual Behaviour*, Proceedings of the 15th Annual Symposium of the Eugenics Society, London, 1978 (Eds. W. Armytage, R. Chester, and J. Peel), Academic Press, London.

Morse, B. (1963). *The Sexually Promiscuous Female*, Pamar, New York.

Moser, J. (1980). *Prevention of Alcohol-Related Problems: an International Review of Preventive Measures, Policies, and Programmes*, Alcoholism and Drug Addiction Research Foundation, Toronto.

Mosher, D. (1972). Interaction of Fear and Guilt in Inhibiting Unacceptable Behavior, in *Applications of a Social Learning Theory of Personality* (Eds. J. Rotter *et al.*), Holt, Rinehart & Winston, New York.

Mulford, H. and Miller, D. (1960). Drinking in Iowa. III: A Scale of Definitions of Alcohol Related to Drinking Behavior, *Quarterly Journal of Studies on Alcohol*, **21**, 267–278.

Murray, R. (1977). Screening and Early Detection Instruments for Disabilities Related to Alcohol Consumption, in Alcohol-Related Disabilities (Eds. G. Edwards, M. Gross, M. Keller, J. Moser, and R. Room), World Health Organization, Geneva.

Murray, R. (1981). The Context of our Current Concern, in *The Misuse of Psychotropic Drugs* (Eds. R. Murray, H. Ghodse, C. Harris, D. Williams, and P. Williams), Gaskell, The Royal College of Psychiatrists, London.

Murray, R. and Stabenau, J. (1982). Genetic Factors in Alcoholism Predisposition, in *Encyclopedic Handbook of Alcoholism* (Eds. E. Pattison and E. Kaufman), Gardner Press, New York.

Myerson, A. (1940). Alcohol: A Study of Social Ambivalence, *Quarterly Journal of Studies on Alcohol*, **1**, 13–20.

Nalven, F. (1967). Some Perceptual Decision-making Correlates of Repressive and Intellectualizing Defenses, *Journal of Clinical Psychology*, **23**, 446–448.

National Health Examination Survey (U.S.A.) (1964). *Blood Pressure, Height and Selected Body Dimensions, United States, 1960–1962*, PHS, No. 1000, Series 11, No. 8 (cited by Ley, 1980).

Negrete, J. (1980). The Andean Region of South America: Indigenous Coca Chewing in the Rural Areas and Coca Paste Smoking in the Cities, in *Drug Problems in the Sociocultural Context: a Basis for Policies and Programme Planning* (Eds. G. Edwards and A. Arif), World Health Organization, Geneva.

Nesbitt, P. (1969). Smoking, Physiological Arousal, and Emotional Response, Unpublished Doctoral Dissertation, Columbia University (cited by Schachter, 1973).

Newman, O. (1972). *Gambling: Hazard and Reward*, Athlone Press, London.

Nisbett, R. (1972). Hunger, Obesity and the Ventromedial Hypothalamus, *Psychological Review*, **79**, 433–453.

Nunnally, J. (1961). Content analysis of the world of confession magazines, in *Popular Conceptions of Mental Health: Their Development and Change* (Ed. J. Nunnally), Holt, Rinehart & Winston, New York.

O'Connor, J. (1978). *The Young Drinkers: A Cross-national Study of Social and Cultural Influences*, Tavistock, London.

Ogborne, A. (1974). Two Types of Heroin Reactions, *British Journal of Addiction*, **69**, 237–242.

Okel, E. and Mosher, D. (1968). Changes in Affective States as a Function of Guilt over Aggressive Behavior, *Journal of Consulting and Clinical Psychology*, **32**, 265–270.

Oliven, J. (1974). *Clinical Sexuality: a Manual for the Physician and the Professions*, Lippincott, Philadelphia.

O'Neill, E. (1941). *Long Day's Journey into Night*, Jonathan Cape, London.

Orbach, S. (1978). *Fat is a Feminist Issue*, Paddington Press, London.

Orcutt, J. (1976). Ideological Variations in the Structure of Deviant Types: a Multivariate Comparison of Alcoholism and Heroin Addiction, *Social Forces*, **55**, 419–435 (cited by Orcutt and Cairl, 1979).

Orcutt, J. and Cairl, R. (1979). Social Definitions of the Alcoholic: Reassessing the Importance of Imputed Responsibility, *Journal of Health and Social Behaviour*, **20**, 290–295.

Orford, J. (1971a). Aspects of the Relationship between Alcohol and Drug Abuse, in *Alcoholism and Drug Dependence*, Proceedings of the 29th International Congress, Sydney, Australia, February 1970 (Eds. L. Kiloh and D. Bell), Butterworth, Australia.

Orford, J. (1971b). The Assessment of Personality and its Influence on the Outcome of Treatment, in *Homosexual Behavior: Therapy and Assessment* (Eds. M. Feldman and M. MacCulloch), Pergamon, Oxford.

Orford, J. (1975). Observations at a Small Hostel for Compulsive Gamblers, Unpublished paper, Addiction Research Unit, London.

Orford, J. (1976). Aspects of the Relationship between Alcohol and Drug Abuse, in *Drugs and Drug Dependence* (Eds. G. Edwards, M. Russell, D. Hawks, and M. MacCafferty), Saxon House, Westmead, Hants.

Orford, J. (1978). Hypersexuality: Implications for a Theory of Dependence, *British Journal of Addiction*, **73**, 299–310.

Orford, J. (1980). Understanding Treatment: Controlled Trials and Other Strategies, in *Alcoholism Treatment in Transition* (Eds. G. Edwards and M. Grant), Croom Helm, London.

Orford, J. and Edwards, G. (1977). *Alcoholism: a Comparison of Treatment and Advice, with a Study of the Influence of Marriage*, Oxford University Press, Oxford.

Orford, J., Guthrie, S., Nicholls, P., Oppenheimer, E., Egert, S., and Hensman, C. (1975). Self-reported Coping Behaviour of Wives of Alcoholics and its Association with Drinking Outcome, *Journal of Studies on Alcohol*, **36**, 1254–1267.

Orford, J. and Keddie, A. (1984). Abstinence or Controlled Drinking in Clinical Practice: Sex Differences, Paper submitted for publication.

Orford, J., Oppenheimer, E., and Edwards, G. (1976). Abstinence or Control: the Outcome of Excessive Drinking Two Years after Consultation, *Behaviour Research and Therapy*, **14**, 409–418.

Orford, J., Waller, S., and Peto, J. (1974). Drinking Behavior and Attitudes and their Correlates among University Students in England, *Quarterly Journal of Studies on Alcohol*, **35**, 1316–1374.

Ostrom, T. (1969). The Relationship between the Affective, Behavioral and Cognitive Components of Attitude, *Journal of Experimental Social Psychology*, **5**, 12–30.

Otto, S. (1975). Women Alcoholics: the Fallen Angel, *Camberwell Council on Alcoholism Journal on Alcoholism*, **3**, 7–10.

Otto, S. and Orford, J. (1978). *Not Quite Like Home: Small Hostels for Alcoholics and Others*, Wiley, Chichester.

Owen, P. and Butcher, J. (1979). Personality Factors in Problem Drinking: a Review of the Evidence and Some Suggested Directions, in *Psychiatric Factors in Drug Abuse* (Eds. R. Pickens and L. Heston), Grune and Stratton, New York.

Paolino, T. and McCrady, B. (1977). *The Alcoholic Marriage: Alternative Perspectives*, Grune and Stratton, New York.

Parsons, T. (1951). *The Social System*, Routledge & Kegan Paul, London (cited by Davies, 1979).

Patoprsta, G. *et al.* (1976). [Compulsive Hedonism Syndrome], *Ceskoslovenska Psychiatrie*, **72**, 225–227. (summary in English).

Pattison, E., Sobell, M., and Sobell, L. (1977). *Emerging Concepts of Alcohol Dependence*, Springer, New York.

Paxton, R. (1980). The Effects of Different Deposit Contracts in Maintaining Abstinence from Cigarette Smoking, Unpublished Ph.D. thesis, University of London.

Pearson, M. (1972). *The Age of Consent: Victorian Prostitution and its Enemies*, David and Charles, Newton Abbot.

Pechacek, T. (1979). Modification of Smoking Behavior, in *Smoking and Health, Report by the Surgeon General*, U.S. Dept of Health, Education and Welfare, Rockville, Maryland.

Peele, S. (1977). Redefining Addiction I Making Addiction a Scientifically and Socially Useful Concept, *International Journal of Health Services*, **7**, 103–123.

Peele, S. and Brodsky, A. (1975). *Love and Addiction*, Taplinger, New York.

Phares, E. (1972). A Social Learning Theory Approach to Psychopathology, in *Applications of a Social Learning Theory of Personality* (Eds. J. Rotter *et al.*), Holt, Rinehart & Winston, New York.

Pickens, R. and Thompson, T. (1971). Characteristics of Stimulant Drug Reinforcement, in *Stimulus Properties of Drugs* (Eds. T. Thompson and R. Pickens), Appleton-Century-Crofts, New York (cited by Kumar and Stolerman, 1977).

Plant, M (1975). *Drugtakers in an English Town*, Tavistock, London.

Pliner, P. and Cappell, H. (1974). Modification of Affective Consequences of Alcohol: a Comparison of Social and Solitary Drinking, *Journal of Abnormal Psychology*, **83**, 418–425.

Polivy, J. (1976). Perception of Calories and Regulation of Intake in Restrained and Unrestrained Subjects, *Addictive Behaviors*, **1**, 237–243.

Popham, R. (1970). Indirect Methods of Alcoholism Prevalence Estimation: a Critical Evaluation, in *Alcohol and Alcoholism* (Ed. R. Popham), University of Toronto Press, Toronto.

Premack, D. (1970). Mechanisms of Self-control, in *Learning Mechanisms in Smoking* (Ed. W. Hunt), Aldine, Chicago.

Quaade, F. (1978). Intestinal Bypass for Severe Obesity, a Randomized Trial. A Report from the Danish Obesity Group, in *Recent Advances in Obesity Research, II*, Proceedings of the Second International Congress on Obesity, October 1977, Washington D.C. (Ed. G. Bray), Newman, London.

Rachman, S. and Teasdale, J. (1969). *Aversion Therapy and Behaviour Disorders: an Analysis*, Routledge & Kegan Paul, London.

Radin, S. (1972). The Don Juan, *Sexual Behaviour*, **December, 1972**, 4–9.

Rado, S. (1933). The Psychoanalysis of Pharmacothymia (drug addiction), *Psychoanalytic Quarterly*, **2**, 1–23 (reprinted in Shaffer and Burglass, 1981).

Ramey, J. (1972). Emerging Patterns of Behaviour in Marriage: Deviations or Innovations?, *Journal of Sex Research*, **8**, 6–30.

Rank, O. (1922). Die Don Juan Gestalt, *Imago*, **8**, 142–196 (cited by Robbins, 1956).

Rathod, N., Gregory, E., Blows, D., and Thomas, G. (1966). A Two-Year Follow-up Study of Alcoholic Patients, *British Journal of Psychiatry*, **112**, 683–692.

Raw, M. (1977). The Psychological Modification of Smoking, in *Advances in Medical Psychology* (Ed. S. Rachman), Pergamon, Oxford.

Ray, C. (1981). Pain, in *Psychology and Medicine* (Ed. D. Griffiths), Macmillan, London.

Reinert, R. (1968). The Concept of Alcoholism as a Bad Habit, *Bulletin of the Menninger Clinic*, **32**, 35–46.

Ries, J. (1977). Public Acceptance of the Disease Concept of Alcoholism, *Journal of Health and Social Behaviour*, **18**, 338–344 (cited by Orcutt and Cairl, 1979).

Robbins, L. (1956). A Contribution to the Psychological Understanding of the Character of Don Juan, *Bulletin of the Menninger Clinic*, **20**, 166–180.

Robins, L. (1966). *Deviant Children Grown Up: a Sociological and Psychiatric Study of Sociopathic Personality*, Williams and Wilkins, Baltimore.

Robins, L., Davis, D., and Wish, E. (1977). Detecting Predictors of Rare Events: Demographic, Family and Personal Deviance as Predictors of Stages in the Progression toward Narcotic Addiction, in *The Origins and Course of Psychopathology: Methods of Longitudinal Research* (Eds. S. Strauss, H. Babigian, and M. Roff), Plenum, New York.

Robinson, D. (1972). The Alcohologist's Addiction: Some Implications of Having Lost Control over the Disease Concept of Alcoholism, *Quarterly Journal of Studies on Alcohol*, **33**, 1028–1042.

Robinson, D. (1979). *Talking Out of Alcoholism: the Self-Help Process of Alcoholics Anonymous*, Croom Helm, London.

Rodin, J. (1978). Has the Distinction between Internal versus External Control of Feeding Outlived its Usefulness? in *Recent Advances in Obesity Research, II*, Proceedings of the Second International Congress on Obesity, Washington D.C., October 1977 (Ed. G. Bray), Newman, London.

Roget's Thesaurus of English Words and Phrases (1966), Penguin, Harmondsworth, Middlesex.

Roizen, R., Cahalan, D., and Shanks, P. (1978). Spontaneous Remission among Untreated Problem Drinkers, in *Longitudinal Research on Drug Use: Empirical Findings and Methodological Issues* (Ed. D. Kandel), Hemisphere, Washington.

Rolleston, H. (1926a). Medical Aspects of Tobacco, *The Lancet*, **i**, 961–965 (cited by Jaffe, 1977).

Rolleston, H. (1926b). *Report of the Departmental Committee on Morphine and Heroin Addiction*, London (cited by Berridge, 1979, p.68).

Roman, P. and Trice, H. (1968). The Sick Role, Labelling Theory, and the Deviant Drinker, *International Journal of Social Psychiatry*, **12**, 245–251 (cited by Orcutt and Cairl, 1979).

Rook, K. and Hammen, C. (1977). A Cognitive Perspective on the Experience of Sexual Arousal, *Journal of Social Issues*, **33**, 7–29.

Room, R. (1977). Measurement and Distribution of Drinking Patterns and Problems in General Populations, in *Alcohol-Related Disabilities* (Eds. G. Edwards, M. Gross, M. Keller, J. Moser, and R. Room), World Health Organization, Geneva.

Rosen, G. and Orenstein, H. (1976). A Historical Note on Thought-stopping, *Journal of Consulting and Clinical Psychology*, **44**, 1016–1017.

Roth, L. (1978). *I'll Cry Tomorrow*, Chivers, Bath.

Rotter, J. (1954). *Social Learning and Clinical Psychology*, Prentice-Hall, New York.

Rowntree, B. (1905). *Betting and Gambling: a National Evil*, Macmillan, London.

Royal College of Physicians of London (1977). *Smoking or Health*, Pitman Medical, Tunbridge Wells.

Royal College of Psychiatrists (1979). *Alcohol and Alcoholism: the Report of a Special Committee of the College*, Tavistock, London.

Rubington, E. and Weinberg, M. (1968). *Deviance, the Interactionist Perspective: Text and Readings in the Sociology of Deviance*, Collier–Macmillan, London.

Rush, B. (1943, orig. 1785). An Inquiry into the Effects of Ardent Spirits upon the Human Body and Mind with an Account of the Means of Preventing and of the Remedies for Curing them. Reprinted with an introduction by the Editor, *Quarterly Journal of Studies on Alcohol*, **4**, 321–341.

Rushing, W. (1969). Deviance, Interpersonal Relations and Suicide, *Human Relations*, **22**, 61–76.

Russell, A. (1932). *For Sinners Only*, Hodder & Stoughton, London.

Russell, J. and Mehrabian, A. (1978). Environmental Effects on Drug Use, *Environmental Psychology and Non-verbal Behavior*, **2**, 109–123.

Russell, M. (1971). Cigarette Smoking: Natural History of a Dependence Disorder, *British Journal of Medical Psychology*, **44**, 1–16.

Russell, M. (1973). Changes in Cigarette Price and Consumption by Men in Britain, 1946–1971: a Preliminary Analysis, *British Journal of Preventive and Social Medicine*, **27**, 1–7.

Russell, M. (1974). Realistic Goals for Smoking and Health: a Case for Safer Smoking, *The Lancet*, **16 February, 1974**, 254–258.

Russell, M., Armstrong, E., and Patel, U. (1976). Temporal Contiguity in Electric Aversion Therapy for Cigarette Smoking, *Behaviour Research and Therapy*, **14**, 103–123.

Russell, M., Peto, J., and Patel, U. (1974). The Classification of Smoking by Factorial Structure of Motives, *Journal of the Royal Statistical Society*, **137**, 313–346.

Russell, M., Wilson, C., Feyerabend, C., and Cole, P. (1976). Effect of Chewing Gum in Smoking Behaviour and as an Aid to Cigarette Withdrawal, *British Medical Journal*, **ii**, 391–393.

Russell, M., Wilson, C., Taylor, C., and Baker, C. (1979). Effect of General Practitioners' Advice against Smoking, *British Medical Journal*, **ii**, 231–235.

Ryan, F. (1973). Cold Turkey in Greenfield, Iowa: a Follow-up Study, in *Smoking Behavior: Motives and Incentives* (Ed. W. Dunn), Wiley, New York.

Sadava, S. (1975). Research Approaches to Illicit Drug Use: a Critical Review, *Genetic Psychology Monographs*, **91**, 3–59.

Sadava, S. and Forsythe, R. (1977). Person–Environment Interaction and College Student Drug Use: Multivariate Longitudinal Study, *Genetic Psychology Monographs*, **96**, 211–245.

Sagarin, E. (1969). *Odd Man In: Societies of Deviants in America*, Quadrangle, Chicago.

Salvation Army (1974). *In Darkest England Now: a Salvation Army Survey of Religious and Social Conditions in Britain Eighty Years after William Booth's Blue-print for Salvation*, Hodder & Stoughton, London.

Samsonowitz, V. and Sjoberg, L. (1981). Volitional Problems of Socially Adjusted Alcoholics, *Addictive Behaviors*, **6**, 385–398.

Sarbin, T. and Nucci, L. (1973). Self-Reconstitution Processes: a Proposal for Reorganizing the Conduct of Confirmed Smokers, *Journal of Abnormal Psychology*, **81**, 182–195.

Sargent, M. (1979). *Drinking and Alcoholism in Australia: a Power Relations Theory*, Longman Cheshire, Melbourne.

Saunders, W. and Kershaw, P. (1979). Spontaneous Remission from Alcoholism—a Community Study, *British Journal of Addiction*, **74**, 251–266.

Saxon, S., Blaine, J., Dennett, C., and Gerstein, D. (1978). Multiple Binds of Drug Treatment Personnel, in *Drug Abuse: Modern Trends, Issues and Perspectives* (Eds. A. Schecter, H. Alksne, and E. Kaufman), Marcel Dekker, New York.

Schachter, S. (1964). The Interaction of Cognitive and Physiological Determinants of Emotional State, in *Advances in Experimental Social Psychology, Vol. 1* (Ed. L. Berkowitz), Academic Press, New York.

Schachter, S. (1971) *Emotion, Obesity and Crime*, Academic Press, New York.

Schachter, S. (1973). Nesbitt's Paradox, in *Smoking Behavior: Motives and Incentives* (Ed. W. Dunn), Wiley, New York.

Schachter, S. (1982) Recidivism and Self-cure of Smoking and Obesity, *American Psychologist*, **37**, 436–444.

Schachter, S., Goldman, R., and Gordon, A. (1968). Effects of Fear, Food Deprivation and Obesity on Eating, *Journal of Personality and Social Psychology*, **10**, 91–97.

Schachter, S., Kozlowski, L., and Silverstein, B. (1977). Effects of Urinary pH on Cigarette Smoking, *Journal of Experimental Psychology: General*, **106**, 13–19.

Schachter, S. and Singer, J. (1962). Cognitive, Social and Physiological Determinants of Emotional State, *Psychological Review*, **69**, 379–399.

Schaefer, J. (1979). Ethnic Differences in Response to Alcohol, in *Psychiatric Factors in Drug Abuse* (Eds. R. Pickens and L. Heston), Grune & Stratton, New York.

Schecter, A. (1978). *Treatment Aspects of Drug Dependence*, CRC Press, W. Palm Beach, Florida.

Schmidt, D. and Sigusch, B. (1973). Women's Sexual Arousal, in *Contemporary Sexual Behaviour: Critical Issues in the 1970s* (Eds. J. Zubin and J. Money), Johns Hopkins University Press.

Schmidt, W. (1977). Cirrhosis and Alcohol Consumption: an Epidemiological Perspective, in *Alcoholism: New Knowledge and New Responses* (Eds. G. Edwards and M. Grant), Croom Helm, London.

Schofield, M. (1968). *The Sexual Behaviour of Young People*, Pelican, London.

Schuckit, M., Goodwin, D., and Winokur, G. (1972). A Study of Alcoholism in Half-siblings, *American Journal of Psychiatry*, **128**, 1132–1136.

Schuman, L. (1977). Patterns of Smoking Behavior, in *Research on Smoking Behavior* (Eds. M. Jarvik, J. Cullen, E. Gritz, T. Vogt, and L. West), National Institute on Drug Abuse Research Monograph 17, U.S. Dept. of Health, Education and Welfare, NIDA, Rockville, Maryland.

Schuster, C. and Thompson, T. (1969). Self-administration of and Behavioral Dependence on Drugs, *Annual Review of Pharmacology*, **9**, 483–502 (cited by Kumar and Stolerman, 1977).

Schuster, C. and Woods, J. (1968). The Conditioned Reinforcing Effects of Stimuli Associated with Morphine Reinforcement, *International Journal of the Addictions*, **3**, 223–230 (cited by Kumar and Stolerman, 1977).

Scodel, A. (1964). Inspirational Group Therapy: a Study of Gamblers Anonymous, *American Journal of Psychotherapy*, **18**, 115–125.

Seeley, J. (1962). Alcoholism is a Disease: Implications for Social Policy, in *Society, Culture and Drinking Patterns* (Eds. D. Pittman and C. Snyder), Wiley, New York.

Seevers, M. (1962). Medical Perspectives on Habituation and Addiction, *Journal of the American Medical Association*, **181**, 92–98.

Shaffer, H. and Burglass, M. (Eds.) (1981). *Classic Contributions in the Addictions*, Brunner/Mazel, New York.

Shaw, S. (1979). A Critique of the Concept of the Alcohol Dependence Syndrome, *British Journal of Addiction*, **74**, 339–348.

Shaw, S., Cartwright, A., Spratley, T., and Harwin, J. (1978). *Responding to Drinking Problems*, Croom Helm, London.

Shiff, N. (1961). *Diary of a Nymph*, Lyle Stuart, New York.

Silverstone, J. (1968). Obesity, *Proceedings of the Royal Society of Medicine*, **61**, 371–375.

Silverstone, J. (1969). Psychological Factors in Obesity, in *Obesity: Medical and Scientific Aspects* (Eds. I. Baird and A. Howard), Livingstone, Edinburgh.

Singer, K. (1974). The Choice of Intoxicant among the Chinese, *British Journal of Addiction*, **69**, 257–268.

Sjoberg, L. (1980). Volitional Problems in Carrying Through a Difficult Decision, *Acta Psychologica*, **45**, 123–132.

Sjoberg, L. and Johnson, T. (1978). Trying to Give up Smoking: a Study of Volitional Breakdowns, *Addictive Behaviors*, **4**, 339–359.

Skog, O. (1977). On the Distribution of Alcohol Consumption, in *The Ledermann Curve*, Report of a Symposium held in London, January, Alcohol Education Centre, London.

Slater, E. and Woodside, M. (1951). *Patterns of Marriage: a Study of Marriage Relationships in the Urban Working Classes*, Cassell, London.

Slochower, J. (1976). Emotional Labelling and Overeating in Obese and Normal Weight Individuals, *Psychosomatic Medicine*, **38**, 131–139 (cited by Ley, 1980).

Smart, R. (1971). Illicit Drug Use in Canada: a Review of Current Epidemiology with Clues for Prevention, *International Journal of the Addictions*, **6**, 383–405.

Smith, J. and Smith, L. (1970). Co-marital Sex and the Sexual Freedom Movement, *Journal of Sex Research*, **6**, 131–142.

Solomon, R. (1980). The Opponent—Process Theory of Acquired Motivation: the Costs of Pleasure and the Benefits of Pain, *American Psychologist*, **35**, 691–712.

Solomon, R. and Corbit, J. (1973). An Opponent—Process Theory of Motivation. II: Cigarette Addiction, *Journal of Abnormal Psychology*, **81**, 158–171.

Solomon, R. and Corbit, J. (1974). An Opponent—Process Theory of Motivation. I: Temporal Dynamics of Affect, *Psychological Review*, **81**, 119–145.

Sonnedecker, G. (1958). Emergence and Concept of Opiate Addiction, in *Narcotics and Drug Addiction Problems* (Ed. R. Livingston), Public Health Service Publication No. 1050, U.S. Dept. of Health, Education and Welfare, Washington D.C. (cited by Kurland, 1978, pp. 1–2).

Spencer, J. and Fremouw, W. (1979). Binge Eating as a Function of Restraint and Weight Classification, *Journal of Abnormal Psychology*, **88**, 262–267.

Squires, P. (1937). Fyodor Dostoevsky: a Psychopathographical Sketch, *Psychoanalytical Review*, **24**, 365–388.

Srole, L., Langner, T., Michael, S., Opler, M., and Rennie, T. (1962). *Mental Health in the Metropolis*, McGraw-Hill, New York.

Staats, G. (1978). An Empirical Assessment of Controls Affecting Marijuana Usage, *British Journal of Addiction*, **73**, 391–398.

Staffieri, J. (1967). A Study of Social Stereotypes of Body Image in Children, *Journal of Personality and Social Psychology*, **7**, 101–104.

Steinmetz. *Gaming Table, Vol. I* (cited by France, 1902).

Stekel, W. (1924). *Peculiarities of Behaviour: Wandering Mania, Dipsomania, Cleptomania, Pyromania and Allied Impulsive Acts*, English Publication 1938, Bodley Head (trans. J. Van Teslaar), London.

Sterne, M. and Pittman, D. (1965). The Concept of Motivation: a Source of Institutional and Professional Blockage in the Treatment of Alcoholics, *Quarterly Journal of Studies on Alcohol*, **26**, 41–57.

Stimson, G. (1973). *Heroin and Behaviour: Diversity among Addicts Attending London Clinics*, Irish University Press, Shannon.

Stimson, G. (1978). Clinics: Care or Control?, *News Release*, **1978**, 14–16.

Stimson, G., Oppenheimer, E., and Thorley, A. (1978). Seven-Year Follow-up of Heroin Addicts: Drug Use and Outcome, *British Medical Journal*, **i**, 1190–1192.

Stockwell, T., Hodgson, R., Rankin, H., and Taylor, C. (1982). Alcohol Dependence, Beliefs and the Priming Effect, *Behaviour Research and Therapy*, **20**, 513–522.

Stone, L. (1979). *The Family, Sex and Marriage in England 1500–1800*, Penguin, Harmondsworth, Middlesex (orig. unabridged version, Weidenfeld and Nicolson, 1977).

Straits, B. (1965). Sociological and Psychological Correlates of Adoption and Discontinuation of Cigarette Smoking, University of Chicago, mimeo. (cited by Bernstein, 1970).

Strickland, L. and Grote, F. (1967). Temporal Presentation of Winning Symbols and Slot-machine Playing, *Journal of Experimental Psychology*, **74**, 10–13.

Stuart, R. (1967). Behavioural Control of Overeating, *Behaviour Research and Therapy*, **5**, 357–365.

Stunkard, A. (1958). The Management of Obesity, *New York State Journal of Medicine*, **58**, 79–87 (cited by Foreyt and Frohwirth, 1977).

Stunkard, A. (1959). Eating Patterns of Obesity, *Psychiatric Quarterly*, **33**, 284–295.

Stunkard, A. (1978). Behavioral Treatment of Obesity: the First Ten Years, in *Recent Advances in Obesity Research, II*, Proceedings of the Second International Congress on Obesity, Washington D.C., October 1977 (Ed. G. Bray), Newman, London.

Stunkard, A. and McLaren-Hume, M. (1959). The Results of Treatment for Obesity, *Archives of Internal Medicine*, **103**, 79–85 (cited by Bray, 1978, and by Leon, 1976).

Sutherland, E. and Cressey, D. (1970). *Criminology*, Lippincott, Philadelphia.

Sutton, S. (1979). Interpreting Relapse Curves, *Journal of Consulting and Clinical Psychology*, **47**, 96–98.

Swanson, D. and Dinello, F. (1969). Therapeutic Starvation in Obesity, *Diseases of the Nervous System*, **30**, 669–674.

Swinson, R. and Eaves, D. (1978). *Alcoholism and Addiction*, MacDonald & Evans, Plymouth.

Szasz, T. (1978). A Dialogue about Drug Education, *Psychiatric Opinion*, **15**, 10–14.

Szasz, T. and Hollender, M. (1956). *Archives of Internal Medicine*, **97**, 586 (cited by Davies, 1979).

Teasdale, J. (1973). Conditioned Abstinence in Narcotic Addicts, *International Journal of the Addictions*, **8**, 273–292.

Tedeschi, J. (Ed.) (1972). *The Social Influence Processes*, Aldine–Atherton, Chicago.

Terry, C. and Pellens, M. (1928). *The Opium Problem*, for the Committee on Drug Addictions in Collaboration with the Bureau of Social Hygiene, Inc., New York (cited by Kurland, 1978, p.23).

Thoresen, C. and Mahoney, M. (1974). *Behavioral Self-Control*, Holt, Rinehart & Winston, New York.

Thorley, A., Oppenheimer, E., and Stimson, G. (1977). Clinic Attendance and Opiate Prescription Status of Heroin Addicts over a Six-Year Period, *British Journal of Psychiatry*, **130**, 565–569.

Thorner, I. (1953). Ascetic Protestantism and Alcoholism, *Psychiatry*, **16**, 167–176.

Tiebout, H. (1944). Therapeutic Mechanisms of Alcoholics Anonymous, *American Journal of Psychiatry*, **100**, 468–473.

Tiebout, H. (1961). Alcoholics Anonymous—an Experiment of Nature, *Quarterly Journal of Studies on Alcohol*, **22**, 52–68.

Todd, J. (1882). *Drunkenness a Vice, Not a Disease*, Case, Lockwood & Brainard, Hartford, Conn. (cited by Jellinek, 1960, pp.207–210).

Tomkins, S. (1965). In *Factors Related to Successful Abstinence from Smoking, Final Report* (Ed. J. Guilford), American Institute for Research, Los Angeles.

Tomkins, S. (1968). A Modified Model of Smoking Behavior, in *Smoking, Health and Behavior* (Eds. E. Borgatta and R. Evans), Aldine, Chicago.

Toomey, M. (1972). Conflict Theory Approach to Decision Making Applied to Alcoholics, *Journal of Personality and Social Psychology*, **24**, 199–206.

Trevelyan, G. (1967, orig. 1942). *English Social History: a Survey of Six Centuries, Chaucer to Queen Victoria*, Penguin, Harmondsworth, Middlesex.

Trotter, T. (1804). *An Essay Medical, Philosophical, and Chemical on Drunkenness, and its Effects on the Human Body*, Longman, London (cited by Edwards, 1971).

Tuchfeld, B. (1977). Comment on 'Alcoholism: a Controlled Trial of Treatment and Advice', *Journal of Studies on Alcohol*, **38**, 1803–1813.

Tuchfeld, B. (1981). Spontaneous Remission in Alcoholics: Empirical Observations and Theoretical Implications, *Journal of Studies on Alcohol*, **42**, 626–641.

Tucker, J., Vuchinich, R., and Sobell, M. (1979). Differential Discriminative Stimulus Control of Non-Alcoholic Beverage Consumption in Alcoholics and in Normal Drinkers, *Journal of Abnormal Psychology*, **88**, 145–152.

Vaillant, G. (1973). A 20-year Follow-up of New York Narcotic Addicts, *Archives of General Psychiatry*, **29**, 237 (cited by Kurland, 1978).

Vaillant, G. (1980). The Doctor's Dilemma, in *Alcoholism Treatment in Transition* (Eds. G. Edwards and M. Grant), Croom Helm, London.

Vallance, M. (1965). A Two-year Follow-up Study of Patients Admitted to the Psychiatric Department of a General Hospital, *British Journal of Psychiatry*, **111**, 348–356.

Van Lancker, J. (1977). Smoking and Disease, in *Research on Smoking Behavior* (Eds. M. Jarvik, J. Cullen, E. Gritz, T. Vogt, and L. West), National Institute on Drug Abuse Research Monograph 17, U.S. Dept. of Health, Education and Welfare, NIDA, Rockville, Maryland.

Volkman, R. and Cressey, D. (1968). Differential Association and the Rehabilitation of Drug Addicts, in *Deviance, the Interactionist Perspective: Text and Readings in the Sociology of Deviance* (Eds. E. Rubington and M. Weinberg), Macmillan, London.

Vuchinich, R. and Tucker, J. (1980). A Critique of Cognitive Labelling Explanations of the Emotional and Behavioral Effects of Alcohol, *Addictive Behaviors*, **5**, 179–188.

Vuchinich, R., Tucker, J., and Sobell, M. (1979). Alcohol, Expectancy, Cognitive Labelling and Mirth, *Journal of Abnormal Psychology*, **88**, 641–651.

Walster, E., Berscheid, E., and Walster, B. (1970). The Exploited: Justice or Justification?, in *Altruism and Helping Behavior* (Eds. J. Macaulay and L. Berkowitz), Academic Press, New York.

Wardle, J. (1980). Dietary Restraint and Binge Eating, *Behaviour Analysis and Modification*, **4**, 201–209.

Wardle, J. and Beinart, H. (1981). Binge Eating: a Theoretical Review, *British Journal of Clinical Psychology*, **20**, 97–109.

Warnock, J. (1903). Insanity from Hasheesh, *Journal of Mental Science*, **49**, 96–110 (cited by Edwards, 1976).

Wasserman, M. (1982). Alcohol No! Gambling, Yes: a Matter of Survival in Aztec Society, *British Journal of Addiction*, **77**, 283–286.

Watson, S. and Akil, H. (1979). Endorphins: Clinical Issues, in *Psychiatric Factors in Drug Abuse* (Eds, R. Pickens and L. Heston), Grune & Stratton, New York.

Weinstein, D. and Deitch, L. (1974). *The Impact of Legalised Gambling: the Socioeconomic Consequences of Lotteries and Off-Track Betting*, Praeger, New York (cited by Cornish, 1978).

Wesson, D. and Smith, D. (1977). *Barbiturates: Their Use, Misuse, and Abuse*, Human Sciences Press, New York.

Westemeyer, J. (1978). Social Events and Narcotic Addiction: the Influence of War and Law on Opium Use in Laos, *Addictive Behaviors*, **3**, 57–62.

Wheeler, L. (1966). Toward a Theory of Behavioural Contagion, *Psychological Review*, **73**, 179–192.

Wijesinghe, B. (1977). Massed Electrical Aversion Treatment of Compulsive Eating, in *Behavioral Treatments of Obesity* (Ed. J. Foreyt), Pergamon, Oxford.

Wikler, A. (1973). Dynamics of Drug Dependence: Implications of Conditioning Theory for Research and Treatment, *Archives of General Psychiatry*, **28**, 611.

Wilkins, L. (1964). *Social Deviance: Social Policy, Action and Research*, Tavistock, London.

Wilkins, R. (1974). *The Hidden Alcoholic in General Practice*, Elek, London.

Wilkinson, R. (1970). *The Prevention of Drinking Problems: Alcohol Control and Cultural Influences*, Oxford University Press, New York.

Wille, R. (1978). Preliminary Communication: Cessation of Opiate Dependence: Processes Involved in Achieving Abstinence, *British Journal of Addiction*, **73**, 381–384.

Willems, P., Letemendia, F., and Arroyave, F. (1973). A Two-year Follow-up Study Comparing Short- with Long-stay In-patient Treatment of Alcoholics, *British Journal of Psychiatry*, **122**, 637–648.

Williams, A. (1966). Social Drinking, Anxiety, and Depression, *Journal of Personality and Social Psychology*, **3**, 689–693.

Williams, P. (1981). Trends in the Prescribing of Psychotropic Drugs, in *The Misuse of Psychotropic Drugs* (Eds. R. Murray, H. Ghodse, C. Harris, D. Williams, and P. Williams), Gaskell, The Royal College of Psychiatrists, London.

Wilsnack, R. and Wilsnack, S. (1978). Sex Roles and Drinking Among Adolescent Girls, *Journal of Studies on Alcohol*, **39**, 1855–1874.

Wilsnack, S. (1973). Sex Role Identity in Female Alcoholism, *Journal of Abnormal Psychology*, **82**, 253–261.

Wilson, A., Davidson, W., and White, J. (1978). Disulfiram Implantation: a Placebo-controlled Trial with Two-year Follow-up, *Journal of Studies on Alcohol*, **39**, 809–818.

Wilson, C. (1982). The Impact on Children, in *Alcohol and the Family* (Eds. J. Orford and J. Harwin), Croom Helm, London.

Wilson, G. (1982). How Useful is Meta-analysis in Evaluating the Effects of Different Psychological Therapies?, *Behavioural Psychotherapy*, **10**, 221–231.

Winick, C. (1962). Maturing Out of Narcotic Addiction, *Bulletin of Narcotics*, **14**, 1.

Wise, J. and Wise, S. (1979). *The Overeaters: Eating Styles and Personality*, Human Sciences Press, New York.

Wiseman, J. (1970). *Stations of the Lost: the Treatment of Skid Row Alcoholics*, Prentice-Hall, Englewood Cliffs, New Jersey.

Wolcott, H. (1974). *The African Beer Gardens of Bulawayo: Integrated Drinking in a Segregated Society*, Rutgers Centre of Alcohol Studies, New Brunswick, New Jersey.

World Health Organization (1952). *Technical Report*, Series No. 48, Expert Committee on Mental Health, Alcohol Sub-Committee, Second Report, WHO, Geneva.

World Health Organization (1964a). *Thirteenth Report*, WHO Expert Committee on Addiction-Producing Drugs Technical Report Series No. 273, WHO, Geneva.

World Health Organization (1964b). *Technical Report*, Series No. 116, Expert Committee on Drug Dependence, WHO, Geneva.

Wray, I. and Dickerson, M. (1981). Cessation of High Frequency Gambling and 'Withdrawal Symptoms', *British Journal of Addiction*, **76**, 401–405.

Yates, F. and Norris, H. (1981). The Use made of Treatment: an Alternative Approach to Evaluation, *Behavioural Psychotherapy*, **9**, 291–309.

Young, J. (1971). *The Drugtakers: The Social Meaning of Drug Use*, Paladin, London.

Zimbardo, P. (Ed.) (1969). *The Cognitive Control of Motivation; the Consequences of Choice and Dissonance*, Scott, Foresman, Glenview, Illinois.

Zinberg, N. (1975). Addiction and Ego Function, *Psychoanalytic Study of the Child*, **30**, 567–588 (Reprinted in *Classic Contributions in the Addictions*, Eds. H. Shaffer and M. Burglass, Brunner/Mazel, New York, 1981).

Zinberg, N., Harding, W., and Winkeller, M. (1977). A Study of Social Regulatory Mechanisms in Controlled Illicit Drug Users, *Journal of Drug Issues*, **7**, 117–133 (Reprinted in *Classic Contributions in the Addictions*, Eds. M Shaffer and M. Burglass, Brunner/Mazel, New York, 1981).

Zinberg, N. and Jacobson, R. (1976). The Natural History of 'Chipping', *American Journal of Psychiatry*, **133**, 37–40.

Author Index

Subject Index